Acknowledgments

I would like to thank the authors who have (with only a small amount of prompting from me) written the excellent chapters that appear in this book. The study of endocrine–immune interactions (including cytokines) has grown by leaps and bounds in the past few years and now has attracted investigators from wide ranging disciplines and diverse areas. I have attempted to incorporate those most current areas here, with the intention that the finished product will supply both background and recent knowledge for the reader. I would also like to thank Piero Foà, MD, the editor for the Endocrinology & Metabolism series, and Springer-Verlag for their invaluable assistance on this project.

Charles J. Grossman
Cincinnati, Ohio

Charles J. Grossman

Editor

Bilateral Communication Between the Endocrine and Immune Systems

With 29 Illustrations

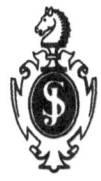

Springer-Verlag

New York Berlin Heidelberg London Paris
Tokyo Hong Kong Barcelona Budapest

Charles J. Grossman, Ph.D.
Department of Biology
Xavier University
and
Research Service
Veterans Affairs Medical Center
Cincinnatti, OH 45220, USA

Library of Congress Cataloging-in-Publication Data
Bilateral communication between the endocrine and immune systems/
  [edited by] Charles J. Grossman.
      p. cm.—(Endocrinology and metabolism; 7)
    Includes bibliographical references and index.
    1. Immunity—Endocrine aspects. 2. Hormones—Immunology.
  I. Grossman, Charles J. II. Series: Endocrinology and metabolism
  (New York, N.Y.); 7.
      [DNLM: 1. Endocrine Glands—physiology. 2. Immune System—
  physiology. 3. Nervous System—physiology. W1 EN396SN v.7/WL
  102 B595 1994]
  QR182.B55 1994
  612.4'—dc20
  DNLM/DLC   93-26904

Printed on acid-free paper.

© 1994 Springer-Verlag New York Inc.
Softcover reprint of the hardcover 1st edition 1994

Production coordinated by Chernow Editorial Services, Inc., and managed by Natalie Johnson; manufacturing supervised by Genieve Shaw.
Typeset by Best-set Typesetter Ltd., Hong Kong.

9 8 7 6 5 4 3 2 1

ISBN-13: 978-1-4612-7608-1   e-ISBN-13: 978-1-4612-2616-1
DOI: 10.1007/978-1-4612-2616-1

Contents

Contributors

ISTVAN BERCZI
Department of Immunology, Faculty of Medicine, University of Manitoba, Winnipeg, Manitoba R3C, Canada

FRANK BERKENBOSCH
Department of Pharmacology, Medical Faculty, Free University, 1081 BT, Amsterdam, The Netherlands

JOHN C. CHAPMAN
Department of Biological Sciences, State University of New York at Binghamton, Binghamton, New York 13902-6000, USA

MIREILLE DARDENNE
Hospital Necker, CNRS URA 1461, 75743 Paris 15, France

ROEL DERIJK
Department of Intramural Research Programs, National Institute of Mental Health, Clinical Neuroendocrinology Branch, Bethesda, Maryland 20892, USA

NICOLA FABRIS
Research Department, Immunology Center, INRCA, 60100 Ancona, Italy

CHARLES J. GROSSMAN
Department of Biology, Xavier University, and Research Service, Veterans Affairs Medical Center, Cincinnati, Ohio 45220, USA

SUDHIR GUPTA
Division of Basic and Clinical Immunology, California College of Medicine, University of California, Irvine, California 92717, USA

CHARU KAUSHIC
Department of Physiology, Dartmouth Medical School, Lebanon, New Hampshire 03756-0001, USA

ALAN B. McCRUDEN
Department of Immunology, University of Strathclyde, Glasgow G4 0NR, Scotland

SANDRA D. MICHAEL
Department of Biological Sciences, State University of New York at Binghamton, Binghamton, New York 13902-6000, USA

JAN RICHARDSON
Department of Physiology, Dartmouth Medical School, Lebanon, New Hampshire 03756-0001, USA

CATHERINE RIVIER
The Clayton Foundation Laboratories for Peptide Biology, The Salk Institute, La Jolla, California 92037, USA

WILSON SAVINO
Department of Immunology, The Oswaldo Cruz Foundation, Rio de Janiero, Brazil

WILLIAM H. STIMSON
Department of Immunology, University of Strathclyde, Glasgow G4 0NR, Scotland

CHARLES R. WIRA
Department of Physiology, Dartmouth Medical School, Lebanon, New Hampshire 03576-0001, USA

1
The Role of Sex Steroids in Immune System Regulation

CHARLES J. GROSSMAN

In 1979 when we published the first reports describing the presence of sex steroid receptors in thymic tissue,[1-3] the area of immuno-endocrinology did not exist. Endocrinologists and immunologists were worlds apart, and scientific societies inadvertently fostered this separatism because of specialization and insulation of the fields. Certainly clinicians had previously made the observation that certain autoimmune diseases were more prevalent in one sex or the other but the underlying mechanism was unknown.

Surprisingly, the earliest observation supporting a linkage between the immune and endocrine systems had been made by the Italian scientist Calzolari in 1898[4] when he reported in his article entitled 'Rescherches experimentales sur un rapport probable entre la function du thymus et celle des testicules' that the thymus of rabbits castrated before sexual maturity was larger than that of noncastrated controls. This observation, falling in the fallow soil of that time probably stimulated little if any interest. In 1940 Chiodi made a similar observation with respect to the effects of castration on thymic weight,[5] and these findings, coupled with the later reports of sex steroid receptors in thymic tissue,[1-3] strongly suggested that the changes in thymic weight observed after castration were mediated by these receptors. The additional observation that in vivo replacement of estrogen reversed this castrate-induced thymic hypertrophy[2] strongly suggested that these thymic sex steroids were mediating this response.

Today we find great interest in the area of hormones and immune system interactions, as demonstrated by the presence of specific societies (such as the International Society for Neuroimmunomodulation founded in 1987) as well as specialty journals (such as Progress in NeuroEndcrin-Immunology). Active research is expanding in this area, with new findings continually being reported. Areas of investigation include (but are not limited to) mechanisms involved in sex steroid and immune system interaction, immunological sexual dimorphism, regulation of autoimmune diseases by sex steroids, adrenal–gonadal interactions regulating stress and immunity, the interaction of cytokines, steroid hormones and im-

1

munity, pituitary hormones and immune function, the effects of aging on hormones and immunity, circadian rhythm and immunity, production of classic hormones [i.e., adrenocorticotropic hormone (ACTH), growth hormone (GH), etc.] by immune effector cell populations, and direct innervation and regulation of immune tissues by elements of the autonomic nervous system. While a number of these topics will be covered in detail in the following chapters, I would initially like to introduce the reader to some of the more pertinent points regarding the effects of sex hormones and immune response.

Steroid Receptors and the Immune System

As mentioned above, the presence of classic steroid binding receptors for estrogen and androgen were initially demonstrated in reticuloepithelial (RE) cells of the thymus.[1-3] However, in these early studies such receptors were not measurable in thymic lymphocyte populations due to the limited sensitivity of the early Scatchard plot kinetic assays. Whereas later investigators were indeed able to demonstrate that such sex steroid receptors actually did exist in various subpopulations of lymphocytes (see below), our inability to measure them was in a peculiar way serendipitous. This was because it forced us to hypothesize an alternate mechanism by which sex steroids could act through the RE cell receptors to modulate effector lymphocyte responses. According to this mechanism, sex steroids (estrogen, androgen) would bind to the appropriate steroid receptors present on RE cells, and this would then alter the release of thymic hormones from the RE cells that would then regulate T cell function. We tested this hypothesis in early studies[6,7] by demonstrating that serum prepared from castrate rats stimulated blastogenic transformation of thymocytes in culture. However, serum prepared from castrated rats that had been treated by in vivo injection with physiological levels of estradiol lost this stimulatory property. In addition, serum prepared from castrate thymectomized rats lost its stimulatory properties, suggesting that the source of the stimulatory factor in the serum was the thymus, and that estrogen was able to modulate its release.

In support of these results Dardeene et al.[8] reported that adrenalectomy and castration altered the secretion of the hormone thymulin and its inhibitory factor. Further support for a linkage between the RE cell sex steroid receptors and thymulin secretion was forthcoming in the work of a Japanese group[9,10] who were able to demonstrate histochemically that the RE cells within the thymus, which possess receptors for estrogen and progestin, were identical to the cells that secreted this thymic hormone. These studies thus supported the view that the sex steroid hormones were involved in regulating the secretion of thymulin. While the function of thymic hormones remains under investigation, it would seem logical that these hormones might be involved in both thymocyte development within the thymic microenvironment and regulation of mature T lymphocytes in locations distant from the thymus.

Since the time of our early work, a number of investigators have reported that sex steroid receptors were present in populations of lymphocytes. This almost certainly implies that sex steroids can directly affect lymphocyte function. For example, estrogen, receptors are present in human thymocytes,[11] fetal thymus tissue[12] large immature thymocytes,[13] and in human peripheral blood mononuclear cells.[11,14] In addition to the lymphocyte estrogen receptors, androgen receptors are also present in lymphocyte populations within the thymus that are also apparently glucocorticoid resistant.[15] Additionally, it has been reported that while androgen receptors were not present in mature blood lymphocytes or thoracic duct T cells, such receptors might function during cell development, since they mediated a reduction in interleukin-2 (IL-2) in cultures of thymocytes exposed to dihydrotestosterone.[16] However, in another study,[17] androgen treatment of NZB mice enhance IL-2 production in vivo. These findings would seem to support the suggestion of Ahmed[18] that sex steroids may affect lymphocytes both during development and later as adult effector cells. Since sex steroid receptors for estrogen,[1,2] androgen,[3,15] and progestin[19,20] have also been identified within the reticuloepithelial matrix of the thymus, it would appear that sex steroids can regulate immune system function both by a direct route (via lymphocyte steroid receptors) and indirectly (via release of other factors such as thymic hormones).

Sex Steroids and Indirect Regulation of Immunity

Given the fact that sex steroids can bind to RE receptors in thymic tissue, one of the possible outcomes of this binding is to modulate release of thymic factors. Since these thymic substances then regulate effector lymphocyte responses, an indirect linkage between gonads and effector lymphocytes is thus established. We have termed these type of pathways as 'hormonal axes,' and outlined two that involve steroid hormone-producing tissues. These are the hypothalamic-pituitary-gonadal-thymic (HPGT) axis, and the hypothalamic-pituitary-adrenal-thymic (HPAT) axis.[21-23] Both of these axes can modulate lymphocyte action through direct regulation with steroid hormones (sex steroids by the HPG pathway, and cortisol by the HPA pathway), and in addition, both probably regulate these effector lymphocytes indirectly by regulating release of thymic hormones. Furthermore, Rebar et al.,[24-26] utilizing an in vitro perfusion system, demonstrated that one of Allan Goldstein's thymic hormones, thymosin-B4, could release gonadotropin-releasing hormone (GnRH) from the hypothalamus, and this, in turn, could release luteinizing hormone (LH) and follicle-stimulating hormone (FSH) from the pituitary. If such a thymic–hypothalamic linkage also exists in vivo, its physiological function might be to increase sex steroid production and release from the gonads. Since elevated levels of sex steroids down-regulate the release of thymic hormones, this arm of the HPGT axis might be considered as a nonclassical, negative feedback loop involving the thymus, hypothalamus, pituitary, and gonads. A similar nonclassical, negative feedback loop involving the thymus, hypothalamus, pituitary, and adrenal has also been hypothesized.

It is interesting to note that at the time Rebar was involved in these studies, Michael[27-29] had demonstrated that early thymectomy of female mice resulted in delayed vaginal opening. She had hypothesized that thymosin was involved in direct regulation of the gonadal production of sex hormones. Thus, in removing the thymus, the absence of thymosin delayed puberty in these female mice. However, Rebar's findings suggested that Michael's observation was not due to a direct effect of thymus on gonads, but instead, to indirect modulation of gonadal function via the HPGT axis. More recently, such a thymic–gonadal link may still be proposed because an age-dependent factor elaborated by the thymus now appears able to regulate the binding of human chorionic gonadotropin (hCG) in rat testis.[30-32] Since hCG and LH possess closely related structures, it is conceivable that the presence of this thymic factor might act to modulate LH binding, and thus effect secretion of sex steroids by the gonads. Thus, thymic–gonadal interactions may proceed both via the more indirect hypothalamus–pituitary link, and additionally, by a direct path from thymus to gonads.

Another indirect pathway that may be effected by sex (and adrenal) steroids probably involves cytokines. For example, Besadovsky[33] has demonstrated that a factor generated by activated lymphocytes in culture (a lymphokine he named glucocorticoid increasing factor or GIF) is capable of stimulating the release of cortisol from the adrenal gland, as mediated through corticotropin-releasing factor (CRH) and ACTH increase. Such a pathway would act to down-regulate an ongoing immune response via the adrenal axis (and theoretically also might impact on the HPAT axis, and involve thymic hormones). In addition to GIF, the classic monokine IL-1, generated by monocyte/macrophages, has also been reported to stimulate cortisol increase from the adrenal axis via CRH and ACTH, and thus also down-regulate an ongoing immune response.[34] Since increasing CRH not only up-regulates the adrenal axis but also inhibits GnRH, this cytokine feedback on CRH may inhibit the gonadal axis, thereby reducing levels of sex steroids while elevating levels of glucocorticoids.[35-37]

In addition to direct thymic modulation of gonadal function, a lymphokine-like factor generated by mitogen-stimulated T cells from the spleen or by allogenic peripheral blood lymphocytes is of interest. This substance has been reported to increase progesterone (P) production through a direct effect on granulosa cells.[38,39] Since sex steroids at elevated levels are immunoinhibitory, if this factor is capable of significantly increasing circulating levels of P (probably in conjunction with other mechanisms), it may assist in quenching an ongoing immune response.

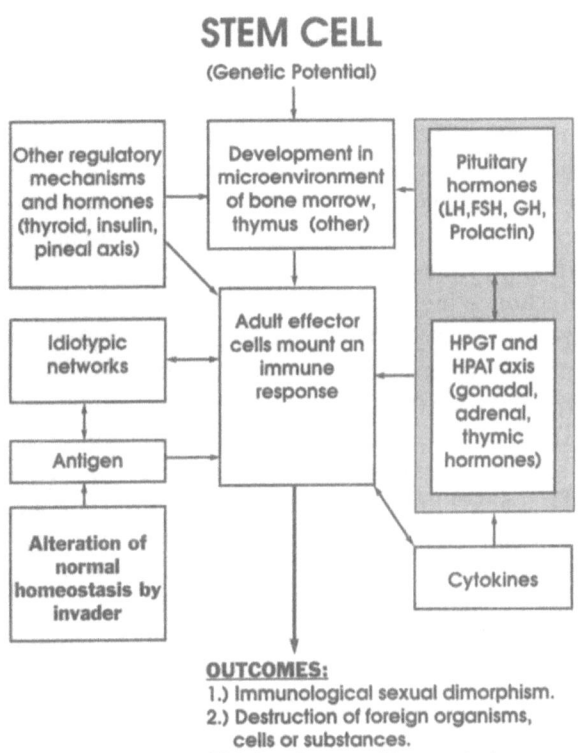

FIGURE 1.1. Interactions between gonadal steroids and various elements of the immune system are outlined. Stem cells destined to form elements of the immune system are programmed initially by genetic potential to develop within the microenvironment of fetal liver, or later in bone marrow, but the stages in the developmental process are modified by hormones present at this time. Formed immunological elements then migrate to the thymus, or remain within the primary lymphatic tissues of the bone marrow, where they undergo further development (also controlled by hormones) to generate pre-adult T and B lymphocytes. These cells then migrate into the secondary lymphatic tissues of the lymph nodes and spleen where they colonize the appropriate areas. Adult effector lymphocytes (primarily T cells) are also found circulating. Upon antigen stimulation, the various steps in clonal formation are activated, leading to the fully functional effector lymphocyte subclass. Such activation into the clone is probably also under the control of hormones. Finally, hormones probably affect the ability of the adult effector cells to mount an immune response against the invader.

Sex Steroids and Immunological Sexual Dimorphism

In females, both the humoral- and cell-mediated immune responses are generally more active (i.e., response threshold may be lower, peak levels of product, such as antibody, greater, and duration of response longer) as compared to males. One apparent outcome of this immunological sexual dimorphism (ISD) is the well-accepted fact that females are more susceptible to autoimmune diseases than are males.[40] Why this should be true, and what benefit this imparts to the female, remains largely unknown. However, it is certain that a functional immune system is centrally responsible for maintenance of homeostasis. It has been suggested that ISD may promote this homeostasis in females because it may facilitate development and nurturing of offspring, which places the female under greater physiological stress than the male.[35,41] It is also interesting to note that, during pregnancy, ISD expression is reduced, probably to prevent rejection of the fetus. This reduction in immune response in the pregnant female is largely due to the presence of elevated levels of estrogen (E) and P. Taking this one step further, it has been suggested that the presence of ISD in the nonpregnant female is due to the sexually dimorphic secretion of a variety of hormones.[35] These include (but are certainly not limited to) differences in circulating levels or patterns of secretions of estrogen, growth hormone, and prolactin, and possible differences in the secretion of cytokines.

One might envision that the genetic potential of a particular stem cell is activated by exposure to sexually dimorphic factors within the microenvironment of the bone marrow or thymus. Upon migration to the secondary lymphatic tissues, the final immunological potential of these effector cells is then further developed after clonal stimulation, during which the cells are exposed to additional hormones, cytokines, and thymic factors. Finally, the adult effector cell response may be further modified by the sexually dimorphic endocrine environment. The outcome is thus to promote differences in the development or activation of subpopulations of T-helper and T-suppressor lymphocytes, other immunological effector cells, and B cells, leading to immunological sexual dimorphism (Figure 1.1).

Sex Steroids and T-Lymphocyte Subpopulations

Since sex steroids clearly alter immune system function, it is not surprising to learn that individual subpopulations are probably specifically targeted by specific types of steroids. For example, 2- to 3-month-old female C57BL/6 mice treated in vivo with estradiol (E) and testosterone (T) for 2 weeks demonstrated a reduction in total lymphocytes recovered from thymus and spleen, but not from bone marrow or lymph nodes.[42] This would appear to support the assumption that lymphocytes in these locations are targets for sex steroids. Also, in mice after short-term in vivo treatment with estradiol, the CD4$^+$ (T-helper) and to a lesser extent the CD8$^+$ (T-suppressor) populations were increased, while the CD4$^+$/CD8$^+$ double positive sub-populations were significantly depleted.[43] In addition, in estradiol deficient human patients (vs. patients with normal levels of estradiol), a significantly lower CD4/CD8 ratio has been reported (1.15, n = 19 vs. 1.80, n = 24), and with reduced estrogen the CD8 (T-suppressor/cytotoxic) cells were significantly increased.[44]

Generally, these findings are in agreement with our own results from castrated male and female rats.[45,46] After separating splenocytes by His-topaque centrifugation, and labeling the individual lymphocyte subpopulations with a fluorescent marker conjugated to specific monoclonal antibodies, we counted the labeled cells by means of a fluorescent cell sorter. We reported that castration increased the numbers of CD5 (total T cells), CD4 (T-helper), and CD8 (T-suppressor) cells in both male and female rats. As expected, the CD4/CD8 ratio was also elevated after castration for both male and female rats. Furthermore, in these studies we replaced E and DHT in the castrate male and female rats, and observed changes in the T-cell subpopulations. The main effect of such steroid replacement was that E appeared to depress the CD4/CD8 ratio in males, while increasing it in females. In addition, dihydrotestosterone (DHT) appeared to increase the number of T-helper and T-suppressor cells in females to a greater extent than in males.[46] Additional studies are currently in progress.

Some corroboration for these results can be found in a study in which animals were treated with the androgen testosterone cypionate (Depo-Testosterone). Here the CD4 and CD8 subpopulations were seen to increase in the thymus, and CD8 cells increased in the spleen after treatment with the androgen.[47] Additionally, castration has also been reported to shift the balance within the T-cell subpopulations towards CD4 cells, while testosterone treatment increased the CD8 population.[48] Furthermore, in male mice, in vivo E treatment has been reported to increase the CD4 and CD8 subpopulations of thymocytes.[49]

These findings may partly explain the observation that expression of certain autoimmune diseases can be reduced by androgen treatment and exacerbated by estrogen replacement. The underlying mechanism depends on activation of T-suppressor cells by androgens, and T-helper cells (or B-cells) by estrogens, thereby modifying the disease process.[40] The observation that androgens target subsets of T-suppressor cells[50] supports this conclusion because this subclass is functionally able to immunosuppress other effector lymphocyte subclasses. In the event that this immunosuppression is lost, autoimmune disorders may be one result. It is not unreasonable to suggest hypothetically that T-suppressor lesions (which may be genetically predetermined) are brought to fruition by events within the microenvironment during development and programming of lymphocyte subclasses. Certainly multiple effects can be elicited in the microenvironment by steroid hormones and thymic hormones, and sex steroid hormones target effector lymphocytes at various points in the functional immune networks (Figure 1.1).

In conclusion, the sex steroids affect T lymphocytes either directly or indirectly. Direct effects are believed to be mediated classically through nuclear steroid receptors, whereas indirect regulation is accomplished through membrane-bound receptors that interact with cytokines and thymic hormones, as well as many other substances such as growth hormone, prolactin, thyroid hormone, insulin, neurotransmitters, etc. An additional level of control between lymphocytes and the endocrine system may exist via the release of cytokines exerting negative feed back through the adrenal axis, or directly at the level of the gonads. The complexity of these interactions is truly amazing, but they are certainly involved in maintaining a disease-free homeostasis in the organism.

References

1. Grossman CJ, Sholiton LJ, Nathan P. Rat thymic estrogen receptor. I. Preparation, location, and physiochemical properties. J Steroid Biochem 1979; 11:1233–1240.
2. Grossman CJ, Sholiton LJ, Blaha GC, Nathan P. Rat thymic estrogen receptor. II. Physiological properties. J Steroid Biochem 1979; 11:1241–1246.
3. Grossman CJ, Nathan P, Taylor BB, Sholiton LJ. Rat thymic dihydrotestosterone receptor: Preparation, location, and physiochemical properties. Steroids 1979; 34:539–553.
4. Calzolari A. Rescherches experimentales sur un rapport probable entre la function du thymus et celle des testicules. Arch Ital Biol 1898; 30:71.
5. Chiodi H. The relationship between the thymus and the sexual organs. Endocrinology 1940; 26:107.
6. Grossman CJ, Sholiton LJ, Roselle GA. Dihydrotestosterone regulation of thymocyte function in the rat—mediation by serum factors. J Steroid Biochem 1983; 19:1459–1467.
7. Grossman CJ, Sholiton LJ, Roselle GA. Estradiol regulation of thymic lymphocyte function in the rat: Mediation by serum thymic factors. J Steroid Biochem 1982; 16:683–690.
8. Dardeene M, Savino W, Duval D, Kaiserlian D, Hassid J, Bach J-F. Thymic hormone-containing cells. VII. Adrenals and gonads control the in vivo secretion of thymulin and its plasmatic inhibitor. J Immunol 1986; 136: 1303–1308.
9. Sakabe K, Kawashima I, Seiki K, Fujii-Hanamoto H. Hormone and immune response, with special reference to steroid hormone 2. Sex steroid receptors in rat thymus. Tokai J Clin Med 1990; 15:201–211.
10. Kawashima I, Sakabe K, Seiki K, Fujii-Hanamoto H, Akatsuka A, Tsukamoto H. Localization of sex steroid receptor cells, with special reference to thymulin (FTS)-producing cells in female rat thymus. Thymus 1991; 18:79–93.
11. Weusten JJAM, Blankenstein MA, Gemlig-Meyling FHJ, Schuurman HJ, Kater L, Thijssen JHH. Presence of oestrogen receptors in human blood mononuclear cells and thymocytes. Acta Endocrinology 1986; 112:409–414.

12. Screpanti I, Gulino A, Pasqualini JR. The fetal thymus of guinea pig as an estrogen target organ. Endocrinology 1982; 111:1552–1561.
13. Gulino A, Screpanti I, Torrisi MR, Frati L. Estrogen receptors and estrogen sensitivity of fetal thymocytes are restricted to blast lymphoid cells. Endocrinology 1985; 117:47–54.
14. Danel L, Souweine G, Monier JC, Saez S. Specific estrogen binding sites in human lymphoid cells and thymic cells. J Steroid Biochem 1983; 18:559–563.
15. Pearce PB, Khalid AK, Funder JW. Androgens and the thymus. Endocrinology 1981; 109:1073–1077.
16. Kovacs WJ, Olsen NJ. Androgen receptors in human thymocytes. J Immunol 1987; 139:490–493.
17. Dauphinee MJ, Kipper S, Roskos K, Wofsky D, Talal N. Androgen treatment of NZB/W mice enhances IL-2 production. Archritis Rheum 1981; 24(suppl):S64.
18. Ahmed AS, Penhale WJ, Talal N. Sex hormones, immune response, and autoimmune disease. Am J Path 1985; 121:531–551.
19. Pearce PT, Khalid BAK, Funder JW. Progesterone receptors in rat thymus. Endocrinology 1983; 113:1287–1291.
20. Fujii-Hanamoto H, Grossman CJ, Roselle GA, Mendenhall CL. Nuclear progestin receptors in rat thymic tissue. Thymus 1990; 15:31–45.
21. Grossman CJ. Regulation of the immune system by sex steroids. Endocr Rev 1984; 3:436–455.
22. Grossman CJ. Interactions between the gonadal steroids and the immune system. Science 1985; 227:257–261.
23. Grossman CJ, Roselle GA. The control of immune response by endocrine factors and the clinical significance of such regulation. Prog Clin Biochem Med 1986; 4:9–55.
24. Rebar RW, Miyaka A, Low TLK, Goldstein AA. Thymosin stimulates secretion of luteinizing hormone-releasing factor. Science 1981; 214:669.
25. Rebar RW, Morandini IC, Silva da Sa MF, Erickson GF, Petze JE. The importance of the thymus gland for normal reproductive function in mice. In: Schwartz NB, Hunzicker-Dunn M, eds. Dynamics of Ovarian Function. New York: Raven Press; 1981:285.
26. Rebar RW, Miyaka A, Erickson GF, Low TLK, Goldstein AL. The influence of the thymus gland on reproductive function: A hypothalamic site of action. In: Greenwald GS, Terranova PF, eds. Factors Regulating Ovarian Function. New York: Raven Press; 1983:465.
27. Michael SD, Taguchi O, Nishizuka Y, McClure JE, Goldstein AL, Barkley MS. The effects of neonatal thymectomy on early follicular loss and circulating levels of corticosterone, progesterone, estradiol, and thymosin. In: Schwartz NV, Hunzicker-Dunn M, eds. Dynamics of Ovarian Function. New York: Raven Press; 1981:279.
28. Michael SD, Taguchi O, Nishizuka Y. Effects of neonatal thymectomy on ovarian development and plasma LH, FSH, GH, and PRL in the mouse. Biol Reprod 1980; 22:343.
29. Kosiewqicz MM, Michael SD. Neonatal thymectomy affects follicle populations prior to the onset of autoimmune oophoritis in B6A mice. J Reprod Fertil 1990; 88:427–440.

30. Hiriat M, Romano MC. Human chorionic gonadotropin binding to rat testis receptors is inhibited by a thymic factor. Life Sci 1986; 38:789–795.
31. Aguilera G, Romano MC. Influence of the thymus on steroidogenesis by rat ovarian cells in vitro. J Endocrinol 1989; 123:367–376.
32. Reyes-Esparza JA, Romano MC. An age-dependent thymic secretion modulates testicular function. J Steroid Biochem 1989; 34:541–545.
33. Besedovsky HO, Del Ray A, Sorkin E, Lotz W, Schwulera U. Lymphoid cells produce an immunoregulatory glucocorticoid increasing factor (GIF) acting through the pituitary gland. Clin Exp Immunol 1985; 59:622–628.
34. Berkenbosch F, van Oers J, Del Ray A, Tilders F, Besedovsky H. Corticotropin-releasing factor-producing neurons in the rat activated by interleukin-1. Science 1987; 238:524–526.
35. Grossman C. Possible underlying mechanisms of sexual dimorphism in the immune response, fact and hypothesis. J Steroid Biochem 1989; 34:241–251.
36. Petragalia F, Sutton S, Vale W, Plotsky P. Corticotropin-releasing factor decreases plasma luteinizing hormone levels in female rats by inhibiting gonadotropin-releasing hormone release into hypophysial-portal circulation. Endocrinology 1987; 120:1083–1088.
37. Grossman CJ. Stress and the immune response: Interactions of peptides, gonadal steroids, and the immune system. Weiner H, Florin I, Murison R, Hellhammer D, eds. Frontiers of Stress Research. Toronto, New York, Bern, Stuttgart: Hans Huber; 181–190.
38. Hughes FM, Pringle CM, Gorospe WC. Production of progestin-stimulating factors(s) by enriched populations of rat T and B lymphocytes. Biol Reprod 1991; 44:922–926.
39. Emi N, Kanzaki H, Yoshida M, Takakura K, Kariya M, Okamoto N, Imai K, Mori T. Lymphocytes stimulate progesterone production by cultured human granulosa luteal cells. Am J Obstet Gynecol 1991; 165:1469–1474.
40. Grossman CJ, Roselle GA, Mendenhall CL. Sex steroid regulation of autoimmunity. J Steroid Biochem Molec Biol 1991; 40:649–659.
41. Rheins LA, Karp RD. Effect of gender on the inducible humoral immune response in honeybee venom in the American cockroach (Periplaneta americana). Dev Comp Immunol 1985; 9:41–49.
42. Ahmed SA, Dauphinee MJ, Talal N. Effects of short-term administration of sex hormones on normal and autoimmune mice. J Immunol 1985; 134:204–210.
43. Screpanti I, Morrone S, Meco D, Santoni A, Gulino A, Paolini R, Crisanti A, Mathieson BJ, Frati L. Steroid sensitivity of thymocyte subpopulations during intrathymic differentiation. Effects of 17β-estradiol and dexamethasone on subsets expressing T-cell antigen receptor of IL-2 receptor. J Immunol 1989; 142:3378–3383.
44. Ho P-C, Tang GWK, Lawton JWM. Lymphocyte subsets in patients with oestrogen deficiency. J Reprod Immunol 1991; 20:85–91.
45. Grossman CJ, Neinaber MA. Bidirectional communication between the immune and endocrine systems—mediation by hormones of the gonads. Hans Selye Symposia in Neuroendocrinology, Advances in Psychoneuroimmunology, Satellite meeting of the 8th International Congress of Immunology, 1992, Budapest, Hungary, (In press).

46. Grossman CJ. Bidirectional communication between the immune and endocrine system: The sex steroid influence on thymic lymphocytes. Am J Reprod Immunol 1992; 27:21.

47. Aboudkhil S, Bureau JP, Garrelly L, Vago P. Effects of castration, Depotestosterone and cyproterone acetate on lymphocyte T-subsets in mouse thymus and spleen. Scand J Immunol 1991; 34:647–653.

48. Olsen NJ, Watson MB, Henderson GS, Kovacs WJ. Androgen deprivation induces phenotypic and functional changes in the thymus of adult male mice. Endocrinology 1991; 129:2471–2476.

49. Screpanti I, Meco D, Morrone S, Gulino A, Mathieson BJ, Frati L. In vivo modulation of the distribution of thymocyte subsets: Effects of estrogen on the expression of different T-cell receptor VB gene families in CD4⁻, CD8⁻ thymocytes. Cell Immunol 1991; 134:414–426.

50. Weinstein Y, Berkovich Z. Testosterone effect on bone marrow, thymus, and suppressor T cells in the (NZB × NZW) F_1 mice: Its relevance to autoimmunity. J Immunol 1981; 126:998–1002.

2
Hormonal and Immunologic Interactions Between Thymus and Ovary

JOHN C. CHAPMAN AND SANDRA D. MICHAEL

Thymic Involvement in Reproductive Development: A Historical Perspective

The first indication of a relationship between reproduction and the thymus gland was in 1898 when Calzolari[1] reported that castration of male rabbits resulted in an increase in the mass of the thymus gland. This was later verified by Chiodi in 1940,[2] and more recently by Fitzpatrick et al.[3] and Greenstein et al.,[4] who each extended their studies to show that the effects of castration on the thymus could be reversed through injections of gonadal steroids. Still later, it was shown that gonadectomy in aged rats and mice not only resulted in hypertrophy of the thymus, but also caused a partial restoration of immune function.[5] The fundamental importance of the thymus as a regulator of reproductive development was demonstrated through studies of the nude mouse and the neonatally thymectomized mouse. Studies of the congenitally athymic female nude (nu/nu) mouse revealed that the animal had delayed sexual maturation, decreased oocyte and follicular growth rates, increased follicular atresia, low circulating concentrations of gonadotropins, decreased levels of gonadal steroids, and premature ovarian failure, all of which resulted in a low incidence of fertility.[6-17] Nude mice given an intact thymus were reproductively competent[16,17] The actual time in which the thymus is most critical to reproductive development was determined by thymectomizing various euthymic strains of rats and mice, starting at birth. This procedure established that the thymus gland exerts its most profound effects on reproductive development in these rodents shortly after they are born. For example, thymectomy performed on female mice and rats prior to 7 days of age results in delayed sexual maturation and ovarian dysgenesis.[18-22] Thymic ablation after this timepoint has no effect on reproductive development. The onset of ovarian dysgenesis is characterized by a disruption in follicular growth patterns, increased follicular degeneration, and extensive changes in circulating levels of gonadotropic hormones.[18,23–26] In addition, there is an alteration in ovarian steroidogenesis, as indicated by abnormally high serum androgen concentrations and low levels of circulating progesterone.[27–30] By the time the thymectomized female reaches the normal age of puberty, its ovaries are dysfunctional and the animal is reproductively incompetent.[18,19,31] However, ovarian dysgenesis can be prevented by thymic implant or by an infusion of thymic derived, Lyt-1$^+$ (CD4) lymphocytes.[31–34] In primates, the critical period for thymic contribution to reproductive development is in utero, rather than postnatally, as shown when fetal thymectomy in monkeys induces ovarian dysgenesis.[35] In human females born with a congenital absence of the thymus, there is no reproductive development. Ovaries from these individuals show a complete lack of functioning follicles.[36]

Thymus Gland: The Cellular and Molecular Level

The increase in thymic mass due to castration is the result of an enlargement in both cortex and medulla, and an increase in overall lymphocyte cellularity.[37] In opposition to castration, estrogen has been shown to reduce thymic mass, disorganize thymic architecture, and promote thymocyte destruction, especially of cortical thymocytes.[37] This occurs regardless of whether the thymus is enlarged due to castration, or is normal in size. In either event, this suggests that these tissues are specific targets for estrogen. Indeed, Screpanti et al. reported that fetal thymus tissue[38] and large immature thymocytes[39] contain receptors for estrogen. In addition, reticuloepithelial (RE) cells of the thymus also contain receptors for estrogen,[40,41] as well as for androgen[42,43] and progestin.[44,45] The presence of sex steroid receptors in both developing lymphocytes and RE cells suggests that the gonadal steroids feed back information to the thymus via these receptors. From this, the end result is a modulation of thymic weight, thymic structure, and thymocyte maturation. In regard to the latter, treatment of thymocytes with androgen during their maturation is reported to alter the thymocytes' ability to produce interleukin-2 (IL-2).[46,47] In a like vein, thymus glands from castrated animals have increased numbers of glucocorticoid-sensitive cells, whereas the number of cortisone-resistent cells remains unchanged,[48] suggesting that removal of gonadal steroids via castration allows for an increased production of thymic lymphocytes from precursor cells.[48]

The evidence that gonadal steroids exert a direct control of the thymus suggests that the hypothalamus/hypophysis may play only a secondary role in regulating immune function, and this via its control of gonadal steroid production. While the latter is true, the hypothalamus also has additional channels of communication between thymic/immune and gonadal functions. This is demonstrated by the observation that the ovaries,[49–51] thymus,[52–54] and thymic-derived lymphocytes[55–57] all have specific receptors for the hypothalamic decapeptide, luteinizing hormone-releasing hormone (LHRH). This releasing hormone is critical to the maturation of ovaries and thymus, as indicated by the observation that neonatal treatment with an LHRH antagonist not only delays sexual maturation, but additionally inhibits the development of the cell-mediated response and alters thymus morphology.[58] The latter is manifested by decreased thymic weight, a specific reduction of cortex area, a diminished epithelial microenvironment, and reduced thymocyte volume. In a recent study it was shown that agonists of LHRH restored thymic weight and function in aged rodents,[53] thereby indicating their involvement in thymic physiology well after puberty. Lymphocytes with LHRH receptors have the ability to synthesize luteinizing hormone (LH),[59] thus providing a potentially direct input into immune modulation of gonadal steroidogenesis. Thymic contribution to this particular control loop is via the mediation of thymic peptides, such as thymosin-β4 acting directly on the hypothalamus to cause the secretion of LHRH.[60,61] The resultant LH subsequently stimulates the synthesis of ovarian steroids, which in turn acts at the thymus to inhibit lymphocyte development, and thymic hormone release.[48]

In vivo it has been shown that thymosin-β4 levels vary throughout the estrous cycle in pigs.[62] Progesterone appears to be the interactive steroid in this instance, since progesterone implants cause a decrease in circulating levels of thymosin-β4.[63] The control of circulating levels of thymosin-α1, on the other hand, appears to be due to estradiol. This is indicated by a report that thymosin-α1 concentrations in adult mice are inversely related to circulating levels of estradiol.[64] In addition, when estradiol was injected into these animals, the levels of circulating thymosin-α1 were decreased.[64]

Other thymic hormones appear to act on gonadal function outside of the hypothalamic control loop. For example, thymulin has been shown to stimulate the proliferation of oogonia in rat fetal ovaries in vitro.[65] In addition, there have been recent reports that thymic humoral factor(s) inhibit human chorionic gonadotropin- (hCG) stimulated steroidogenesis in rat ovarian cells in vitro.[66] It has also been proposed that sex steroids function not just at the level of the stem cell, pre-T, and possibly pre-B lymphocytes, but that the steroids also directly and indirectly regulate adult T cells and monocytes.[67] In regard to direct control, a number of reports indicate that human peripheral blood mononuclear cells contain estrogen and androgen receptors.[68–72] A possible role of the steroid receptors in these cells is the regulation of mRNA transcription for the production of lymphokines. For example, estrogen and progesterone have both been shown to depress interleukin-1β (IL-1B) mRNA levels in cultures of activated monocytes and macrophages.[73] This results in a steroid modulation of IL-1 levels, as measured in cultured monocytes[74] and circulating blood.[75,76] Further, lymphocytes isolated from preovulatory follicles of human ovaries also contain estrogen receptors.[77,78] Estrogen may act on these intrafollicular lymphocytes to regulate the production of lymphokines. Evidence suggesting this is provided by the finding that intrafollicular levels of these lymphocytes are directly correlated with the presence of interferon-γ.[78] This particular lymphocyte population has been characterized as the CD8 (cytotoxic/suppressor) subset;[71,72] thus, this subset is implicated in major histocompatibility complex (MHC) Class I immunologic reactions. These immunologic reactions do not involve monocyte/antigen presenting cells. Instead, the CD8 lymphocytes are stimulated directly by target cells expressing MHC Class I antigens. Granulosa cells in atretic follicles in rat ovaries express Class I antigen.[79] Indirect regulation of extrathymic lymphocyte function by sex steroids is suggested by reports that estrogen and androgens act on the thymus to cause the secretion of soluble serum factor(s) that function, in turn, as inhibitory or excitatory modulators of specific effector lymphocytes.[80-82]

Steroid receptors in thymic reticular epithelial cells are also very likely involved in the regulation and/or release of thymic hormones. This concept is suggested by reports demonstrating via histochemical analyses that the RE cells containing receptors for estrogen and progestin are the same cells that secrete thymulin (FTS).[83,84] FTS is one of approximately 50 individual thymic polypeptide hormones. Its actual role in intrathymic regulation has not been fully elucidated and requires further research. However, it is possible that it, as well as other thymic hormones, are involved in both thymocyte development, and the extrathymic regulation of mature T lymphocytes. Evidence for the latter is tentatively suggested by a report indicating that components of thymosin fraction V are located in the thecal layer of ovarian follicles.[85] In this location, the thymic peptides may play a role in intraovarian lymphocyte regulation. Evidence suggesting this possibility is provided by the observation that lymphocytes with the CD8 antigenic marker have been detected in the thecal layer of growing follicles in mouse ovary (Kosiewicz and Michael, unpublished), as well as isolated from human preovulatory follicles.[77,78] This is the same subset that is reported to contain estrogen receptors.[71,72]

Immune Involvement in Ovarian Physiology

An ever increasing number of immunologic components have been implicated in ovarian physiology. For example, monocytes/antigen presenting cells (APCs) have been detected in growing follicles,[79,86] and have been suggested to be required for follicular maturation. Macrophages, on the other hand, have been identified in follicular fluid,[87] and in the corpus luteum.[88,89] Atretic follicles contain immune cells with the antigenic marker of natural killer function.[79,86] In the corpus luteum, macrophages are involved in the secretion of progesterone[90,91] and in heterophagic luteolysis.[89] Prostaglandins (PGs) have also been implicated in the latter process, as well as in ovulation, and are thought to be products of both macrophages and T lymphocytes.[92,93] Prostaglandins have been shown to inhibit mitogen- and antigen-induced T-lymphocyte proliferation, lymphokine production, and T-helper and T-cytotoxic function.[94] Mast cells are present near perifollicular capillaries, and increase in number during the latter stages of follicular maturation.[94] At the LH surge prior to ovulation, these mast cells degranulate and release histamine. From this, localized hyperemia occurs, with the result that eosinophils and T lymphocytes migrate into the corpus luteum.[95,96] Here, the T lymphocytes become activated and they, in turn, are thought to mobilize and activate luteal macrophages.[97-99] The activated macrophages subsequently produce additional cytokines.

Cytokines are thought to be involved in a number of intraovarian regulatory processes. In most instances the cytokines either modulate, or are modulated by, gonadal steroids. Implicated under these conditions are cytokines such as IL-1, IL-2, and tumor necrosis factor (TNF), as well as IFN-γ.[100-110] As an example, IL-1, suggested to be in follicular fluid,[111] inhibits the FSH-induced expression of LH/hCG receptors, suppresses progesterone secretion in cultured granulosa cells,[112] and inhibits luteinization of granulosa cells.[113] In the same context, IFN-γ, a lymphokine that attracts monocytes/macrophages, has been identified in preovulatory follicles of human ovaries.[78] Its existence in these follicles is correlated with the appearance of CD8 lymphocytes;[77,78] therefore, it is suggested that these lymphocytes may be the source of the IFN-γ. IFN-γ production by T cells is reported to be increased via estradiol stimulation.[108] Since preovulatory follicles are known to contain high levels of estrogen,[114] the possibility exists that the combination of this steroid and the CD8 lymphocytes may be a means of control for ovarian macrophages and/or other white blood cells (WBCs). In addition, lymphokines may be involved in the actual synthesis of steroids. Two recent reports indicate that mitogen-activated T cells and allogenic blood lymphocytes secrete lymphokine-like factor(s) that stimulate the production of progesterone by granulosa cells.[115,116]

Further indications of cytokine control of ovarian functions also exist. For example, granulosa cells in growing follicles are normally negative for MHC Class II antigens.[78] However, their expression can be induced by IFN-γ,[117] setting the stage for follicular atresia. As previously discussed for IL-1, IFN-γ is also reported to inhibit both the FSH-stimulated granulosa cell production of progesterone and estradiol, and the FSH induction of LH/hCG receptor formation.[118] This, too, could select out those follicles destined for atresia. In any event, evidence that IFN-γ is important to ovarian physiology is indicated by the observation that cyclosporin A, an inhibitor of IFN-γ production,[119] causes impaired ovarian function.[120] The cytokine TNF-α has been isolated from rabbit corpora lutea.[89] Its occurrence there is correlated with the presence of macrophages and T lymphocytes. Those corpora lutea undergoing luteolysis produce the highest levels of TNF-α.[89]

A Specific Focus on Lymphocyte Involvement in Follicular Growth and Atresia

Subpopulations of T lymphocytes appear to be specifically affected by steroids. For example, in an early study Kalland[121] reported that neonatal injections of estrogen into female mice resulted in a lowering of the maturation rate of the Lyt-1$^+$ lymphocytes, and an increase in levels of immature thymocytes. In contrast, Novotony et al.[122] found that castrated adult mice given estrogen injections had significantly lower levels of Lyt-2$^+$ thymocytes. A more recent report indicated that treatment of 2- to 3-month-old female mice with either estradiol or testosterone reduced all thymocyte and splenocyte populations.[123] However, in this instance estradiol preferentially depleted the Lyt-2$^+$ supressor/cytotoxic thymocytes. Others have reported that short-term in vivo treatment with estradiol results in a significant depletion of the immature CD4/CD8 double-positive thymocyte subpopulation.[124] In addition, this group also indicated that estradiol caused an increase in the CD4 and, to a lesser extent, the CD8 subpopulations. Mathur et al.[125] examined WBC populations over the course of the human menstrual cycle and reported that there was a negative correlation in lymphocyte counts with estrogen levels. The lowest levels of circulating lymphocytes coincided with the preovulatory surge of estrogen. Most recently, Ho et al.[126] examined CD4/CD8 lymphocyte ratios in women with idiopathic premature ovarian failure and found a positive correlation between circulating estrogen levels and CD4/CD8 ratios. This correlation was the result of a preferential depression of CD8 lymphocytes by estradiol. In a study of estrogen deficient women, it was reported that these individuals had a lowered CD4/CD8 lymphocyte ratio relative to that found in normal women.[127] The lowered CD4/CD8 ratio resulted from elevated levels of CD8 lymphocytes, thus indicating a negative correlation with estrogen levels. Recently, Grossman[128] reported that estradiol treatment increased the CD4/CD8 ratio in both intact and castrate female rats, due to a preferential decrease in the CD8 subset.

Injections of antithymocyte serum given to female rats results in the disruption of follicular maturation.[129] Experimentally induced lymphopenia in cattle causes luteal dysfunction.[130] Together, these results tentatively suggest lymphocyte involvement in follicular maturation and/or ovulation. Corroborating evidence for this is: (1) reproductive dysfunctions, such as idiopathic premature ovarian failure and estrogen deficiency, are correlated with altered levels of CD8 lymphocytes;[126,127] (2) injections of estrogen preferentially decrease the CD8 lymphocyte subset;[122,123,128] (3)

CD8 lymphocytes are found in preovulatory ovarian follicles;[77,78] (4) CD8 lymphocytes have estrogen receptors;[71,72] and (5) intrafollicular estrogen levels are highest in those follicles destined for ovulation.[114] In toto, this suggests the possibility that CD8 lymphocytes are involved in follicular maturation, and are under the control of intrafollicular estrogen.

Neonatal Steroid Injections Disrupt Reproductive Development

The usual consequence of neonatal injections of testosterone and estrogen given to rats and mice is anovulation and sterility.[131-135] From earlier studies this was interpreted to be the result of steroid damage to the immature hypothalamus so that it never develops the ability to initiate a preovulatory surge of LH/FSH,[133-135] suggesting that the gland is the site of the estrogen-induced positive feedback mechanism. In subsequent years it was found that testosterone injections, given neonatally, caused morphological changes in the hypothalamus.[136,137] More recently, Naftolin et al.[138] reported that estrogen alters synaptic density postsynaptic membrane structure of neurones within the arcuate nucleus. Within the framework of this belief, the anterior pituitary, the site of LH/FSH release, is considered to have been unaffected by the injected steroids.[133-135] Also, estrogen is considered the active steroid, with testosterone being effective only because it is aromatized to estrogen in the steroid-injected animal.[138] Over the years a number of studies have challenged this concept.[139-143] In a series of rather elegant experiments using the female rhesus monkey, Knobil and his group provided evidence to suggest that the hypothalamus may not even be the positive feedback center for LH release.[143] Their data strongly suggest that the negative and positive feedback effects of gonadal steroid hormones occur mostly on the anterior pituitary. The contribution of the hypothalamus to the feedback mechanism is a pulsatile release of LHRH. Earlier studies indicated that the anterior pituitary was not damaged by the neonatally injected steroids;[133,134] this suggests that some requisite component other than the hypothalamus/adenohypophysis may be responsible for the anovulation due to the neonatally injected gonadal hormones. As briefly discussed, evidence indicates the possibility that the missing component could very likely be the Lyt-1+ lymphocytes.[121]

Neonatal Steroid Injections: A Model to Study Lymphocyte Involvement in Follicular Maturation

In common with neonatal thymectomy, neonatal steroid injections disrupt reproductive development in laboratory mice and rats.[131-135] The two insults are effective if performed within 7 days postpartum, and both may involve thymic-derived lymphocytes. For example, in the thymectomized female mouse, an infusion of T lymphocytes, characterized as the Lyt-1$^+$ (CD4) subset, prevents the effect of thymectomy.[33,34] Similarly, an infusion of adult thymocytes prior to steroid injection obviates the effect of neonatal testosterone injection.[139] To date, these thymocytes have not been characterized as to their specific subset. In an earlier study, Kalland[121] reported that neonatal estrogen injections caused a reduction in the maturation rate of Lyt-1$^+$ (CD4) lymphocytes. It is also possible that steroid injections may alter the lymphocyte's receptor control mechanism. In a number of recent studies to be discussed next, we began an examination of the relationship between neonatal steroid injections, fertility, and changes in lymphocyte subpopulations.

Neonatal Injections of Estradiol-17β and Testosterone Cause Anovulation by Separate Mechanisms

In the first experiment (Griffin, Chapman, and Michael, unpublished) we examined whether estradiol and testosterone cause the same incidence of infertility when injected into different strains of female mice. The results of this experiment could indicate whether the two steroids have a common pathway of action, a tenet important to the concept of damage to the hypothalamus. In the study, (C57BL × A/J)F_1 (B6A) and (C3H/HeJ × 129/J)F_1 (C31) female mouse pups were injected with either estradiol-17β, testosterone, or both steroids. The injections were given subcutaneously for 4 consecutive days, and either from 0 to 3 days of age, or from 3 to 6 days of age. When the animals were 100 days old, they were placed with a male for 10 days, and all subsequent litters recorded. This mating procedure was repeated twice more. The results of the experiment are shown in Figures 2.1 and 2.2. As indicated, the two steroids did not cause the same incidence of sterility, especially when given from 3 to 6 days of age. In the B6A strain, estrogen injections given from 3 to 6 days of age caused almost complete infertility, whereas testosterone did not. Estradiol given to the C31 animals during this same time period caused the incidence of fertility to increase over time. For example, at 100–125 days of age, 75% of the recipient animals were infertile, whereas at 180–200 days of age, only 25% were infertile. To our knowledge the observation that the effects of neonatal estrogen injections are ameliorated over time has heretofore been unreported. Possibly, the most telling evidence that the two steroids do not have a common mechanism of action is indicated by the results of injecting the two steroids together. As shown in the C31 animals injected with estrogen and testosterone from 3 to 6 days of age, the graph of the incidence of fertility does not compare with the graph of the incidence of fertility of separate injections of either steroid (Figure 2.2). In the estradiol-injected animals the incidence of

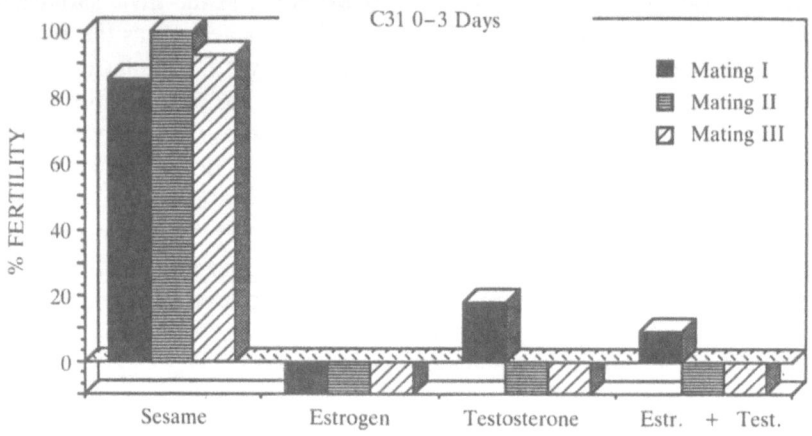

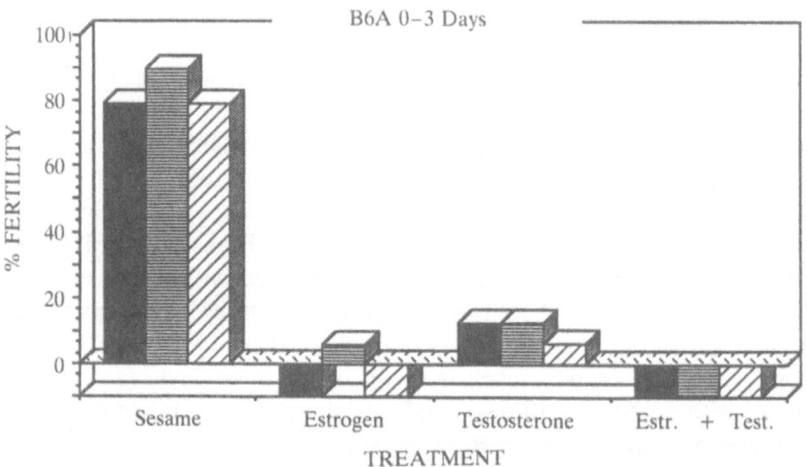

FIGURE 2.1. The incidence of fertility in C31 and B6A female mice injected with either estrogen (estradiol-17β), or testosterone, or estrogen plus testosterone, or sesame oil. Animals were given 20 μg of each steroid for 4 consecutive days, starting at day 0 postpartum. At 100 days of age they were tested for fertility. This consisted of housing 2 females of identical treatment with a fertile male for 10 days, and any subsequent litters were recorded. All females underwent 3 separate fertility tests with different males. Each treatment group consisted of at least 10 females (Griffin, Chapman, and Michael, unpublished).

fertility increases over time, and in the testosterone-injected females the incidence of fertility decreases over time. This suggests that the incidence of fertility caused by the two steroids together is very likely due to the combined results of both steroids, indicating that each steroid has a different mechanism of action in causing anovulation.

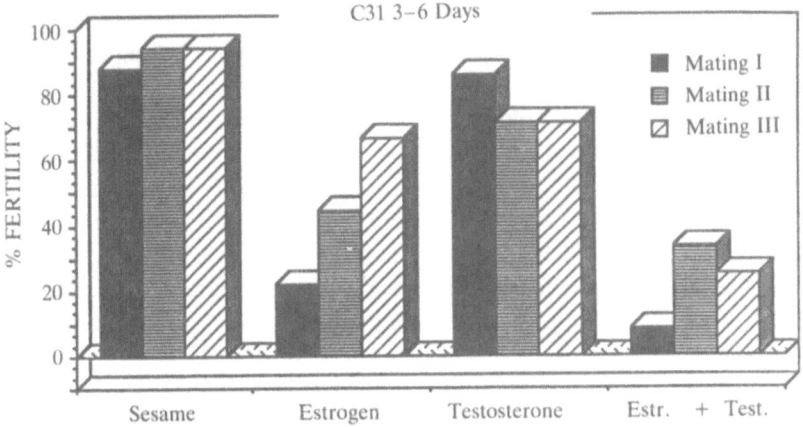

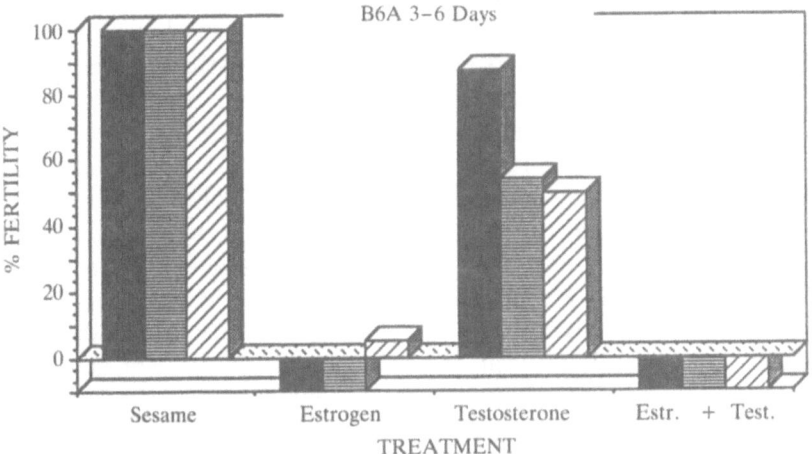

FIGURE 2.2. The incidence of fertility in C31 and B6A female mice injected with either estrogen (estradiol-17β), or testosterone, or estrogen plus testosterone, or sesame oil. Animals were given 4 daily injections of 20 μg of each steroid, starting at day 3 postpartum. Fertility testing was as described in the legend for Figure 2.1. Each treatment group consisted of at least 10 females (Griffin, Chapman, and Michael, unpublished).

Neonatal Estrogen-Induced Changes in Lymphocyte Populations as a Possible Correlate to Anovulation

The observation that neonatal estrogen injections do not cause permanent sterility in the C31 mouse provided the basis for our next study (Deshpande, Chapman, and Michael, unpublished). For this we were interested in determining if the gradual increase in fertility of the mice injected with estrogen from 3 to 6 days of age could be correlated with the eventual establishment of normal numbers of Lyt-1[+] lymphocytes. In the study by Kalland,[121] the estrogen-injected animals were killed at 8 weeks of age, and very likely before ovarian function was restored. As shown in the previous study, fertility in the estrogen-injected animals was extremely low at this age. In our study, female C3H pups were given 4 daily injections of estradiol-17β, either from 0 to 3 days or from 3 to 6 days postnatally. The injected animals were killed at 8, 12, 20, 28, 32, or 40 weeks of age. Spleens and thymuses were removed and evaluated for CD4[+] and CD8[+] lymphocytes via double color labeling and fluorescence-activated cell-sorting (FACS) analysis. This technique takes into account the presence of CD4/CD8 double-positive lymphocytes. In addition, ovaries were removed and examined histologically for the presence of corpora lutea. As a control for the evaluation of lymphocyte subsets, another group of female mice were thymectomized. Previous reports indicate that neonatal thymectomy also affects the Lyt-1[+] subset.[33] Therefore, we wanted to determine whether thymectomy and steroid injection altered this lymphocyte subset by the same degree. The results of neonatal injections of estrogen are shown in Figures 2.3–2.5 and Table 2.1. As indicated in Figure 2.3, the percentage of CD4 lymphocytes was increased over control values at most ages as a result of estrogen injections. In contrast, estrogen injections caused the percentage of CD8 lymphocytes to be lower than control values at all ages (Figure 2.4). Of significance was the gradual change in percentage of CD8 lymphocytes isolated from animals injected with estradiol from 3 to 6 days of age. When these animals reached 32 weeks of age, the percentage of CD8 lymphocytes was close to that of control animals. As shown in Figure 2.5, neonatal estrogen injections cause an elevation over control animals in the CD4/CD8 percentage ratio at all ages, except the 32-week-old animals injected with estradiol from 3 to 6 days of age. In the 32-week-old animals of this treatment group, the CD4/CD8 percentage ratio in both thymus and spleen was virtually identical to the CD4/CD8 percentage ratio in control animals. Of greatest importance to the study was the observation that this was the only group of steroid-injected animals to have ovaries with corpora lutea (Table 2.1). Note that the percentage of CD8 cells isolated from the thymus of C31, 0- to 3-day estrogen-injected animals was extremely low and remained that way throughout the study (Figure 2.4). In the previous experiment (Figure 2.1), none of the animals of the 0- to 3-day estrogen-injected group ever became fertile. In this experiment, none of the animals had ovaries with corpora lutea (Table 2.1).

Shown in Table 2.2 are the results of neonatal thymectomy. As indicated, the surgery caused a reduction in the percentages of both CD4 and CD8 lymphocytes. However, the greatest decrease was in the CD4

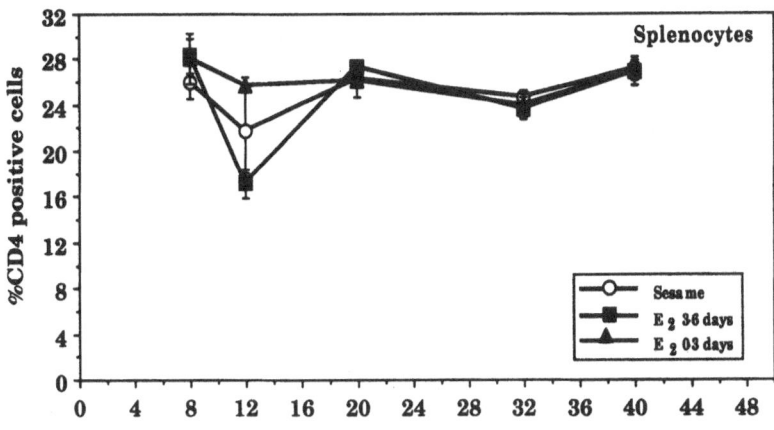

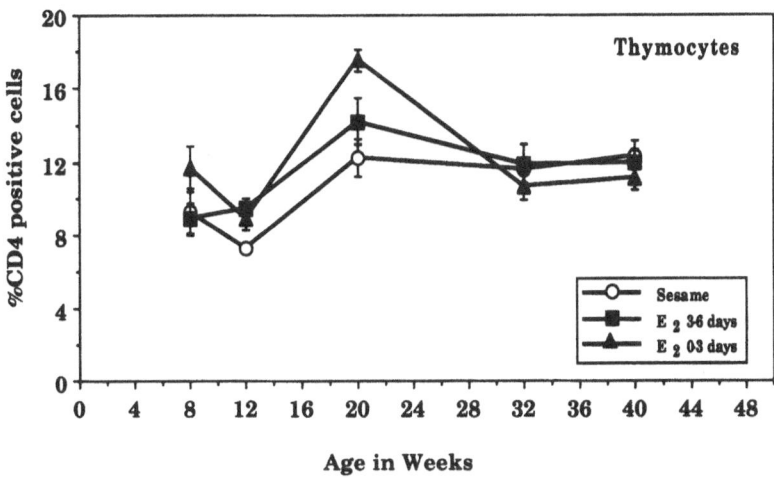

FIGURE 2.3. The effect of estradiol-17β (E_2) injection on the CD4 lymphoid cells in C31 female mice. Groups of animals were given 4 daily injections of 20 µg E, either from 0 to 3 days, or from 3 to 6 days postpartum. One group received injections of sesame oil only. Starting at 8 weeks of age, the animals were killed, spleens and thymuses removed, and lymphocytes analyzed via FACS analysis for the percentages of $CD4^+$ and $CD8^+$ T cells. FACS analysis was via double color label with 20,000 events collected. Each group consisted of 5 mice. Shown are the means ± SEM (Deshpande, Chapman, and Michael, unpublished).

subset. This was not surprising since infusions of CD4 lymphocytes prevented ovarian dysgenesis in neonatally thymectomized mice.[34] Also indicated in Table 2.2, the preferential decrease in the CD4 subset caused by neonatal thymectomy resulted in a lowered CD4/CD8 percentage ratio when compared to control animals. This is in contrast to the effect of

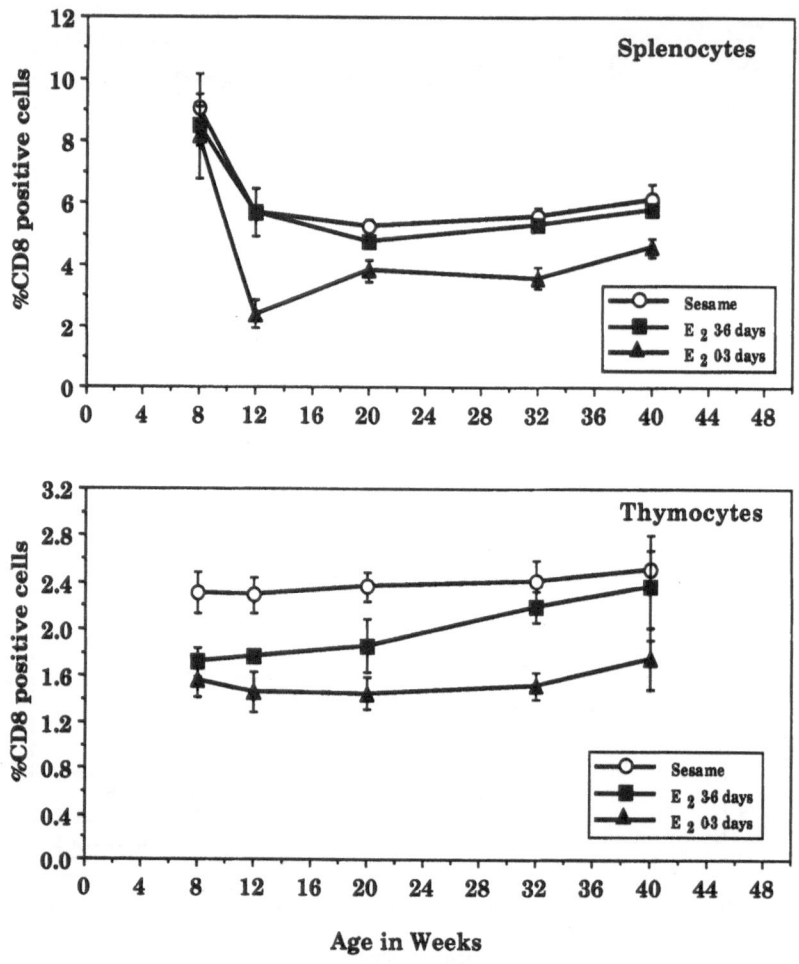

FIGURE 2.4. The effect of estradiol-17β (E_2) injection on the CD8 lymphoid cells in C31 female mice. Procedures are as described in the legend for Figure 2.3. Each group consisted of 5 mice. Shown are the means ± SEM (Deshpande, Chapman, and Michael, unpublished).

neonatal estrogen injections which resulted in an increased CD4/CD8 percentage ratio over that of control animals.

The results of this study strongly suggest that neonatal injections of estradiol-17β preferentially alter the CD8 T-cell subset. This does not corroborate the data of Kalland.[121] Whether this can be attributed to strain differences in mice is not clear at this time. In any event, the literature does contain a number of reports indicating that populations of CD8 lymphocytes are preferentially responsive to levels of estrogen.[122,123,126–128] Further, since reproductive competency can be restored to neonatally thymectomized mice by an infusion of CD4 lymphocytes,[34] it is possible

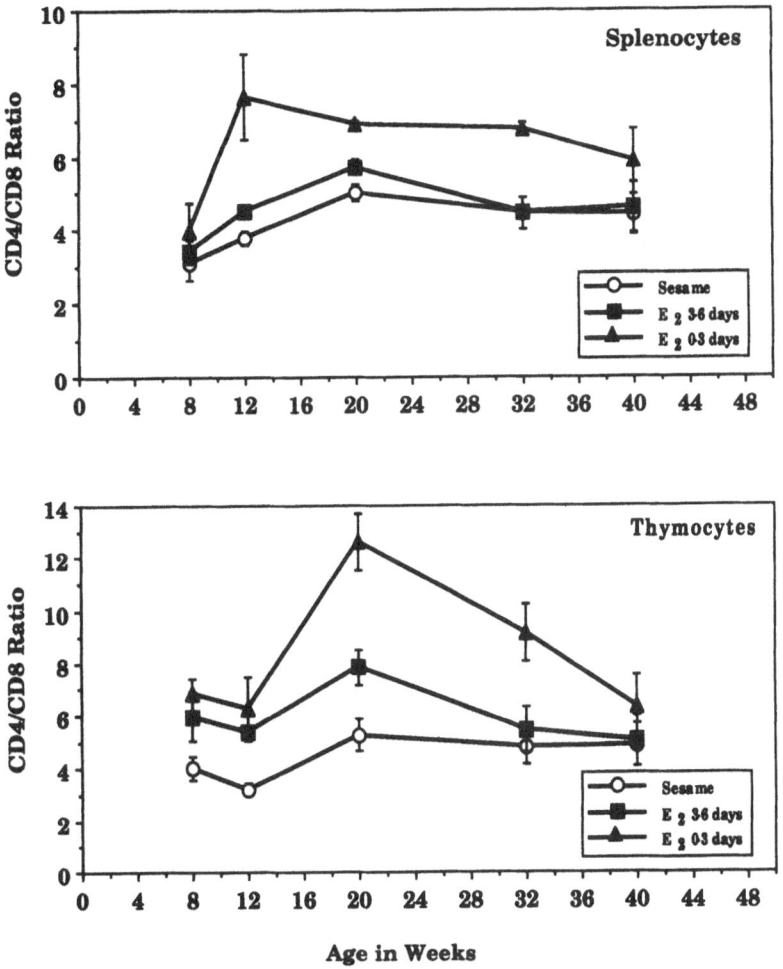

FIGURE 2.5. The effect of estradiol-17β (E_2) injection on CD4/CD8 lymphoid cell ratio in C31 female mice. Individual percentages of lymphoid cells shown as a mean value in Figures 2.3 and 2.4 were recalculated as a ratio of percentage CD4 cells to percentage CD8 cells. Each group consisted of 5 mice. Shown are their means ± SEM (Deshpande, Chapman, and Michael, unpublished).

that anovulation in the estrogen-injected animal can be obviated by an infusion of CD8 lymphocytes.

Conclusions and Future Research

It is becoming increasingly clear that the immune system is essential to female reproduction. Its first critical role is in reproductive development. Animals that are either congenitally athymic or are thymectomized never

TABLE 2.1. Effect of neonatal estradiol injections on corpora lutea formation in the ovaries of C31 female mice.[a]

Injection Treatment	Percentage of animals with ovaries containing corpora lutea at given week of age:				
	8 wks	12 wks	20 wks	32 wks	40 wks
Sesame oil	100%	100%	100%	100%	100%
Estradiol					
0–3 days	0%	0%	0%	0%	0%
3–6 days	0%	0%	0%	40%	40%

[a] Newborn female (C3H/HeJ × 129/J)F$_1$ (C31) mice were injected with sesame oil, or with sesame oil containing 20 µg estradiol-17β for 4 consecutive days, beginning either on day 0 postpartum (0–3 days), or on day 3 (3–6 days). At adulthood, the animals were killed and the ovaries examined histologically for the presence of corpora lutea. Each group consisted of 5 mice (Deshpande, Chapman, and Michael, unpublished).

attain reproductive competence. In euthymic, postpubertal animals, components of the thymic/immune system are involved in several aspects of normal ovarian function. For example, macrophages are a requisite component of corpora lutea, and very likely involved in progesterone synthesis and luteolysis. In addition, lymphocytes have been implicated in luteolysis, as well as in follicular maturation. We have chosen to study the role of lymphocytes in ovarian physiology by examining the effects of neonatal steroid injections on lymphocyte development. So far, a tentative correlation has been made between estrogen depression of the CD8 lymphocyte maturation rate with delayed fertility in the C31 female

TABLE 2.2. The effect of neonatal thymectomy (Tx-3) on %CD4 and %CD8 positive cells isolated from spleens of B6A female mice.[a]

Treatment	%CD4 cells	%CD8 cells	CD4/CD8 ratio
Intact	26.87 ± 0.5	6.82 ± 0.3	3.19 ± 0.1
Tx-3	8.08 ± 0.6	3.22 ± 0.1	2.55 ± 0.2

[a] Intact and neonatally thymectomized 12-week-old female (C57BL × A/J)F$_1$ (B6A) mice were killed and their spleens removed and analyzed via FACS analysis for the percentages of CD4$^+$ and CD8$^+$ splenocytes. FACS analysis was via double color label with 20,000 events collected. Each group consisted of 5 mice (Deshpande, Chapman and Michael, unpublished).

mouse. To make the correlation less tentative, the estrogen-injected animal is to be given an infusion of CD8 lymphocytes to determine if this restores normal ovarian function earlier, rather than later. Following this, the particular CD8 subset will be characterized by analyzing the requisite lymphocytes for suppressor and cytotoxic function. The deleterious effects of testosterone injection on ovarian function are not ameliorated over time. This is in contrast to estrogen injections and suggests that the effects of testosterone are permanent. As to whether testosterone affects the maturation rate of the CD8 lymphocytes similarly to estrogen will be the subject of a future study.

Acknowledgments. We acknowledge the efforts of Dr. Michele Kosiewicz, Mr. William Griffin, Ms. Rohini Deshpande, and Mr. Milo Vassallo. Data taken from their individual research projects were used in this chapter. Financial support for the research projects was provided by the National Institutes of Health through grant #R01-HD2336203.

References

1. Calzolari A. Rescherches experimentales sur un rapport probable entre la function du thymus et cells des testicules. Arch Ital Biol 1898; 30:71–77.
2. Chiodi H. The relationship between the thymus and the sexual organs. Endocrinology 1940; 26:107–116.
3. Fitzpatrick FTA, Kendall MD, Wheeler MJ, Adcock IM, Greenstein BD. Reappearance of thymus of ageing rats after orchidectomy. J Endocrinol 1985; 106:R17–R19.
4. Greenstein BD, Fitzpatrick FTA, Adcock IM, Kendall MD, Wheeler MJ. Reappearance of the thymus in old rats after orchidectomy: Inhibition of regeneration by testosterone. J Endocrinol 1986; 110:417–422.
5. Utsuyama M, Hirokawa K. Hypertrophy of the thymus and restoration of immune functions in mice and rats by gonadectomy. Mech Ageing Dev 1989; 47:175–185.
6. Flanagan SP. (Nude) a new hairless gene with pleiotropic effects in the mouse. Genet Res 1966; 8:295–309.
7. Shire JGM, Pantelouris EM. Comparison of endocrine function in normal and genetically athymic mice. J Comp Biochem Physiol 1974; 47A:93–100.
8. Besedovsky HO, Sorkin E. Thymus involvement in sexual maturation. Nature 1974; 249:356–358.
9. Alten HE, Groscurth P. The postnatal development of the ovary in the nude mouse. Anat Embryol 1975; 148:35–46.
10. Rebar RW, Morandini IC, Erickson GF, Petze JE. The hormonal basis of reproductive defects in athymic mice: Diminished gonadotropin concentrations in prepubertal females. Endocrinology 1981; 108:120–126.
11. Bukovsky A, Presl J, Holub M. Ovarian morphology in congenitally athymic mice. Folia Biol (Praha) 1978; 24:442–444.

12. Lintern-Moore S, Pantelouris EM. Ovarian development in athymic nude mice. I. The size and composition of the follicle population. Mech Ageing Dev 1975, 4:385–390.

13. Sprumont P. Ovarian follicles of normal NMRI mice and homozygous 'nude' mice. 2. Morphometric comparison before puberty and after puberty in various environments. Cell Tissue Res 1978; 188:389–408.

14. Lintern-Moore S, Pantelouris EM. Ovarian development in athymic nude mice. II. The growth of the oocyte and follicle. Mech Ageing Dev 1975; 4:391–398.

15. Rebar RW, Morandini IC, Silva de Sa MF, Erickson GF, Petze JE. The importance of the thymus gland for normal reproductive function in mice. In: Schwartz NB, Hunzicker-Dunn M, eds. Dynamics of Ovarian Function. New York: Raven Press; 1981:285–290.

16. Rebar RW, Morandini IC, Benirschke K, Petze JE. Reduced gonadotropins in athymic mice: Prevention by thymic transplantation. Endocrinology 1980; 107:2130–2135.

17. Pierpaoli W, Besedovsky HO. Role of the thymus in programming of neuro-endocrine functions. Clin Exp Immunol 1975; 20:323–338.

18. Nishizuka Y, Sakakura T. Thymus and reproduction: Sex-linked dysgenesis of the gonad after neonatal thymectomy in mice. Science 1969; 166:753–755.

19. Nishizuka Y, Sakakura T. Ovarian dysgenesis induced by neonatal thymectomy in the mouse. Endocrinology 1971; 89:886–893.

20. Nishizuka Y, Sakakura T. Effect of combined removal of thymus and pituitary on post-natal ovarian development in the mouse. Endocrinology 1971; 89:902–903.

21. Nishizuka Y, Sakakura T. Thymic control mechanism in ovarian development: Reconstitution of ovarian dysgenesis in thymectomized mice by replacement with thymic and other lynphoid tissues. Endocrinology 1972; 90:431–437.

22. Hattori M, Brandon MR. Thymus and the endocrine system: Ovarian dysgenesis in neonatally thymectomized rats. J Endocrinol 1979; 83:101–111.

23. Michael SD. Interactions of the thymus and the ovary. In: Greenwald GS, Terranova PF, eds. Factors Regulating Ovarian Function. New York: Raven Press; 1983:445–464.

24. Kosiewicz MM, Michael SD. Neonatal thymectomy affects follicle populations before the onset of autoimmune oophoritis in B6A mice. J Reprod Fertil 1990; 88:427–440.

25. Michael SD, Taguchi O, Nishizuka Y. Effect of neonatal thymectomy on ovarian development and plasma LH, FSH, GH, and PRL in the mouse. Biol Reprod 1980; 22:343–350.

26. Michael SD, Taguchi O, Nishizuka Y. Changes in hypophyseal hormones associated with accelerated aging and tumorigenesis of the ovaries in neonatally thymectomized mice. Endocrinology 1981; 108:2375–2380.

27. Nishizuka Y, Sakakura T, Tsujimura T, Matsumoto K. Steroid biosynthesis in vitro by dysgenic ovaries induced by neonatal thymectomy in mice. Endocrinology 1973; 93:786–792.

28. Michael SD, Taguchi O, Nishizuka Y, McClure JE, Goldstein AL, Barkley MS. The effect of neonatal thymectomy on early follicular loss and circulating levels of corticosterone, progesterone, estradiol, and thymosin-α1. In:

Schwartz NB, Hunzicker-Dunn M, eds. Dynamics of Ovarian Function. New York: Raven Press; 1981:279–284.

29. Marmor LH, Michael SD. Circulating levels of testosterone in neonatally thymectomized female mice. IRCS Med Sci 1984; 12:1022–1023.

30. Scalzo CM, Michael SD. Sources of high testosterone levels associated with autoimmune ovarian dysgenesis in neonatally thymectomized B6A mice. Biol Reprod 1988; 38:1115–1121.

31. Sakakura T, Nishizuka Y. Thymic control mechanism in ovarian development: Reconstitution of ovarian dysgenesis in thymectomized mice by replacement with thymic and other lymphoid tissues. Endocrinology 1972; 90:431–437.

32. Kojima A, Sakakura T, Tanaka Y, Nishizuka Y. Sterility in neonatally thymectomized female mice: Its nature and prevention by the injection of spleen cells. Biol Reprod 1973; 8:358–361.

33. Sakaguchi S, Takahashi T, Nishizuka Y. Study on cellular events in post-thymectomy autoimmune oophoritis in mice. II. Requirement of Lyt-1 cells in normal female mice for the prevention of oophoritis. J Exp Med 1982; 156:1577–1586.

34. Smith H, Sakamoto Y, Kasai K, Tung KSK. Effector and regulatory cells in autoimmune oophoritis elicited by neonatal thymectomy. J Immunol 1991; 147:2928–2933.

35. Healy DL, Bacher J, Hodgen GD. Thymic regulation of primate fetal ovarian–adrenal differentiation. Biol Reprod 1985; 32:1127–1133.

36. Miller JJ, Chatten J. Ovarian changes in ataxia telangectasia. Acta Paediatr Scand 1967; 56:559–561.

37. Grossman CJ. Interactions between the gonadal steroids and the immune system. Science 1985; 227:257–261.

38. Screpanti I, Gulino A, Pasqualini JR. The fetal thymus of guinea pig as an estrogen target organ. Endocrinology 1982; 111:1552–1561.

39. Gulimo A, Screpanti I, Torrisi MR, Frati L. Estrogen receptors and estrogen sensitivity of fetal thymocytes are restricted to blast lymphoid cells. Endocrinology 1985; 117:47–54.

40. Grossman CJ, Sholiton LJ, Nathan P. Rat thymic estrogen receptor. I. Preparation, location, and physiochemical properties. J Steroid Biochem 1979; 11:1233–1240.

41. Grossman CJ, Sholiton LJ, Blaha GC, Nathan P. Rat thymic estrogen receptor. II. Physiological properties. J Steroid Biochem 1979; 11:1241–1246.

42. Grossman CJ, Nathan P, Taylor BB, Sholiton LJ. Rat dihydrotestosterone receptor. Preparation, location, and physiochemical properties. Steroids 1979; 34:539–553.

43. Pearce P, Khalid BAK, Funder JW. Androgens and the thymus. Endocrinology 1981; 109:1073–1077.

44. Pearce P, Khalid BAK, Funder JW. Progesterone receptors in rat thymus. Endocrinology 1983; 113:1287–1291.

45. Fujii-Hanamoto H, Grossman CJ, Roselle GA, Mendenhall CL. Nuclear progestin receptors in rat thymic tissue. Thymus 1990; 15:31–45.

46. Kovacs WJ, Olsen NJ. Androgen receptors in human thymocytes. J Immunol 1987; 139:490–493.

47. Dauphinee MJ, Kipper S, Roskos K, Wofsky D, Talal N. Androgen treatment of NZB/W mice enhances IL-2 production. Arthritis Rheum 1981; 24(suppl):S64.118.

48. Grossman CJ. The regulation of the immune system by sex steroids. Endocr Rev 1984; 5(3):435–448.

49. Marchetti B, Cioni M, Badr M, Follea N, Pelletier G. Ovarian adrenergic nerves directly participate in the control of luteinizing hormone-releasing hormone and adrenergic receptors during puberty: A biochemical and autoradiographic study. Endocrinology 1987; 121:219–227.

50. Marchetti B, Cioni M. Opposite changes of pituitary and ovarian receptors for LHRH in aging rats: Further evidence for a direct neural control of ovarian LHRH receptor activity. Neuroendocrinology 1988; 48:242–252.

51. Marchetti B, Pelletier G, Cioni M, Badr M, Palumbo G, Scapagnini U. Age-dependent changes of LHRH receptor systems: Role of central and peripheral LHRH in the decline of reproductive function. In: Genanzaani AR, Montemagno U, Nappi C, Petraglia F, eds. The Brain and Female Reproductive Function. Parthenon Press, 1988:207–220.

52. Marchetti B, Guarcello V, Morale MC, Bartoloni G, Farinella Z, Cordaro S, Scapagini U. Luteinizing hormone-releasing hormone binding sites in the rat thymus: Characteristics and biological function. Endocrinology 1989; 125:1025–1036.

53. Marchetti B, Guarcello V, Morale MC, Bartoloni G, Raiti F, Palumbo G, Farinella Z, Cordaro S, Scapagnini U. Luteinizing hormone-releasing hormone (LHRH) agonist restoration of age-associated decline of thymus weight, thymic LHRH receptors and thymocyte proliferative capacity. Endocrinology 1989; 125:1037–1045.

54. Morale MC, Batticane N, Bartoloni G, Guarcello V, Farinella Z, Galasso MG, Marchetti B. Blockade of central and peripheral luteinizing hormone-releasing hormone (LHRH) receptors in neonatal rats with a potent LHRH-antagonist inhibits the morphofunctional development of the thymus and maturation of the cell-mediated and humoral immune responses. Endocrinology 1991; 128:1073–1085.

55. Marchetti B, Guarcello V, Scapagini U. Luteinizing hormone-releasing hormone agonist (LHRH-A) binds to lymphocytes and modulates the immune response. In: Castagnetta L, Nenci I, eds. Biology and Biochemistry of Normal and Cancer Cell Growth. London: Harwood Academic Press; 1988:149–153.

56. Emanuele MA, Tentler J, Kirstein L, Emanuele NV, Lawrence AM. Rat spleen lymphocytes contain an immunoreactive and bioactive luteinizing hormone-releasing hormone (LHRH). 71st Annual Meeting of the Endocrine Society. 1989; 1252.

57. Batticane N, Morale MC, Gallo F, Farinella Z, Marchetti B. Luteinizing hormone-releasing hormone signalling at the lymphocyte involves stimulation of interleuken-2 receptor expression. Endocrinology 1991; 129:277–286.

58. Marchetti B, Cioni M, Palumbo G, Morale MC, Guarcello V, Scapagini U. Neonatal treatment with LHRH antagonist alters thymocyte maturity in mice. 71st Annual Meeting of the Endocrine Society. 1989; 921.

59. Ebaugh MJ, Smith EM. Human lymphocyte production of immunoreactive luteinizing hormone. 72nd Annual Meeting of the Federation of American Society of Experimental Biologists. 1988; 7811.

60. Rebar RW, Miyake A, Low TLK, Golstein AL. Thymosin stimulates secretion of luteinizing hormone-releasing factor. Science 1981; 214:669–671.
61. Hall NR, McGillis JP, Spangelo BL, Palaszynski E, Moody W, Goldstein AL. Evidence for a neuroendocrine thymus axis mediated by thymosin polypeptides. In: Serrou B, Rosenfeld C, Daniels JC, Saunders JP, eds. International Symposium on Current Concepts in Human Immunology & Cancer Immunomodulation: Proceedings of the International Symposium on Current Concepts in Human Immunology & Cancer Immunomodulation. New York: Elsevier North Holland; 1982:653–660.
62. Ford JJ, Vakharia DD, Anderson LL, Klindt J. Thymosin-β4 concentrations during the estrous cycle and after hypophyseal stalk transection of female pigs. Soc Exp Biol Med 1990; 193:185–189.
63. Wise T, Maurer RR. Characterization of thymosin α1 and β4 during the bovine estrous period: Effects of elevated estradiol and progestin. Biol Reprod 1991; 45:57–63.
64. Allen LS, McClure JE, Goldstein AL, Barkley MS, Michael SD. Estrogen and thymic hormone interactions in the female mouse. J Reprod Immunol 1984; 6:25–37.
65. Prepin J. Thymus and thymulin stimulate the proliferation of oogonia in rat fetal ovaries in vitro. C R Acad Sci (Paris) 1991; 313:407–411.
66. Aguilera G, Romano MC. Influence of the thymus on steroidognesis by rat ovarian cells in vitro. J Endocrinol 1989; 123:367–373.
67. Ahmed SA, Penhale WJ, Talal N. Sex hormones, immune responses, and autoimmune diseases. Am J Path 1985; 121:531–551.
68. Weusten JJAM, Blankenstein MA, Gamlig-Meyling FHJ, Schuurman HJ, Kater L, Thijssen JHH. Presence of oestrogen receptors in human blood mononuclear cells and thymocytes. Acta Endocrinol 1986; 112:409–414.
69. Danel L, Souweine G, Monier JC, Saez S. Specific estrogen binding sites in human lymphoid cells and thymic cells. J Steroid Biochem 1983; 18:559–563.
70. Pearce PB, Khalid AK, Funder JW. Androgens and the thymus. Endocrinology 1981; 109:1073–1077.
71. Cohen JHM, Danel L, Cordier G, Saez S, Revillard J-P. Sex steroid receptors in peripheral T cells: Absence of androgen receptors and restriction of estrogen receptors to OKT-8 positive cells. J Immunol 1983; 131:2767–2771.
72. Stimson WH. Oestrogen and human T lymphocytes: Presence of specific receptors in the T-suppressor/cytoxic subset. Scand J Immunol 1988; 28:345.
73. Polan ML, Loukides J, Nelson P, Carding S, Diamond M, Walsh A, Bottomly K. Progesterone and estradiol modulate interleukin-1β messenger ribonucleic acid levels in cultured human peripheral monocytes. J Clin Endocrinol Metab 1989; 69:1200–1206.
74. Polan ML, Kuo KA, Loukides J, Bottomly K. Cultured human luteal monocytes secrete increased levels of interleukin-1. J Clin Endocrinol Metab 1990; 70:480–484.
75. Pacifici R, Rifas L, McCracken R, Vered I, McMurtry C, Avioli LV, Peck WA. Ovarian steroid treatment blocks a postmenopausal increase in blood interleukin-1 release. Proc Natl Acad Sci USA 1989; 86:2398–2402.
76. Cannon JC, Dinarello CA. Increased plasma interleukin-1 activity in women after ovulation. Science 1985; 227:1247–1250.
77. Hill JA, Barbieri RL, Anderson DJ. Detection of T8 (suppressor/cytotoxic) lymphocytes in human ovarian follicular fluid. Fertil Steril 1987; 47:114–117.

78. Grasso G, Muscettola M. Possible role of interferon-gamma in ovarian function. Ann NY Acad Sci 1992; 650:191.

79. Bukovsky A, Presl J, Holub M. The ovarian follicle as a model for the cell-mediated control of tissue growth. Cell Tissue Res 1984; 236:717–724.

80. Grossman CJ, Sholiton LJ, Roselle GA. Dihydrotestosterone regulation of thymocyte function in the rat: Mediation by serum factors. J Steroid Biochem 1983; 19:1459–1467.

81. Luster MI, Hayes HT, Korach K, Tucker AN, Dean JH, Greenlee WF, Boorman GA. Estrogen suppression is regulated through estrogenic responses in the thymus. J Immunol 1984; 133:110–116.

82. Grossman CJ, Sholiton LJ, Roselle GA. Estradiol regulation of thymocyte function in the rat: Mediation by serum thymic factors. J Steroid Biochem 1982; 16:683–690.

83. Sakabe K, Kawashima I, Seiki K, Fujii-Hanamoto H. Hormone and immune response, with special reference to steroid hormone. 2. Sex steroid receptors in rat thymus. Tokai J Clin Med 1990; 15:201–211.

84. Kawashima I, Sakabe K, Seiki K, Fujii-Hanamoto H, Akatsuka A, Tsukamoto H. Localization of sex steroid receptor cells, with special reference to thymulin (FTS)-producing cells in female rat thymus. Thymus 1991; 18:79–93.

85. Bukovsky A, Presl J, Holub M, Mancal P, Krabec Z. The localization of brain–thymus shared antigen (Thy-1) and thymosin 5 within the adult rat ovary. IRCS Med Sci 1982; 10:69–70.

86. Presl J, Bukovsky A. Role of Thy-1$^+$ and Ia$^+$ cells in ovarian function. Biol Reprod 1986; 34:159–169.

87. Loukides JA, Loy RA, Edwards R, Honig J, Visintin I, Polan ML. Human follicular fluids contain tissue macrophages. J Clin Endocrinol Metab 1990; 71:1363–1367.

88. Hume DA, Halpin D, Charlton H, Gordon S. The mononuclear phagocyte system of the mouse defined by immunohistochemical localization of antigen F4/80: Macrophages of endocrine organs. Proc Natl Acad Sci 1984; 81:4174–4177.

89. Bagavandoss P, Kunkel SL, Wiggins RC, Keyes, PL. Tumor necrosis factor-a (TNF-a) production and localization of macrophages and T lymphocytes in the rabbit corpus luteum. Endocrinology 1988; 122:1185–1187.

90. Kirsch TM, Friedman AC, Vogel RL, Flickinger GL. Macrophages in corpora lutea of mice: Characterization and effects on steroid secretion. Biol Reprod 1981; 25:629–638.

91. Kirsch TM, Vogel RL, Flickinger GL. Macrophages: A source of luteotropic cybernins. Endocrinology 1983; 113:1910–1912.

92. Goodwin JS, Ceuppens JL, Gualde N. Control of the immune response in humans by prostaglandins. In: Advances in Inflammation Research, Vol 7. Otterness I, Capetola RJ, Wong S, eds. New York: Raven Press; 1984:79–92.

93. Hadden JW. Neuroendocrine modulation of the thymus-dependent immune system. In: Jankovic BD, Markovic BM, Spector NH, eds. Neuroimmune interactions: Proceedings of the Second International Workshop on Neuroimmunomodulation. Ann NY Acad Sci 1987; 496:39–48.

94. Adashi EY. The potential relevance of cytokines to ovarian physiology: The emerging role of resident ovarian cells of the white blood cell series. Endocr Rev 1990; 11:454–464.

95. Azad N, Agrawal L, Emanuele MA, Kelley MR, Mohagheghpour N, Lawrence AM, Emanuele NV. Advances in neuroimmuno-endocrinology. Am J Reprod Immunol 1991; 26:160–172.

96. Espey LL. Ovulation as an inflammatory reaction—a hypothesis. Biol Reprod 1980; 22:73–106.

97. De Weger RA, Pels E, Den Otter W. The induction of lymphocytes with the capacity to render macrophages cytoxic in an allogeneic murine system. Immunology 1982; 47:541.

98. Pels E, Deweger RA, Den Otter W. Lymphocyte induced macrophage cytotoxicity: Characterization of the macrophage cytotoxicity-inducing lymphocyte. Immunobiology 1984; 166:84.

99. Reinherz EL, Kung PC, Pesando JR, Ritz J, Goldstein C, Schlossman SF. Ia determinants on human T-cell subsets defined by monoclonal antibody. Activation stimuli required for expression. J Exp Med 1979; 150:1472.

100. Warren DW, Pasupuleti V, Lu Y, Platler BW, Horton R. Tumor necrosis factor and interleukin-1 stimulate testosterone secretion in adult male rat Leydig cells in vitro. J Androl 1990; 11:353–360.

101. Hurwitz A, Payne DW, Packman JN, Andreani CL, Resnick CE, Hernandez ER, Adashi EY. Cytokine-mediated regulation of ovarian function: Interleukin-1 inhibits gonadotropin-induced androgen biosynthesis. Endocrinology 1991; 129:1250–1256.

102. Feinberg BB, Tan NS, Gonik B, Brath PC, Walsh SW. Increased progesterone concentrations are necessary to suppress interleukin-2-activated human mononuclear cell cytotoxicity. Am J Obstet Gynecol 1991; 165:1872–1876.

103. Suzuki T, Suzuki N, Daynes RA, Engleman EG. Dehydroepiandrosterone enhances IL-2 production and cytotoxic effector function of human T cells. Clin Immunol Immunopathol 1991; 61:202–211.

104. Adashi EY, Resnick CE, Croft CS, Payne DW. Tumor necrosis factor alpha inhibits gonadotropin hormonal action in nontransformed ovarian granulosa cells. J Biol Chem 1989; 264:11591–11597.

105. Gaillard RC, Turnill D, Sappino P, Muller AF. Tumor necrosis factor alpha inhibits the hormonal response of the pituitary gland to hypothalamic releasing factors. Endocrinology 1990; 127:101–106.

106. Adashi EY, Resnick CE, Packman JN, Hurwitz A, Payne DW. Cytokine-mediated regulation of ovarian function: Tumor necrosis factor α inhibits gonadotropin-supported progesterone accumulation by differentiating and luteinizing murine granulosa cells. Am J Obstet Gynecol 1990; 162:889–899.

107. Ralston SH, Russell RGG, Gowen M. Estrogen inhibits release of tumor necrosis factor from peripheral blood mononuclear cells in postmenopausal women. J Bone Miner Res 1990; 5:983–998.

108. Grasso G, Muscettola M. The influence of beta-estradiol and progesterone on interferon gamma production in vitro. Int J Neurosci 1990; 51:315–317.

109. Ishikawa R, Bigley NJ. Sex hormone modulation of interferon (IFN) alpha/beta and gamma production by mouse spleen cell subsets following picornavirus infection. Viral Immunol 1990; 3:225–236.

110. Fox HS, Bond BL, Parslow TG, Estrogen regulates the IFN-γ promoter. J Immunol 1991; 146:4362–4367.

111. Khan SA, Schmidt K, Hallin P, Pauli R, Degeyter CH, Nieschlag E. Human testis cytosol and ovarian follicular fluid contain high amounts of interleukin-1-like factor(s). Mol Cell Endocrinol 1988; 58:221–230.
112. Gottshall PE, Uehara A, Talbott-Hoffman S, Arimura A. Interleukin-1 inhibits follicle stimulating hormone-induced differentiation in rat granulosa cells in vitro. Biochem Biophys Res Commun 1987; 149:502–507.
113. Fukuoka M, Mori T, Taii S, Yasuda K. Interleukin-1 inhibits luteinization of porcine granulosa cells in culture. Endocrinology 1988; 122:367–369.
114. McNatty KP, Smith DM, Makris A, Osathanondh R, Ryan KJ. The microenvironment of the human antral follicle: Interrelationships among the steroid levels in antral fluid, the population of granulosa cells, and the status of the oocyte in vivo and in vitro. J Clin Endocrinol Metab 1979; 49:851–860.
115. Hughes FM, Pringle CM, Gorospe WC. Production of progestin-stimulating factor(s) by enriched populations of rat T and B lymphocytes. Biol Reprod 1991; 44:922–926.
116. Emi N, Kanzaki H, Yoshida M, Takakura K, Kariya M, Okamoto N, Imai K, Mori T. Lymphocytes stimulate progesterone production by cultured human granulosa luteal cells. Am J Obstet Gynecol 1991; 165:1469–1474.
117. Hill JA, Welch WR, Faris HMP, Anderson DJ. Induction of class II major histocompatibility complex antigen expression in human granulosa cells by interferon-gamma: A potential mechanism contributing to autoimmune ovarian failure. Am J Obstet Gynecol 1990; 162:534–540.
118. Gorospe WC, Tuchel T, Kasson G. γ-Interferon inhibits rat granulosa cell differentiation in culture. Biochem Biophys Res Commun 1988; 157: 891–897.
119. Espevik T, Figari IS, Shalaby MR, Lackides GA, Lewis GD, Shepard HM, Palladino Jr MA. Inhibition of cytokine production by cyclosporin A and transforming growth factor. J Exp Med 1987; 166:571–576.
120. Al-Chalabi HA. Effect of cyclosporin A on the morphology and function of the ovary and fertility in the rabbit. Int J Fertil 1984; 29:218–223.
121. Kalland TK. Decreased and disproportionate T-cell population in adult mice after neonatal exposure to diethylstibestrol. Cellular Immunol 1980; 51:55–63.
122. Novotny EA, Raveche ES, Sharrow S, Ottinger M, Steinberg AD. Analysis of thymocyte subpopulations following treatment with sex hormones. Clin Immunol Immunopathol 1983; 28:205–217.
123. Ahmed SA, Dauphinee MJ, Talal N. Effects of short-term administration of sex hormones on normal and autoimmune mice. J Immunol 1985; 134:204–210.
124. Screpanti I, Morrone S, Meco D, Santoni A, Gulino A, Paolini R, Crisanti A, Mathieson BJ, Frati L. Steroid sensitivity of thymocyte subpopulations during intrathymic differentiation. Effects of 17β-estradiol and dexamethasone on subsets expressing T-cell antigen receptor or IL-2 receptor. J Immunol 1989; 142:3378–3383.
125. Mathur S, Mathur RS, Goust JM, Williamson HO, Fudenberg HH. Cyclic variation in white cell subpopulations in the human menstrual cycle: Correlations with progesterone and estradiol. Clin Immunol Immunopathol 1979; 13:246–253.

126. Ho PC, Tang GWK, Fu KH, Fan MC, Lawton JWM. Immunologic studies in patients with premature ovarian failure. Obstet Gynecol 1988; 71:622–626.
127. Ho PC, Tang GWK, Lawton JWM. Lymphocyte subsets in patients with oestrogen deficiency. J Reprod Immunol 1991; 20:85–91.
128. Grossman CJ. Bidirectional communication between the immune and endocrine systems: Sex steroid influence on thymic lymphocytes. Am J Reprod Immunol 1992; 27:21.
129. Bukovsky A, Presl J, Krabec Z, Bednarik T. Ovarian function in rats treated with antithymocyte serum. Experimentia 1977; 33:280–281.
130. Alila HW, Hansel W. Induction of lymphopenia causes luteal dysfunction in cattle. Biol Reprod 1984; 31:671–678.
131. Barraclough CA, Leathem JH. Infertility induced in mice by a single injection of testosterone propionate. Proc Soc Exp Biol Med 1954; 85:673–674.
132. Barraclough CA. Production of anovulatory, sterile rats by single injections of testosterone propionate. Endocrinology 1961; 68:62–67.
133. Barraclough C, Gorski RA. Evidence that the hypothalamus is responsible for androgen-induced sterility in the female rat. Endocrinology 1961; 68:68–79.
134. Gorski RA. Modification of ovulatory mechanisms by postnatal administration of estrogen to the rat. Am J Physiol 1963; 205:842–844.
135. Gorski RA, Barraclough CA. Effects of low dosages of androgen on the differentiation of hypothalamic regulatory control of ovulation in the rat. Endocrinology 1963; 73:210–216.
136. Gorski RA. Steroid-induced sexual characteristics in the brain. In: Muller EE, MacLeod RM, eds. Neuroendocrine Function. Amsterdam: Elsvier Science Publishers; 1983; 2:1–35.
137. Gorski RA. Sexual differentiation of the brain: Comparative aspects. In: Grumbach MM, Sizonenko PC, Aubert ML, eds. Control of the Onset of Puberty. Baltimore: Williams and Wilkins Publishers; 1990:231–250.
138. Naftolin F, Garcia-Segura LM, Feefe D, Leranth C, Maclusky NJ, Brawer JR. Estrogen effects on the synaptology and neural membranes of the rat hypothalamic arcuate nucleus. Biol Reprod 1990; 42:21–26.
139. Kincl FA, Oriol A, Folch Pi A, Maqueo M. Prevention of steroid-induced sterility in neonatal rats with thymic cell suspension. Proc Soc Exp Biol Med 1965; 120:252–253.
140. Forsberg JG. Treatment with different antiestrogens in the neonatal period and effects in the cervicovaginal epithelium and ovaries of adult mice: A comparison to estrogen-induced changes. Biol Reprod 1985; 32:427–441.
141. Kincl FA. Influence of steroid treatment during neonatal life on sexual maturation. Proc Royal Soc Med 1966; 59:817–818.
142. Arai Y. A possible process of the secondary sterilization: Delayed anovulation syndrome. Experimentia 1971; 27:463–464.
143. Knobil E. On the neuroendocrine control of the menstrual cycle. Recent Prog Horm Res 1980; 36:53.

3
Effects of Estrogens/Androgens on the Immune Response

ALAN B. McCRUDEN AND WILLIAM H. STIMSON

The effects of sex steroids on the immune system had remained largely undetermined because the model for steroid action was taken to be the glucocorticoid system, which is easily examined in a wide range of in vitro assay systems. The action of practically any immune cell can be modified by either physiological or pharmacological concentrations of this class of hormone; a good dose–response relationship can also be seen in these systems. These actions could then be extrapolated to the desirable anti-inflammatory properties seen in vivo. Receptor affinity and potency measurements for synthetic analogues led to the development of a range of synthetic glucocorticoids with improved properties. Thus dexamethasone, for instance, has a higher anti-inflammatory action but a lower mineralocorticoid effect than cortisol. The distribution of glucocorticoid receptors throughout the body is universal and, therefore, an effect can be expected in any tissue.

Sex steroid receptor distribution was thought to be confined to those tissues immediately concerned with reproduction and secondary sex characteristics, together with components of the central nervous system. However, when it began to be suspected that the sex steroids may have a role in the apparent immunological tolerance of the mother towards the fetus during pregnancy, workers turned toward the type of in vitro assay system that had proved so useful in the analysis of glucocorticoid action. However, attempts to correlate sex steroid concentrations with the responses of isolated leucocytes in vitro were unsuccessful.[1] There have even been recent attempts to do this sort of experiment again, without success.[2,3] It is now believed that tolerance in pregnancy is mediated by antigen-specific mechanisms, but there is good evidence that the sex steroids are responsible for some of the immunological changes during gestation and, perhaps more importantly, for the sex differences that are a feature of the majority of autoimmune diseases. The failure of in vitro experiments to show any direct effects on leucocytes led us to suggest that the effects in vivo proceeded by indirect routes, as indeed might be expected, given the distributed architecture of the immune system in lymphoid tissue, as well as in the form of effector leucocytes.[4,5] More complete understanding began to emerge as we and others identified specific androgen and estrogen receptors in primary lymphoid tissues, and, more recently, in leucocyte subpopulations, which had previously defied analysis. This chapter will review how these direct and indirect effects on immune system cells contribute to the physiological action of sex steroids on the immune system, as well as considering their possible role in the pathology of certain diseases.

Sex differences in immunological responses have been extensively documented. Plasma immunoglobulin levels are higher in females,[6-8] as are the primary and secondary responses to a number of pathogens, including brucella, hepatitis B, and rubella.[9-11] Cell-mediated immunity (CMI) is possibly also higher in females, although this may depend on how it is measured; graft rejection is certainly more vigorous.[12-14] This increased reactivity may be a reflection of the higher incidence of autoimmune disease seen in women; these include rheumatoid arthritis, systemic lupus erythematosus, and autoallergic thyroiditis.[15,16] It is also interesting to note that allergies are more common in males until puberty, after which the prevalence is greater in females.[17]

Immunological Effects of Androgen

Testosterone can increase susceptibility to infection,[18] inhibit the development of autoallergic thyroiditis in male animals, and ameliorate the effects of adjuvant arthritis,[19,20] It has been shown to reduce cellular invasion of the lacrimal glands in a mouse model of Sjogren's syndrome.[21] It can cause changes in $CD^+/CD8^+$ lymphocyte distribution in animals in experiments involving castration and restoration with exogenous hormone.[22] This change could be expected to reduce immune responsiveness, as would the increase in suppressor cell activity reported by Holdstock et al.[23] A profound effect of sex steroids on immunity in vivo can be seen in the (NZB × NZW) F_1 mouse, which is regarded as a good model for the human autoimmune disease systemic lupus erythematosus (SLE). This occurs in a female/male ratio approaching 14:1, which is reflected in the increased incidence and severity in female NZB/NZW animals.[24] Androgenic hormones such as testosterone or 5α-dihydrotestosterone can be used as a prophylactic measure in young animals and, importantly, can give therapeutic benefit in older animals with established disease. Estrogen has an opposite effect, giving rise to early and severe symptoms, even in male animals;[25-27] these effects are at least partially dependent on the presence of the thymus.[26] Huston et al.[28] demonstrated that the thymic epithelium was important to the development of the autoantibodies that are a characteristic feature of this disease.

Thymic atrophy occurs at puberty in both sexes. Testosterone itself can cause this effect. Gregoire[29] showed that the reduction in size of the gland, following treatment, was largely due to the loss of cortical thymocytes, but in addition indicated that the thymic epithelial cells were involved in this process. Definitive evidence for the involvement of the thymic epithelium came when a number of workers identified specific androgen receptors located there, in animals[30–33] and in human thymus.[34,35] The epithelial cells, which produce thymopoietin and various other thymic hormones, also participate in the very important localized processing of T lymphocytes.[36,37] Antireceptor antibodies have recently been used to confirm receptor distribution.[38] These results provide an explanation as to why many immunomodulatory effects are seen only in the whole animal and can be abolished by prior removal of the thymus. Androgen receptors have not so far been demonstrated on any type of lymphocyte, so it seems likely that the effects reported above are mediated indirectly. Testosterone does seem to be able to modify surface marker expression on leucocyte subpopulations in vivo. In idiopathic hypogonadotrophic hypogonadism, $CD4^+$ (helper phenotype) cells are elevated and the number of $CD16^+$ (non-T, non-B) cells is reduced compared to normal controls; following treatment, to restore normal testosterone levels, the two populations also normalized. Natural killer cell activity was normal in these individuals and was unaffected by treatment.[39]

The thymus is only one part of the primary lymphoid system. The bursa of Fabricius in birds and its presumed mammalian equivalent in the bone marrow must also be considered as a possible route of action; bursal size is susceptible to hormonal manipulation in a way similar to the thymus.[40–43] Sullivan and Wira[44] demonstrated a bursal androgen receptor. In thymus-independent areas of peripheral lymphoid tissue, testosterone can be shown to cause histological changes, presumably following upon some bursal effect. This was thought to involve a reduction in the number of progenitor cells that would commit to the B cell lineage.[45–47] As well as influencing differentiation events within primary lymphoid tissue, such as bursa/bone marrow and thymus, androgen has been shown to elicit the production of soluble immunoregulatory factors by the thymic epithelial cells referred to above.[48,49] While such factors may be important in the local processing of immature cells, they probably also influence, via the circulation, peripheral blood lymphocytes and lymph node cells; thymocytes and mature lymphocytes certainly respond to these epithelial cell culture supernatants.[49] A circulating thymic factor had previously been elicited by estrogen treatment of rats.[5] It seems likely that androgen can elicit similar factors, in the light of the epithelial culture results. Testosterone has also been shown to antagonize the increase in antibody response to sheep red blood cells caused by injected thymosin fraction 5.[50] Curiously, a direct effect from testosterone, using isolated leucocytes, has also been noted in a system using pokeweed mitogen-driven B-cell proliferation.[51] It may be that some as yet unidentified subpopulation of lymphocytes is directly sensitive to this hormone.

The remarkable therapeutic effect of androgen in the NZB/NZW mouse led a number of workers to carry out trials on patients with SLE. Estrogen did appear to exacerbate the condition, but the effects of androgen were variable.[52-54] An early trial of the anabolic steroid nandrolone (19-nor-testosterone-decanoate) had a marginal effect in the improvement of the suppressor/helper T-cell ratio.[55] This steroid had been shown to have good affinity for the thymic androgen receptor in the rat and is less virilizing than testosterone itself. Pharmacokinetic data did show that the necessary plasma steroid concentration had not been maintained in this study (Bergink 1983, unpublished data). A recent trial with 19-nor-testosterone showed no effect on female patients and appeared to worsen the condition in males.[56] It may be that a steroid with a greater affinity for the thymus may prove more useful. The male patients' testosterone level declined, which might be expected if the synthetic steroid was causing feedback inhibition in the hypothalamus. There is evidence that a degree of thymus targeting can be achieved by modifying steroid structure. Receptor affinity data in both rat and human have indicated that the 5α-dihydro form of 19-nor-testosterone has an even higher affinity for the thymus, together with a lower affinity for a classical androgen dependent tissue, the prostate.[35,57] While this steroid would be expected to have an even lower virilizing capacity, it is not clear that this would prevent the undesirable effects noted in males in the recent study. Human SLE probably has a number of possible etiological factors, whereas an inbred mouse strain represents only one possible set of circumstances. Another model of human autoimmunity, the MRL lpr/lpr mouse, shows a different pattern of response to steroids, with some pathological events being ameliorated by estrogen, but others, as in the NZB/NZW model, made worse.[58] A better understanding of which particular pathology is dominant is a given patient may allow better selection of steroid treatment. In addition, there is some evidence that thymic hormones can be important in the induction of suppressor cell activity in SLE.[52]

A large part of immune system development takes place during fetal life, at a time when it is known that sex steroids play an important role in the regulation of differentiation in the reproductive organs and the brain. A number of reports suggest that the immune system is also influenced at this early stage. A connection between fetal androgen exposure, left handedness, and impaired immune regulation has been suggested. Statistics show that there is a higher incidence of autoimmune disease in dyslexic or left-handed individuals, and an elevated fetal androgen concentration has been implicated.[59,60] Effects on cerebral development and immunity in adult life have been produced by testosterone treatment.[59]

Naturally left-handed women have been shown to have lower natural killer cell activity than right-handed controls,[61] and similar effects have been shown in mice.[62] In contrast, T-cell mitogen responsiveness is higher in 'left-handed' mice.[63] Fetal estrogen exposure has also been reported to influence immunity[64] and there is evidence that immunodeficient mice have cognitive defects.[65]

Immunological Effects of Estrogen

The immune response is often considered in terms of a dichotomy between humoral and cell-mediated mechanisms. The response to estrogen appears to be split in this way, in that cell-mediated immunity is depressed[66-69] and humoral immunity enhanced,[5,70] as are the responses to certain mitogens.[71] This may be of value during pregnancy, where a degree of CMI depression is offset by an improved humoral response.

As previously mentioned, SLE occurs mainly in women, and estrogens have been shown to worsen the disease in both animal models and patients. Aberrant steroid metabolism has been found in patients, resulting in the production of high levels of 16α-hydroxyestrone, even in males.[72,73] This steroid has a high receptor affinity and its concentration could reduce suppressor cell-like function and promote autoantibody production in a way similar to estradiol. Elevated estrogen production is also a feature of Klinefelter's syndrome, which is associated with a higher risk of SLE development.[52,73,74] Sex steroid concentrations show considerable variation throughout the menstrual cycle and this is reflected in cyclical alterations in SLE disease severity. The worst symptoms often coincide with the luteal phase.[75] The effect of hormonal changes in pregnancy is unclear, with published work reporting either improvement or worsening of symptoms.[76-80] Estrogen-containing oral contraceptives do exacerbate the disease,[81-83] but there is little evidence that they can actually trigger SLE in healthy individuals.[84,85] Receptor blockage with tamoxifen, a competitive estrogen antagonist, did not help patients in a single study.[86] Antigonadotropic therapy with cyproterone acetate was found to be helpful, although its mode of action was unclear. At the dose used, it reduced plasma estradiol without affecting testosterone concentration, so its effect may have been attributable to this alone.[87]

Rheumatoid arthritis (RA), in contrast to SLE, and despite its shared higher prevalence in women, responds favorably to pregnancy,[88,89] the menstrual cycle luteal phase,[90,91] and to oral contraceptives.[89,92] Evidence has been advanced that oral contraceptive use reduces the risk of succumbing to rheumatoid arthritis.[93-95] Progesterone effects cannot be excluded from these data, and comparison of pathological events with SLE is certainly not appropriate. Different factors operate in the triggering phase from those in the chronic period of the disease process. It is possible to suggest that humoral events are more important in SLE, and cell-mediated immunity is more important in rheumatoid arthritis. This would accord with the dichotomous effects of estrogen on the two arms of the immune system. In the mouse collagen-induced arthritis model, estrogen was shown to reduce both the incidence and severity of disease;[96] CMI and levels of anti-type II collagen IgG antibodies fell in these animals, although IgM did increase. Beneficial effects from estrogen were demonstrated in the rat by the same workers, however, this time without any change in the anti-type II collagen antibodies.[97] This does support the idea that CMI is more important than humoral immunity in the disease process. The role of androgen is uncertain, but there have been reports of altered metabolism.[98,99] Male RA patients have been shown to have low serum testosterone levels compared to normal controls,[100] and the androgen could be anti-arthritic by interacting with the macrophage-like synoviocytes within joints, reducing their antigen presentation activity.[101]

Estrogen receptors have been identified in rat thymus,[102-107] mouse thymus,[108] and in human thymus.[109,110] Thymic epithelial cell culture supernatants were shown to contain immunoregulatory factors following treatment with physiological concentrations of estrogen. The effect was inhibitory to the mitogen-driven proliferation of bone marrow cells, as opposed to the stimulatory effect of testosterone-treated culture supernatant.[49] As already mentioned, a thymic-dependent factor was found in estradiol-treated rat serum.[5,111] Other workers also demonstrated an indirect effect on CMI by estrogen.[112] Antireceptor antibodies have recently been used to confirm receptor distribution within thymus tissue, showing that, like the androgen receptor, the estrogen receptor is associated with the epithelial portion, including cells producing thymic hormone.[38] More controversially, A small quantity of mRNA for estrogen receptor has recently been found in the lymphocyte component of the thymus, as well as in the epithelial portion.[113] It may be that the antibody[38] or radioligand[102-107] based methods are too insensitive to show binding to thymic lymphocytes or that the cells containing mRNA are preparing to synthesise receptor molecules, as part of the maturation process.

Chick bursa contains estrogen receptors, and it seems likely that they will permit indirect effects on lymphocytes. In birds, processing of B lymphocytes occurs in the bursa of Fabricius in a manner analogous to thymic processing of T lymphocytes. The sex hormones influence bursal size in much the same way as they do the thymus.[40,41] Human spleen has also been shown to contain estrogen receptors,[114] although they were found in lymphoid cells. Since then, estrogen receptors have been identified in circulating lymphocytes, but only in a small proportion. These were the CD8+ cells, i.e., those of the suppressor/cytotoxic lineage.[115] Human spleen cells of the same phenotype have also been shown to contain the same receptor.[116] The precursors of these may well have been the thymocytes described by Gulino et al.[117] and also Kawashima et al.[38,113] In support of this possibility for direct action of estrogen on lymphocytes, Paavonen et al.[118] showed modification of suppressor cell function in vitro. These cells were apparently inhibited, allowing a greater production of immunoglobulin by pokeweed mitogen-stimulated B cells. In a similar system, testosterone was found to reduce antibody production, provided that the concentration of pokeweed mitogen was carefully chosen.[51] Rheumatoid factor production is inhibited by estrogen, the likely route of action involving the suppressor cells.[119]

The macrophage has also emerged as a direct and indirect target for sex steroid action. It had been known for a considerable time that estrogen can promote the clearance of colloidal carbon in mice.[120] This presumably involves all the cell types of the reticuloendothelial system, such as liver Kupfer cells, as well as macrophages, and does not indicate a direct effect. Isolated macrophages in vitro do increase both phagocytosis and lysosomal enzyme release in response to physiological concentrations of estrogen.[121] This was clearly a direct effect and led to the recent discovery of estrogen receptors in rat peritoneal macrophages as well as in the human monocyte-derived cell line J111.[122] The data appear to describe two independent binding sites with a Kd of 2.5×10^{-9} M and 8.7×10^{-11} M respectively, a similar picture to that found in the chick oviduct.[123] It is interesting to note that macrophages respond to estrogen in two separate time frames. Phagocytic activity can be promoted after only one hour's exposure[121], which is too rapid for classical steroid-mediated events seen in other tissues such as oviduct. On the other hand, enhanced secretion of interleukin-1 and interleukin-6 takes place over a period on the order of 24 hours, which is sufficient for gene activation events.[122] Production of other cytokines may also be modified and work is continuing to identify this. Relative receptor affinity data also indicated that the binding selectivity in the macrophage is different from that in other estrogen-dependent tissues. In particular, diethylstilbestrol has a much higher affinity for the macrophage, which raises the possibility of selective intervention directed towards the immune system, perhaps minimizing potential feminizing side effects. Recent work in our laboratory has also shown that estradiol inhibits macrophage nitric oxide production. Androgen, on the other hand, promotes nitric oxide release, although no specific binding in a radio-receptor assay could be demonstrated (Ronald & Stimson, unpublished observation). This could be because binding to any receptor is reversible under the conditions of the assay. It may be that antibody-based methods will be more successful in identifying receptors, as has recently been shown for certain cell lines derived from the lymphatic and hemopoietic systems.[124]

The androgens and estrogens are only a small part of the network of control mechanisms involved in the regulation of the immune system. When these have been more fully investigated, there will be a new framework for the investigation of a number of disease states. This will improve our understanding of autoimmunity, cancer, and the general defence against infection.

References

1. Schiff RI, Mercier D, Buckley RH. Inability of gestational hormones to account for the inhibitory effects of pregnancy plasmas on lymphocyte responses in vitro. Cell Immunol 1975; 20:69–80.
2. Saleem MA, Jha P, Buckshee K, Farooq A. Studies on the immunosuppressive role of steroid hormones during pregnancy. Immunol Invest 1992; 21:1–10.
3. Van den Brink HR, Van Wijk MJG, Bijlsma JWJ. Influence of steroid hormones on proliferation of peripheral blood mononuclear cells in patients with rheumatoid arthritis. Br J Rheumatol 1992; 31:663–667.
4. Stimson WH, Hunter IC. An investigation into the immunosuppressive properties of oestrogen. J Endocrinol 1976; 69:42–43.
5. Stimson WH, Hunter IC. Oestrogen-induced immuno-regulation mediated through the thymus. J Clin Lab Immunol 1980; 4:27–33.
6. Rowley MJ, MacKay IR. Measurement of antibody producing capacity in man. Clin Exp Immunol 1969; 5:407–418.
7. Eidinger D, Garret TJ. Studies of the regulatory effects of the sex hormones on antibody formation and stem cell differentiation. J Exp Med 1972; 136: 1098–1116.
8. Tartaknovsky B, DeBaetselies P, Feldman M, Segal S. Sex associated differences in the immune response against fetal major histocompatibilty antigens. Transplantation 1981; 32:395–397.
9. Spencer MJ, Cherry JD, Powell KR, Mickey MR, Teraski P, Marcy SM, Sumaya CV. Antibody responses following Rubella immunization analyzed by HLA and ABO types. Immunogenetics 1977; 4:365–372.
10. London WI, Drew JR. Sex differences in the response to Hepatitis B infection among patients receiving chronic dialysis treatment. Proc Natl Acad Sci USA 1977; 74:2561–2563.
11. Kalland T. Decreased and disproportionate T-cell population in adult mice after neonatal exposure to diethylstilbestrol. Cell Immunol 1980; 51:55–63.
12. Brent L, Medawar PB. Quantitative studies on tissue transplantation immunity. Proc Royal Soc 1966; (Ser B) 165:413–423.
13. Graff RJ, Hildemann WH, Snell GD. Histocompatibility genes of mice. Transplantation 1966; 4:425–437.
14. Graff RJ, Lappe MA, Snell GD. The influence of gonads and adrenal glands on the immune response to skin grafts. Transplantation 1969; 7:105–111.
15. Hochberg MC. Adult and juvenile rheumatoid arthritis: Current epidemiological concepts. Epidemiol Rev 1981; 3:27–44.
16. Masi AT. Clinical epidemiologic perspective of systemic lupus erythematosus. In: Lawrence RC, Shulman LE, eds. Epidemiology of the Rheumatic Diseases. New York: Gower Medical Publishing; 1984:145–163.
17. Masi AT, Kaslow RA. Sex effects in SLE: A clue to pathogenesis. Arthritis Rheum 1978; 21:480–484.

18. Levine HB, Madin SH. Enhancement of experimental coccidiomycosis in mice with testosterone and estradiol. Sabouraudia 1962; 2:47–52.
19. Kappas A, Jones HES, Roitt IM. Effects of steroid sex hormones on immunological phenomena. Nature (Lond) 1963; 198:902–904.
20. Schuurs AHWM, Dietrich H, Gruber J, Wick G. Effects of sex steroid analogs on spontaneous autoimmune thyroiditis in obese strain chickens. Int Arch Allergy Immunol 1992; 97(4):337–344.
21. Sato EH, Ariga H, Sullivan DA. Impact of androgen therapy in Sjogren's syndrome: Hormonal influence on lymphocyte populations and Ia expression in lacrimal glands of MRL/Mp-lpr/lpr mice. Invest Ophthalmol Visual Sci 1992; 33:2537–2545.
22. Aboudkhil S, Bureau JP, Garrelly L, Vago P. Effects of castration, Depo-testosterone and cyproterone acetate on T-lymphocyte subsets in mouse thymus and spleen. Scand J Immunol 1991; 34(5):647–53.
23. Holdstock G, Chastenay BF, Krawitt EL. Effects of testosterone, estradiol, and progesterone on immune reaction. Clin Exp Immunol 1992; 47:449–56.
24. Burnet FM, Homes MC. The natural history of the NZB/NZW F_1 mouse: A laboratory model of systemic lupus erythematosus. Austr Ann Med 1965; 14:185–191.
25. Roubinian JR, Papoian R, Talal N. Androgenic hormones modulate auto-antibody responses and improve survival in murine lupus. J Clin Invest 1977; 59:1066–1070.
26. Roubinian JR, Talal N, Greenspan JS, Goodman JR, Siiteri PK. Effect of castration and sex hormone treatment on survival, anti-nucleic acid antibodies, and glomerulonephritis in NZB/NZW F_1 mice. J Exp Med 1978; 147:1568–1583.
27. Verheul HAM, Stimson WH, den Hollander FC, Schuurs AHWM. Prophylactic and therapeutic effects of nandrolone and its decanoate ester (Deca-durabolin) in murine lupus. Int J Pharmacol 1981; 2:230–236.
28. Huston DP, Smathers PA, Steinberg AD. Effect of thymic epithelium on autoantibodies in NZB/NZW F_1 mice. Arthritis Rheum 1980; 23:693.
29. Gregoire C. Sur le mechanisme de l'hypertrophie thymique declanchee par la castration. Arch Int Pharmacodyn Ther 1945; 67:45–77.
30. Grossman CJ, Nathan P, Taylor BB, Sholiton LJ. Rat thymic dihydro-testosterone receptor: Preparation, location, and physiochemical properties. Steroids 1979; 34:539–553.
31. McCruden AB, Stimson WH. Androgen and other sex steroid cytosol receptors in the rat thymus. J Endocrinol 1980; 85:47–48.
32. Raveche ES, Vigersky RA, Rice MK, Steinberg AD. Murine thymic androgen receptors. J Immunopathol 1980; 2:425–434.
33. Sasson S, Mayer M. Effect of androgenic steroids on rat thymus and thymocytes in suspension. J Steroid Biochem 1981; 14:509–517.
34. Grossman CJ, Sholiton LJ, Helmsworth JA. Characteristics of the cytoplasmic and nuclear dihydrotestosterone receptors of human thymic tissue. Steroids 1983; 42:11–22.
35. McCruden AB, Stimson WH. Androgen receptor in the human thymus. Immunol Lett 1984; 8:49–53.
36. Wekerle H, Ketelson UP. Thymic nurse cells Ia-bearing epithelium involved in lymphocyte differentiation. Nature 1980; 283:402–404.

37. Haynes BF. The human thymic microenvironment. Adv Immunol 1984; 36:87–142.
38. Kawashima I, Sakabe K, Seiki K, Fujii-Hanamoto H, Akatsuka A, Tsukamoto H. Localization of sex steroid receptor cells, with special reference to thymulin (FTS)-producing cells in female rat thymus. Thymus 1991; 18(2):79–93.
39. Kiess W, Liu LL, Hall NR. Lymphocyte subset distribution and natural killer cell activity in men with idiopathic hypogonadotrophic hypogonadism. Acta Endocrinol 1991; 124:399–404.
40. Szenberg A. Influence of testosterone on the primary lymphoid organs of the chicken. In: Wolstenholme GE, Knight J, eds. Hormones and the Immune System. (Ciba Foundation Study Group No. 35.) London: Churchill; 1970:42–49.
41. Hirota Y, Suzuki T, Bito Y. The B-cell development independent of the bursa of Fabricius but dependent on the thymus in chickens treated with testosterone propionate Immunology 1980; 39:37–46.
42. Hirota Y, Suzuki T, Bito Y. The development of unusual B-cell functions in the testosterone propionate treated chicken. Immunology 1980; 39:29–36.
43. Mesi Y, Oishi T. Effects of castration and testosterone treatment on the development and involution of the bursa of Fabricius and the thymus in the Japanese quail. Gen Comp Endocrinol 1991; 84:426–433.
44. Sullivan DA, Wira CR. Sex hormone and glucocorticoid receptors in the bursa of Fabricius of immature chicks. J Immunol 1979; 122:2617–2623.
45. Fujii H, Nowa Y, Tsuchiya H, Matsuno K, Fukumoto T, Fukuda S, Kotani M. Effect of a single administration of testosterone on the immune response and lymphoid tissue in mice. Cell Immunol 1975; 20:315–320.
46. Kotani M, Nawa Y, Fujii H. Inhibition by testosterone of immune reactivity and of lymphoid regeneration in irradiated and marrow reconstituted mice. Experientia 1974; 30:1343–1345.
47. Kotani M, Nawa Y, Fujii H. Histological observations of inhibitory effects of testosterone on lymphoid regeneration in the thymus independent areas of mice. Arch Histol Jpn 1975; 38:117–120.
48. Stimson WH, Crilly PJ, McCruden AB. Effect of the sex steroids on the synthesis of immunoregulatory factors by thymic epithelial cell cultures. IRCS Med Sci 1980; 8:263–264.
49. Stimson WH, Crilly PJ. Effects of steroids on the secretion of immunoregulatory factors by thymic epithelial cell cultures. Immunology 1981; 44: 401–407.
50. Catanzano P, Troutaud D, Ardail D, Deschaux PA. Testosterone inhibits the immunostimulant effect of thymosin fraction 5 on secondary immune response in mice. Int J Immunopharmacol 1992; 14:263–268.
51. Sthoeger ZM, Chiorazzi N, Lahita RG. Regulation of the immune response by sex hormones. I. In vitro effects of estradiol and testosterone on pokeweed mitogen-induced human B-cell differentiation. J Immunol 1988; 141:91–98.
52. Horowitz S, Borcherding W, Vishnu Moorthy A, Chesney R, Schulte-Wisserman H, Hong R. Induction of suppressor T cells in systemic lupus erythematosus by thymosin and cultured thymic epithelium. Science 1977; 197:999–1001.

53. Morimoto C. Loss of suppressor T-lymphocyte function in patients with systemic lupus erythematosus. Clin Exp Immunol 1978; 32:125–133.

54. Amor B, Dougados M, Benhamou L, Kuhn JM, Laudat MH. Achec de l'androgentherapie au cours d'une poussee de lupus erythemateux. Presse Med 1983; 12:1726–1734.

55. Hazelton RA, McCruden AB, Sturrock RD, Stimson WH. Hormonal manipulation of the immune response in systemic lupus erythematosus: A drug trial of an anabolic steroid, 19-nor-testosterone. Ann Rheum Dis 1983; 42:155–157.

56. Lahita RG, Cheng CY, Monder C, Bardin CW. Experience with 19-nortestosterone in the therapy of systemic lupus erythematosus: Worsened disease after treatment with 19-nortestosterone in men and lack of improvement in women. J Rheumatol 1992; 19:547–555.

57. McCruden AB, Stimson WH. Androgen binding cytosol receptors in the rat thymus: Physicochemical properties, specificity, and localization. Thymus 1981; 3:105–117.

58. Carlsten H, Nilsson N, Jonsson R, Backman K, Holmdahl R, Tarkowski A. Estrogen accelerates immune complex glomerulonephritis but ameliorates T cell-mediated vasculitis and sialadenitis in autoimmune MRL lpr/lpr mice. Cell Immunol 1992; 144:190–202.

59. Geschwind N, Behan PO. Left-handedness: Association with immune disease, migraine, and developmental learning disorder. Proc Natl Acad Sci USA 1982; 79:5097–5100.

60. Geschwind N, Behan PO. Laterality, hormones, and immunity. In: Geschwind N, Galaburda AM, eds. Cerebral Dominance. Harvard University Press; 1984:211–224.

61. Kang DH, Ershler WB, Davidson RJ, Coe CL, Wheeler RE, Tomarken AJ. Frontal brain asymmetry and immune function. Behav Neurosci 1991; 105:860–869.

62. Betancur C, Neveu PJ, Vitiello S, Le Moal M. Natural killer cell activity is associated with brain asymmetry in male mice. Brain Behav Immun 1991; 5:162–169.

63. Neveu PJ, Betancur C, Barneoud P, Vitiello S, Le Moal M. Functional brain asymmetry and lymphocyte proliferation in female mice: Effects of right and left cortical ablation. Brain Res 1991; 550:125–128.

64. Ansar AS, Dauphinee MJ, Talal N. Prenatal effects of sex hormones (immunologic imprinting) in normal and autoimmune-prone mice. Clin Res 1986; 34:667a.

65. Spencer DG, Lal H. Specific behavioural impairments in associational tasks in mice with an autoimmune disorder. Soc Neurosci Abstr 1983; 9:96.

66. Ablin RJ, Bhatti RA, Guinan PD, Khin W. Modulatory effects of estrogen on immunological responsiveness. II. Suppression of tumour-associated immunity in patients with prostatic cancer. Clin Exp Immunol 1979; 38:83–91.

67. Ablin RJ, Bartkus JM, Gonder MJ. In vitro effects of diethylstilbestrol and the LHRH analogue leuprolide on natural killer cell activity. Immunopharmacology 1988; 15:95–101.

68. Comsa J, Leonhardt H, Wekerle H. Hormonal coordination of the immune response. Physiol Biochem Pharmacol 1982; 92:115–191.

69. Kuhl H, Gross M, Schneider M, Weber W, Mehlis W, Stegmuller M, Taubert M. The effect of sex steroids and hormonal contraceptives upon thymus and spleen in intact female rats. Contraception 1983; 28:587–601.
70. Brick JE, Wilson DA, Walker SE. Hormonal modulation of responses to T-dependent and T-independent antigens in autoimmune NZB/NZW mice. J Immunol 1985; 134:3693–3698.
71. Gilbody JS, Wheeler MJ, Wolstencroft R, Greenstein BD. Dose-related effects of oestradiol on rat thymic and splenic T-lymphocyte responsiveness to mitogens. Int J Immunopharmacol 1992; 14:167–172.
72. Bucala R, Lahita RG, Fishman J, Cerami A. Increased levels of 16α-hydroxyestrone modified proteins in pregnancy and SLE. J Clin Endocrinol Metab 1985; 60:841–847.
73. Talal N. Systemic lupus erythematosus, autoimmunity, sex, and inheritance. N Engl J Med 1979; 301:838.
74. Miller KB, Schwartz RS. Familial abnormalities of suppressor-cell function in SLE. N Engl J Med 1979; 301:803–809.
75. Steinberg AD, Steinberg BJ. Lupus disease activity associated with the menstrual cycle. J Rheumatol 1985; 12:816–817.
76. Jungers P, Dougados M, Pelissier C, Kuttenn F, Tron F, Lesavre P, Bach J-F. Lupus nephropathy and pregnancy. Report of 104 cases in 36 patients. Arch Intern Med 1982; 142:771–776.
77. Spiera H. The clinical picture of connective diseases in pregnancy. Prog Clin Biol Res 1981; 70:303–307.
78. Varner MW, Meehan RT, Syrop CH, Strottman MP, Goplerud CP. Pregnancy in patients with SLE. Am J Obstet Gynecol 1983; 145:1025–1040.
79. Imbasciati E, Surian M, Bottino S, Cosci P, Colussi G, Ambroso GC, Massa E, Minetti L, Pardi G, Ponticelli C. Lupus nephropathy and pregnancy. A study of 26 patients with SLE and nephritis. Nephron 1984; 36:46–51.
80. Rubbert A, Pirner K, Wildt L, Kalden JR, Manger B. Systemic lupus erythematosus and pregnancy. Z Rheumatol 1992; 51:78–86.
81. Chapel TA, Burns RE. Oral contraceptives and exacerbation of lupus erythematous. Am J Obstet Gynecol 1971; 110:366–369.
82. Jungers P, Dougados M, Pelissier C, Kuttenn F, Tron F, Lesavre P, Bach J-F. Influence de la contraception hormonal sur l'evolutivitee des nephropathies lupiques. Nour Presse Med 1982; 11:3765–3768.
83. Jungers P, Dougados M, Pelissier C, Kuttenn F, Tron F, Lesavre P, Bach J-F. Influence of oral contraceptive therapy on the activity of SLE. Arthritis Rheum 1982; 25:618–623.
84. Travers RL, Hughes GRV. Oral contraceptive therapy and SLE. J Rheumatol 1978; 5:448–451.
85. Garovich M, Agudelo C, Pisko E. Oral contraceptives and systemic lupus erythematosus. Arthritis Rheum 1980; 23:1396–1398.
86. Sturgess AD, Evans DTP, MacKay IR, Riglar A. Effect of the oestrogen antagonist Tamoxifen in disease indices in SLE. Clin Lab Immunol 1984; 13:11–14.
87. Jungers P, Kuttenn F, Liote F, Pelissier C, Athea N, Laurent M-C, Viriot J, Dougados M, Bach J-F. Hormonal modulation in SLE. Preliminary clinical and hormonal results with cyproterone acetate. Arthritis and Rheumatism 1985; 8:1243–1250.

88. Lawrence JS. Rheumatoid arthritis: Nature or nurture? Ann Rheum Dis 1970; 29:357–379.
89. Spector TD, Roman E, Silman AJ. The pill, parity, and rheumatoid arthritis. Arthritis Rheum 1990; 33:782–789.
90. Latman NS. Relation of menstrual cycle phase to symptoms of rheumatoid arthritis. Am J Med 1983; 74:957–960.
91. Rudge SR, Kuwanko IC, Druy PL. Menstrual cyclicity of finger joint size and grip strength in patients with rheumatoid arthritis. Ann Rheum Dis 1983; 42:425–430.
92. Gilbert M, Rotstein J, Cunningham C, Estrin I, Davidson A, Pincus G. Norethynodrel and mestranol in the treatment of rheumatoid arthritis. JAMA 1964; 190:235–237.
93. Allebeck P, Ahlbom A, Ljungstron K, Allander E. Do oral contraceptives reduce the incidence of rheumatoid arthritis? Scand J Rheumatol 1984; 13:140–146.
94. Vandenbroucke JP, Valkenberg HA, Boersma JW, Cats A, Festen JJM, Huber-Bruning O, Rasker JJ. Oral contraceptives and rheumatoid arthritis. Further evidence of a preventive effect. Lancet 1982; II:8303:839–842.
95. Hazes JMW, Silman AJ, Brand R, Spector TD, Walker DJ, Vandenbroucke JP. Influence of oral contraception on the occurrence of rheumatoid arthritis in female sibs. Scand J Rheumatol 1990; 19:306–310.
96. Holmdahl R, Jansson L, Meyerson B, Klareskog L. Oestrogen induced suppression of collagen arthritis. I. Long-term oestradiol treatment of DBA/1 mice reduces severity and incidence of arthritis and decreases the anti-type II collagen immune response. Clin Exp Immunol 1987; 70:372–378.
97. Larsson P, Holmdahl R. Oestrogen-induced suppression of collagen arthritis. II. Treatment of rats suppresses arthritis but does not affect the anti-type II collagen humoral response. Scand J Immunol 1987; 26:579–583.
98. Feher GK, Feher T, Zahumensky Z. A study on the inactivation mechanisms of androgens in rheumatoid arthritis: Excretory rate of free and conjugated 17-keto steroids. Endokrinologie 1979; 73:167–172.
99. Masi AT, Josipovic DJ, Jefferson WE. Low adrenal androgenic-anabolic steroids in women with rheumatoid arthritis. GLC indicating reduced 11-deoxy-17ketosteroid excretion. Semin Arthritis Rheum 1984; 14:1–42.
100. Cutolo M, Accardo S. Sex hormones, HLA, and rheumatoid arthritis. Clin Exp Rheumatol 1991; 9:641–646.
101. Cutolo M, Accardo S, Villaggio B, Clerico P, Indiveri F, Carruba G, Fecarotta E, Castagnetta L. Evidence for the presence of androgen receptors in the synovial tissue of rheumatoid arthritis patients and healthy controls. Arthritis Rheum 1992; 35:1007–1015.
102. Reichman ME, Villee CA. Estradiol binding by rat thymus cytosol. Biochemistry 1978; 9:637–641.
103. Grossman CJ, Sholiton LJ, Nathan P. Rat thymic estrogen receptor. I. preparation, location, and physiochemical properties. J Steroid Biochem 1979; 11:1233–1240.
104. Brodie JY, Hunter IC, Stimson WH, Green B. Specific oestradiol binding in cytosols from the thymus glands from normal and hormone-treated male rats. Thymus 1980; 1:337–345.

105. Imanishi Y, Seiki K, Haruki Y. Cytoplasmic estrogen receptor in castrated-rat thymus. Endocrinol Jpn 1980; 27:395–399.
106. Malacarne P, Piffanelli A, Indelli M, Fumero S, Mondino A, Gionchiglia E, Silvestri S. Estradiol binding in rat thymus cells. Horm Res 1980; 12: 224–232.
107. Barr IG, Pyke KW, Pearce P, Toh P-H, Funder JW. Thymic sensitivity to sex hormones develops post-natally: An in vivo and an in vitro study. J Immunol 1984; 132:1095–1099.
108. Detlefson MA, Smith BC, Dickerman HW. A high affinity and low capacity receptor for estradiol in normal and anaemic mouse spleen cytosols. Biochem Biophys Res Commun 1978; 76:1151–1158.
109. Nilsson B, Carlsson S, Damer M-G, Lindholm G, Sodergard R, von Schoultz B. Specific binding of 17-beta-estradiol in human thymus. Am J Obstet Gynecol 1984; 149:544–547.
110. Ranelletti FO, Carmignani M, Marchetti P, Natoli C, Iacobelli S. Estrogen binding by neoplastic human thymus cytosol. Eur J Cancer 1984; 16: 951–955.
111. Grossman CJ, Sholiton LJ, Roselle GA. Estradiol regulation of thymic lymphocyte function in the rat: Mediation by serum thymic factors. J Steroid Biochem 1982; 16:683–690.
112. Myers MJ, Butler LD, Petersen BH. Estradiol-induced alteration in the immune system. Suppression of cellular immunity in the rat is not the result of direct estrogenic action. Immunopharmacology 1986; 11:47–55.
113. Kawashima I, Seiki K, Sakabe K, Ihara S, Akatsuka A, Katsumata Y. Localization of estrogen receptors and estrogen receptor mRNA in female mouse thymus. Thymus 1992; 20:115–121.
114. Danel L, Souweine G, Monier JC, Saez S. Specific estrogen binding sites in human lymphoid cells and thymic cells. J Steroid Biochem 1983; 18: 559–563.
115. Cohen JHM, Danel L, Cordier G, Saez S, Revillard J-P. Sex steroid receptors in peripheral T cells. Absence of androgen receptor and restriction of oestrogen receptor to OKT8 positive cells. J Immunol 1983; 131: 2767–2771.
116. Stimson WH. Oestrogen and human T lymphocytes: Presence of specific receptors in the T-suppressor/cytotoxic subset. Scand J Immunol 1988; 28: 345–350.
117. Gulino A, Screpatini I, Torrisi MR, Frati L. Estrogen receptor and estrogen sensitivity of foetal thymocytes are restricted to blast lymphoid cells. Endocrinology 1985; 117:47–54.
118. Paavonen T, Andersson LC, Adlercreutz H. Sex hormone regulation of in vitro immune responses. Estradiol enhances human B-cell maturation via inhibition of suppressor T-cells in pokeweed mitogen stimulated cultures. J Exp Med 1981; 154:1935–1945.
119. McCruden AB, Stimson WH. Rheumatoid factor production in the mouse: Sex differences and the effect of the sex steroids. Immunopharmacology 1990; 19:33–38.
120. Nicol TD, Bilbey DLJ, Charles LM, Cordingley JL, Vernon-Roberts B. Oestrogen: The natural stimulant of body defense. J Endocrinol 1964; 30:277–91.

121. Stimson WH. Serum proteins, steroids and the maternal immune reponse. In: Wegman TG, Gill TJ, eds. Immunology of Reproduction. Oxford University Press; 1983:281–301.
122. Gulshan S, McCruden AB, Stimson WH. Estrogen receptors in macrophages. Scand J Immunol 1990; 31:691–697.
123. Raymoure WJ, McNaught RW, Smith RG. Reversible activation of nonsteroid binding estrogen receptor. Nature 1985; 314:745–747.
124. Jakob F, Tony HP, Schneider D, Thole HH. Immunological detection of the oestradiol receptor protein in cell lines derived from the lymphatic system and the haematopoietic system: Variability of skpecific hormone binding in vitro. J Endocrinol 1992; 134:397–404.

4
Sex Hormone, Glucocorticoid, and Cytokine Regulation of Mucosal Immunity in the Male and Female Reproductive Tract

CHARLES R. WIRA, JAN RICHARDSON, AND CHARU KAUSHIC

Immune Protection at Mucosal Surfaces

Present throughout the body, the secretory immune system is the first line of defense at mucosal surfaces against bacterial and viral organisms that threaten to disrupt systemic homeostasis (for reviews see[1,2]). Characterized by secretory IgA and IgG in secretions that bathe mucosal surfaces of the respiratory, gastrointestinal, and urogenital tracts, protection is the result of successful interactions between the humoral and cellular components of the immune system. As the predominent immunoglobulin in mucosal secretions, IgA is transported from tissue to lumen through epithelial cells by secretory component (SC), the IgA receptor.[2] Acting through afferent and efferent arms, the mucosal immune system recognizes and responds to antigen through both cell-mediated and humoral immune actions against pathogens.[2,3] Protection at these sites is conferred by T and B lymphocytes, monocytes, and macrophages, as well as other antigen-presenting cells that monitor mucosal surfaces and respond to antigenic challenge with specific antibodies,[1,4] phagocytosis,[5] and cytotoxic mechanisms[6] to destroy and/or contain antigens.

The Mucosal Immune System in the Male Reproductive Tract

As a part of the mucosal immune system, the male reproductive tract has evolved to meet the demands characteristic to this particular surface. For example, the male reproductive tract is an immunologically privileged site that is periodically exposed to potentially dangerous infectious agents that may enter the tract and cause ascending infection.[7] At other times, allogeneic sperm either traverse the reproductive tract or are stored in defined regions for extended periods of time prior to ejaculation. As a result, the immunological status of the male reproductive tract varies with the site analyzed.[8] Immunofluorescence studies have demonstrated that SC is present in epithelial cells at several sites, including the ejaculatory ducts, excretory ducts, and selected glands of the rat reproductive tract.[9] In the rodent, IgA-plasma cells are confined to the urethral gland in the bulbous portion of the urethra. In studies of the human testis, macrophages and lymphocytes are present in the interstitial spaces between the seminiferous tubules, but not in the tubules of normal testes.[10] Antibody levels are reportedly low or undectable in testicular and epididymal fluids.[11] Secretory IgA in seminal fluid is derived primarily from the prostate and may be either of serum origin or produced locally in the prostate.[12]

The Mucosal Immune System in the Female Reproductive Tract

Within the female genital tract, the mucosal immune system protects against both bacterial and viral pathogens.[13,14] Periodically exposed to allogeneic sperm and to a fetal–placental unit which is immunologically unique, the immune system in the uterus, cervix, and vagina is regulated by female sex hormones to optimize maternal and fetal survival.[15,16,17] Depending on the site analyzed and the reproductive state (endocrine balance), immuno-competency of the female reproductive tract may be either plentiful or sparse.[18] For example, in the uterus, whereas some studies have demonstrated the presence of immunocompetent cells, others have reported that IgA and/or IgG lymphocytes are either absent or present in very limited numbers.[19,20,21] In contrast, the cervix and vagina contain significant numbers of IgA and IgG lymphocytes.[20,22]

Previous studies have shown that immunization can lead to the presence of specific antibodies in uterine and vaginal secretions. Ogra and Ogra demonstrated that inactivated polio virus, given either orally or deposited in the uterus or vagina of women, resulted in IgG antibodies in uterine and cervico-vaginal secretions.[23] In other studies, local antibody production in the lower genital tract was demonstrated when antigens were placed in the vagina and/or cervix.[24,25,26,27] That gastrointestinal, intrauterine, and pelvic immunization lead to the accumulation of antibodies in reproductive tract secretions[28,29,30] demonstrates that IgA and IgG antibodies in secretions of the uterus, cervix, and vagina are derived from both distal sites and locally in the reproductive tract.

Physiological states, including sex hormone endocrine balance, glucocorticoid levels, and the presence of selected cytokines, are known to have profound effects on the mucosal immune system in the female reproductive tract. Previously, we and others showed that the levels of total immunoglobulins in the female reproductive tract vary with the stage of the estrous cycle in rodents,[15] and during the menstrual cycle in humans.[16] Estradiol and progesterone regulate uterine and cervico-vaginal levels of IgA, IgG, and SC.[31,32,33] Similar hormone-dependent changes occur within the human reproductive tract. Schumacher et al. demonstrated that cervical IgA and IgG levels are depressed in women who received oral contraceptives.[16] We found that SC levels in uterine secretions were significantly higher during the secretory (postovulatory) phase than those measured during the proliferative phase of the menstrual cycle in women.[34] More recently, glucocorticoids have been shown to redistribute mucosally derived antibodies from secretions into blood.[35] In other studies, cytokines produced locally act during the reproductive cycle, at implantation, and throughout pregnancy to regulate both humoral and cell-mediated immunity in the reproductive tract.[18,36,37] These studies indicate that steroid hormones and cytokines have profound effects on reproductive tract immune protection and reproduction of the species.

In this chapter, we describe studies from our laboratory that define the roles of sex hormones, glucocorticoids, and selected cytokines in regulating the mucosal immune system in the male and female reproductive tract. In studies to be presented, particular attention is paid to the mechanisms whereby hormones and cytokines exert their effects in intact animals and in animals treated with hormones. The data presented indicate that the regulation of reproductive tract mucosal immunity is the result of a precise interplay between androgens, estrogens, and cytokines. Further, it indicates that glucocorticoids have marked effects on mucosal immune function. Lastly, these studies emphasize that endocrine regulation and immune functions at different sites of the male and female reproductive tracts are separate and distinct, and that immune function at each site must be analyzed in the context of the unique contributions that each makes to procreation and to immune protection.

Androgen Effects on the Mucosal Immune System in the Male Reproductive Tract

To characterize the role of sex hormones in the regulation of the immune system in the male reproductive tract, a study was undertaken to identify the sites at which SC is present in the reproductive tract of intact adult male rats.[38] Following saline perfusion, cytosol fractions were prepared which consisted of tissue extract and secretions. This approach was utilized to eliminate the problem of incomplete secretion collection. As shown in Figure 4.1, when measured in the prostate, epididymis, and vas deferens, levels of SC varied markedly with the site analyzed. The SC levels were highest in the prostate, present in the seminal vesicles, and either very low or not measurable in the epididymis, vas deferens, and testes.

To examine the effect of hormone treatment on SC levels in the prostate, animals were castrated prior to hormone treatment. As seen in Figure 4.2, when animals received dihydrotesterone (DHT) or estradiol (E$_2$), SC levels in the prostates of treated animals were significantly

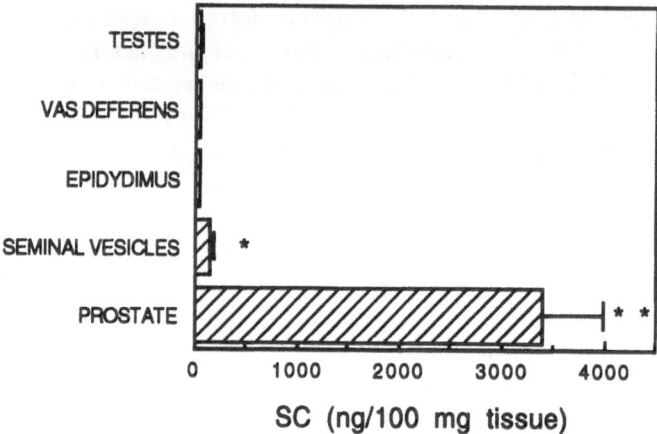

FIGURE 4.1. SC in reproductive tract tissues of male rats. SC levels were measured by radioimmunoassay in reproductive tract tissues of normal male rats. Tissues were perfused, removed, blotted dry, weighed, and prepared for assay of SC. Hatched bars represent the SC levels as the mean ± SEM (3 animals per group). (*), Significantly ($P < 0.02$) greater than testis, vas deferens, and epididymis; (**), significantly ($P < 0.005$) greater than testis, vas deferens, epididymis, and seminal vesicles. (From[38] with permission.)

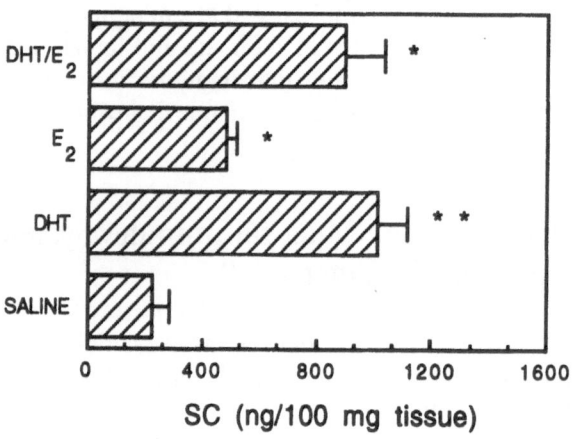

FIGURE 4.2. SC levels in the prostate glands of castrate rats treated with sex hormones. SC was measured by radioimmunoassay in prostatic tissues recovered from hormone-treated castrate rats. Rats were castrated 6–7 days prior to receiving 6 daily injections of either saline (0.1 ml/day), DHT (1 mg/0.1 ml per day), E_2 (2 µg/0.1 ml per day), or a combination of DHT and E_2 (as indicated). Tissues were prepared as described for Figure 4.1. Hatched bars represent the mean ± SE for 5 animals per group. (*), Significantly ($P < 0.01$) greater than saline controls; (**), significantly ($P < 0.001$) greater than saline controls. (From[38] with permission.)

greater than that seen in saline controls. When animals received DHT and E_2, SC levels were not significantly different from those animals that received only DHT. When seminal vesicles were analyzed (not shown), DHT was found to have a significant stimulatory effect (three-fold) on SC levels when compared with saline controls. In contrast, E_2 had no effect on SC levels in seminal vesicles. As a part of these studies, SC levels were also measured in the vas deferens of castrate hormone-treated rats. Irrespective of whether animals received saline, DHT, or E_2, the levels of SC in cytosols from the vas deferens were below the limits of assay sensitivity.

In other studies, we found that sex hormones have a more pronounced effect on SC levels than on IgA levels in the prostate. SC increased in response to both DHT and E_2 treatment, with DHT having the more profound effect. In contrast, only DHT increased IgA. However, when E_2 was given along with DHT, it interfered with the stimulatory effect of DHT on IgA levels in the prostate. These findings indicate that in the male reproductive tract, the SC response of tissue to hormone is more dramatic than that of IgA. These observations suggest that in the male, direct regulation of the immune system by steroid hormones is mediated through the regulation of secretory component, the receptor responsible for transporting IgA from tissue to lumen.

Hormone Regulation of Mucosal Immunity in the Female Reproductive Tract

Figure 4.3 shows results obtained in our laboratory in 1977 demonstrating that IgA and IgG levels in uterine secretions from intact rats fluctuate with the stage of the reproductive cycle. Immunoglobulin levels were higher at the time of ovulation than at any other stage of the cycle.[15] These observations led to the conclusion that estradiol and progesterone are the principle hormones responsible for regulating both IgA and IgG in uterine secretions. When ovariectomized rats were treated with estradiol, IgA and IgG levels in uterine secretions were elevated relative to saline controls.[31] We also found that IgA and IgG levels in cervicovaginal secretions are also under hormonal control, but in contrast to the uterus, levels were lowered in response to estradiol and/or progesterone treatment.[39] These responses are separate, since uterine ligation had no effect on vaginal IgA and IgG responses to estradiol. We also found that the uterine response was specific for estradiol and that progesterone blocks estradiol-stimulated increases in uterine IgA and IgG.

Since IgA was known to be transported from tissues into secretions at mucosal surfaces by SC, the external domain of the polymeric IgA receptor (for review see[2]), studies were undertaken to determine whether

SC was under hormonal control. As seen in Figure 4.4, in response to estradiol given to ovariectomized rats for 3 days, SC and IgA levels increased in parallel in uterine secretions in response to hormone treatment.[33] When SC levels were analyzed in cervico-vaginal secretions, both SC and IgA levels were reduced with estradiol treatment.[39] In other studies, we found that whereas IgA of blood origin enters uterine tissues within 2–4 h after each injection of estradiol, IgA entry into the uterine lumen occured only after epithelial cells were stimulated by estradiol or interferon-γ (IFN-γ) to produce SC.[40,41]

To identify the origins of antibodies and the role of hormones in regulating their presence in reproductive tract secretions, adult female rats were immunized via Peyer's patches (PP) or intraperitoneal (IP) immunization, and boosted 6 days later with sheep red blood cells (SRBCs), a known T-cell dependent antigen.[28] Following two normal estrous cycles, uterine secretions from uterine-ligated animals were analyzed for specific anti-SRBC IgA antibodies. When animals were PP or IP immunized, IgA antibodies were found in uterine and cervico-

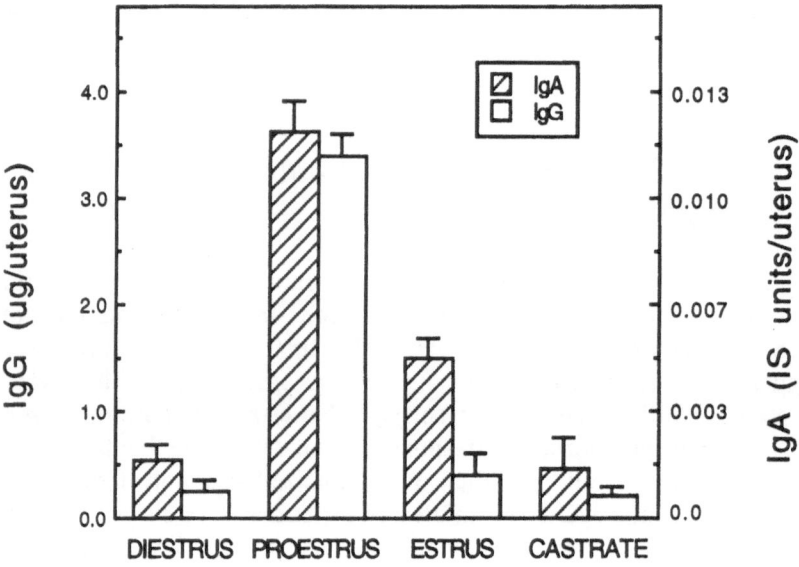

FIGURE 4.3. Immunoglobulin A and G levels in uterine secretions of adult female rats at various stages of the estrous cycle and following castration. Values represent the mean ± SEM of 5–8 rats per group. IgG values are expressed as micrograms per uterus; IgA results as immunocytoma serum (IS) units, where 1.0 IS unit is defined as a concentration of 1 mg of lyophilized immunocytoma serum in 1 ml distilled water. Values of IgA and IgG at proestrus, and IgA at estrus are significantly different from those measured during diestrus and following castration ($P < 0.01$). No significant differences were measured in serum samples. (Adapted from[15] with permission.)

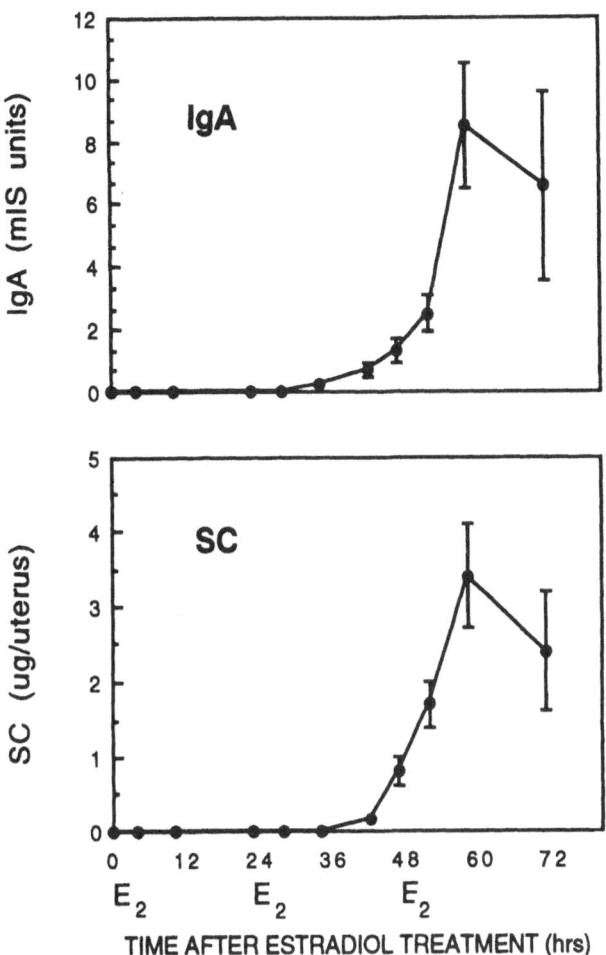

FIGURE 4.4. Time course of the effect of 1, 2, or 3 estradiol treatments on SC and IgA content in uterine secretions of ovariectomized rats. Animals were injected with either estradiol (E_2, $2 \mu g$/day) or saline (controls, indicated as 0 time point). Each value equals the mean $\pm$ SE of 4 (E_2) or 12 (saline) determinations. (From[17] with permission, © The Endocrine Society.)

vaginal secretions. IgG antibodies were found in uterine but not in cervico-vaginal secretions.

To determine whether the presence of specific antibodies in uterine secretions was estradiol-dependent, ovariectomized animals were immunized with SRBC via PP and were then boosted via the same route 13 days later. Rats were treated with estradiol or saline for 3 days before sacrifice on day 13 following the boost. As shown in Figure 4.5, significantly more IgA and IgG anti-SRBC antibodies accumulated in uterine secretions of estradiol-treated rats than in immunized, saline-treated or

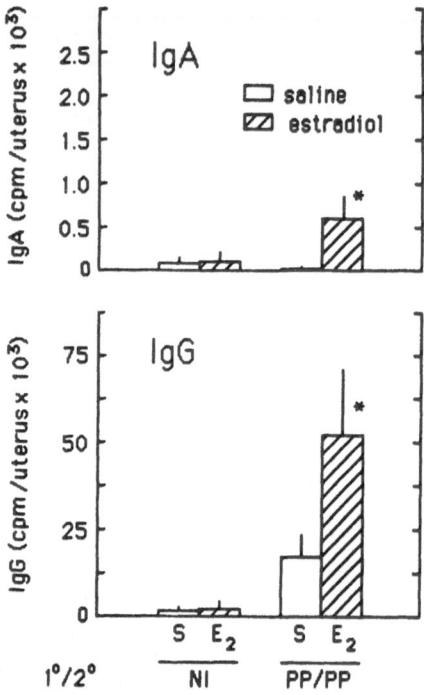

FIGURE 4.5. Effect of estradiol on specific IgA and IgG antibodies in uterine secretions of nomimmunized and immunized animals after the injection (primary; day 0) and boosting (secondary; day 13) by SRBC injection into PP (PP/PP). Nonimmunized rats (NI) were sham-operated. Animals were ovariectomized before immunization and received either estradiol (E_2, 1 μg/day) or saline (S) for 3 days before sacrifice 13 days after boosting. Each *bar* represents the mean ± SE of 4 animals per group. (*), Significantly greater ($P < 0.05$) than control immunized (S, saline injected) and nonimmunized animals. (From[28] with permission.)

nonimmunized, estradiol-treated animals. These findings indicate that specific antibodies in uterine secretions are in part derived from the gastrointestinal tract and that their presence in the uterine lumen is estradiol-dependent.

In other studies, ovariectomized animals were immunized and boosted with SRBC placed directly in the uterine lumen.[29] Under these conditions, we obtained a uterine antibody response that was more pronounced than that seen following PP immunization. In contrast to PP and IP, estradiol treatment of uterine (UT)-immunized animals had no effect on uterine antibody levels. To determine whether immunological information is shared, uterine horns of UT/UT-immunized animals were ligated at the utero-cervical junction at the time of immunization to prevent transfer between horns of uterine fluid and antigen. As seen in Figure 4.6, when animals were treated with saline or estradiol for 3 days prior to sacrifice on day 13 postboost, IgA and IgG antibodies accumu-

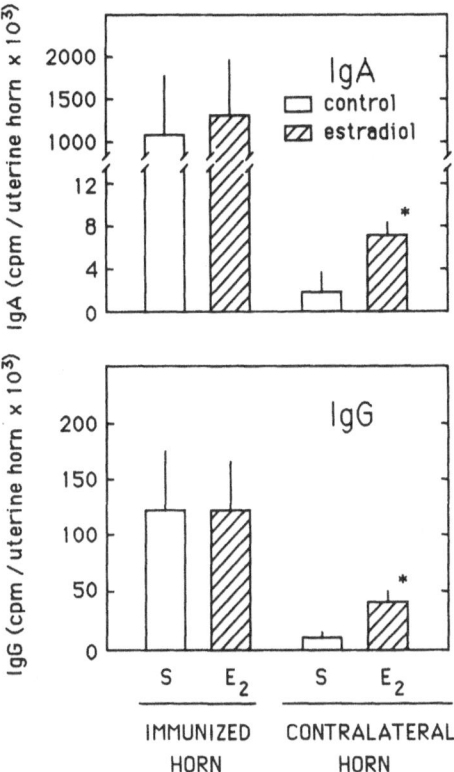

FIGURE 4.6. Effect of immunization and boost in one uterine horn on the presence of antibodies in the nonimmunized contralateral uterine horn. Ovariectomized rats received primary immunization (day 0) by instillation of SRBC (20–30 μl/horn) into one uterine horn. Following injection of SRBC into the lumen, uteri were ligated at the utero–cervical junction to prevent leakage. On the day of boost (day 13), SRBCs were injected into the oviductal end of the immunized horn, which was then ligated. Animals were treated with 0.1 ml of estradiol (E_2, 1 μg/day) or saline (S) for 3 days prior to killing, 24 h after the last injection (day 26 post-primary immunization). *Bars* represent the mean ± SE of 4 animals per group. (*), Significantly ($P < 0.05$) greater than immunized saline controls. (From[29] with permission.)

lated in the nonimmunized (contralateral) horns of estradiol-treated animals. To determine whether immunological information is shared with mucosal surfaces distal to the female genital tract, antibody levels were measured in sera and saliva of UT/UT-immunized rats. Relative to non-immunized controls, UT immunization resulted in anti-SRBC IgG antibodies in both serum and saliva. When estradiol was administered daily for 3 days prior to sample collection, levels of IgG antibody in serum, but not in saliva, were significantly higher than those measured in immunized animals that received saline. When serum and saliva were analyzed for anti-SRBC IgA antibodies, IgA antibodies against SRBCs were present in sera of immunized estradiol-treated rats but were inconsistently found in sera (saline-treated) and saliva of immunized animals. In other experiments, low levels of IgA antibodies have been periodically measured in serum (saline treated) and in saliva following UT/UT immunization. The lack of a consistent response may reflect either the rapid clearance of IgA from serum by hepatocytes, or the migration of limited numbers of IgA-producing lymphocytes to the salivary glands. These studies indicate that UT immunization, in addition to eliciting a pronounced local antibody response, results in immunological information being shared througout as well as at sites distal to the reproductive tract.

Actions of Glucocorticoids on Reproductive Tract Mucosal Immune Responses

To examine the role of glucocorticoids in influencing mucosal immune responses, studies were undertaken to determine whether SC, which is synthesized by rat hepatocytes,[42] was hormonally regulated. As shown in Figure 4.7, when isolated rat hepatocytes were incubated with dexame-

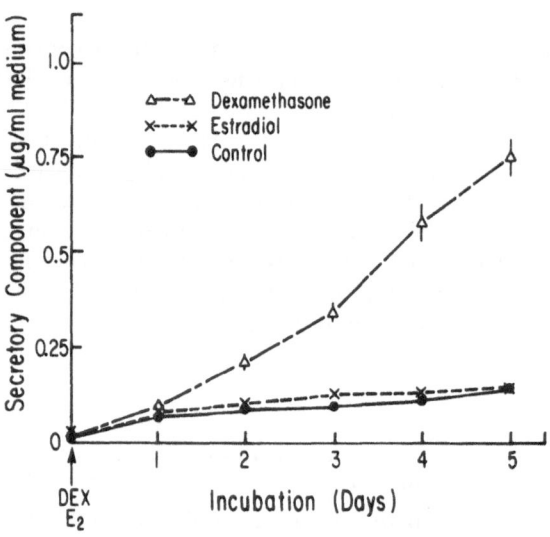

FIGURE 4.7. Time course of the effect of estradiol (X) and dexamethasone (Δ) on SC accumulation in media. Isolated hepatocytes were incubated at 37°C for 24 h. After incubation, nonattached cells were removed by washing, and flasks were reconstituted with incubation media containing either estradiol (10^{-6}M) or dexamethasone (10^{-7}M). Control cells ($\bullet$) received incubation media without hormone. Each value represents the mean $\pm$ SE of five determinations. (From[42] with permission.)

thasone (10^{-7} M), a synthetic glucocorticoid, SC accumulation in media after exposure for 5 days was significantly greater than that seen with control cells. To eliminate the possible effect of dexamethasone on hepatocyte attachment, flasks were incubated for 24 h without hormone, rinsed with media to remove nonadherent cells, and reconstituted with an equal volume of media either with or without dexamethasone. Also shown in Figure 4.7 is the lack of an effect by estradiol (10^{-6} M) on hepatocyte SC release. In other studies (not shown), when estradiol was added at several concentrations (10^{-10} to 10^{-6} M), no significant effect relative to controls could be detected. To assess whether estradiol might antagonize the glucocorticoid effect, estradiol was added along with dexamethasone to the incubation media. Under these conditions, estradiol (10^{-6} M) diminished the glucocorticoid effect on hepatocyte SC production. This finding suggests that estradiol may regulate hepatocyte SC in the presence of glucocorticoids, even though by itself it has no effect on SC production.

Since glucocorticoids given in vitro stimulated hepatocyte SC production, studies were undertaken to determine whether dexamethasone given in vivo influenced the levels of IgA and SC in serum and bile.[35,43] As shown in Figure 4.8, when administered daily for 3 days, dexamethasone had a stimulatory effect on the levels of IgA and SC in serum. IgA levels increased approximately two-fold while SC levels increased six- to seven-fold, relative to saline controls. To examine the effect of dexamethasone on bile IgA and SC, bile ducts were cannulated and bile collected during the second hour of flow. As seen in Figure 4.8, dexamethasone treatment had a significant inhibitory effect on bile IgA levels relative to that seen in saline-treated animals. In contrast, bile SC levels remained unchanged in those animals that were treated with dexamethasone. When bile flow, which was significantly greater in dexamethasone-treated animals, was used to calculate SC production per hour, significantly more SC was produced by dexamethasone-treated animals than by saline controls. The net effect was that SC in bile from dexamethasone-treated animals was approximately 80% greater than that seen in the bile of saline controls, indicating that dexamethasone increases both bile flow and hepatocyte SC production. These findings demonstrate that, in response to dexamethasone, bile IgA is lowered at a time when serum IgA is elevated. Further, it indicates that under the same conditions, serum SC and hepatocyte production of SC measured in bile are increased with glucocorticoid treatment.

To characterize SC in serum, we used high performance liquid chromatography (HPLC) to determine whether SC in serum is associated with IgA.[43] When pooled sera was analyzed, chromatographic separation of serum from both saline- and dexamethasone-treated animals resulted in the appearance of two IgA peaks. The first peak eluted near the column exclusion volume and corresponded in size to polymeric IgA, whereas the second peak eluted in a region that corresponded in size to monomeric

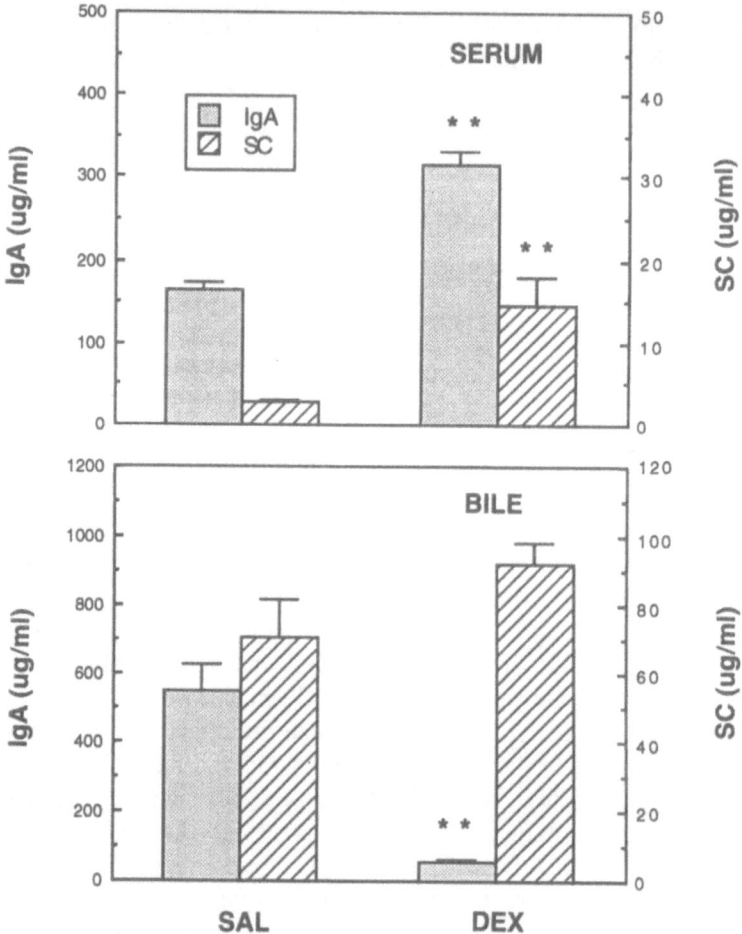

FIGURE 4.8. The effect of dexamethasone on IgA and SC levels in serum and bile. Ovariectomized rats were treated with dexamethasone (2 mg/day) or saline (0.1 ml) for 3 days. Twenty-four hours after the last injection, bile and serum were collected and analyzed for SC and IgA. Each *bar* represents the mean value of seven animals per group. Vertical lines on the bars indicate the SE. (**), Significantly ($P < 0.001$) different than saline group. (From[43] with permission, © The Endocrine Society.)

IgA. When fractions were assayed for SC, a single peak was found only in those fractions that contained polymeric IgA, irrespective of whether serum was from saline- or dexamethasone-treated animals. Since SC in bile and external secretions ranges in size from 50 to 90 kDa (for review see[2]), these findings suggest that all of the SC detected in serum was associated with polymeric IgA.

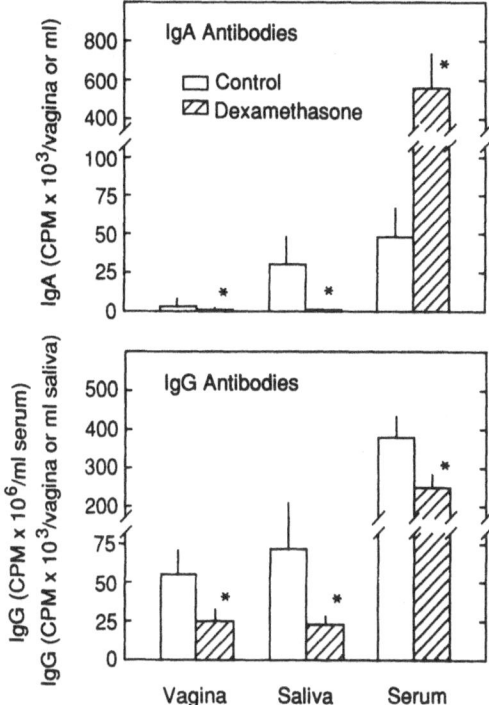

FIGURE 4.9. Effect of dexamethasone on levels of specific IgA and IgG antibodies in vaginal fluid, saliva, and serum of immunized animals after the injection (primary: day 0; Peyer's patches) and boost (secondary: day 13; intrauterine) with SRBCs. Animals were ovariectomized 1 week before immunization and received either dexamethasone (1 mg/day) or saline daily for 3 days prior to sacrifice 24 h after the last injection on day 26 post-primary immunization. *Bars* represent mean ± SE of 4 animals per group. (*), Significantly ($P < 0.01$) different from control groups. (From[35] with permission.)

To determine whether glucocorticoids influence specific antibody responses in vaginal fluid, saliva, and serum, ovariectomized rats were immunized by injecting SRBCs directly into Peyer's patches and then boosting animals by injecting SRBCs into the uterine lumen 13 days later. This approach has been shown by us to elicit specific IgA and IgG antibody responses at selected mucosal surfaces and in serum.[29] Animals received either dexamethasone or saline for 3 consecutive days prior to sacrifice on day 26 after primary immunization. As shown in Figure 4.9, significantly more IgA antibodies were present in the sera of dexamethasone-treated rats than in saline-treated animals. In contrast, in response to dexamethasone, IgA-antibody levels in vaginal and salivary secretions were significantly reduced. These findings indicated that dexamethasone markedly alters specific IgA-antibody levels in serum and secretions in a way that is similar to its effects on total IgA levels. In contrast to IgA, dexamethasone reduced IgG antibodies in vaginal secretions, saliva, and serum. In other studies we found that dexamethasone, administered prior to estradiol treatment, reduced the levels of IgA in uterine secretions.[33]

IgA in external secretions is the body's primary line of defense against bacterial and viral infections.[1] As proposed previously,[43] our findings suggest that IgA, in response to glucocorticoid stimulation, is redistributed away from mucosal surfaces to blood, possibly to enhance systemic immune protection. That mucosally-derived IgA anti-SRBC antibodies, induced by Peyer's patch and intrauterine immunization, increase in serum and decrease at mucosal surfaces following dexamethasone treatment support this hypothesis. Further investigation, however, is needed to determine whether the endogenous glucocorticoids, produced by the adrenal gland in response to bacterial and/or viral infections, enhance systemic humoral immune protection by antibody redistribution from mucosal surfaces.

Influence of Antigen and Cytokines on Female Reproductive Tract Immunity

Several recent studies have demonstrated that selected cytokines including IFNs, TNF, and interleukin (IL)-6 are produced by cells in the female reproductive tract.[44,45,46,47] To examine the role of IFN-γ in uterine immune responses, we undertook to determine whether these cytokines might be involved in regulating SC production. When IFN-γ was placed in the uterine lumen of ovariectomized rats, increasing doses of IFN-γ increased SC levels in uterine secretions.[41] This response was specific for IFN-γ because IFN-α/β at the same dose (5000 Units) had no effect on uterine SC levels.[41] These studies build on the finding of Sollid et al.[48] that IFN-γ added to the incubation media increases the expression of SC of human colon carcinoma cells, which led to the proposal that epithelial cell-mediated SC IgA transport might respond to cytokine stimulation.[49] To test this hypothesis with normal cells, rats were ovariectomized and treated with IFN-γ and/or estradiol. As seen in Figure 4.10, when animals received IFN-γ alone, SC but not IgA levels increased in the uterine lumen. Since tissue IgA levels are low in the absence of estradiol,[40] animals were treated with estradiol for 2 days prior to sacrifice 4 h after the second injection. This time interval of estradiol exposure has previously been shown by us to increase tissue levels of monomeric and polymeric IgA without increasing either SC or IgA levels in uterine secretions.[17,40] When estradiol was given to IFN-γ treated animals, IgA levels increased in uterine secretions relative to those seen in animals that received either estradiol or IFN-γ alone. These findings suggest that stimulation of uterine SC by IFN-γ increases the movement of IgA from

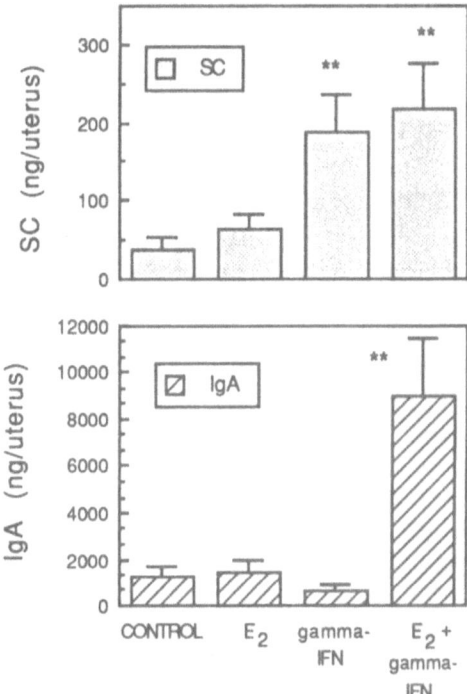

FIGURE 4.10. The effect of IFN-γ and estradiol on SC and IgA levels in the uterine lumen of ovariectomized animals. PBS or IFN-γ (5000 Units/uterus) was placed in the uterine lumen. Animals were given systemically, either saline (0.1 ml) or estradiol (2 μg/day) daily for the last 2 days prior to sacrifice 4–6 h after the second injection on day 7. *Bars* represent the mean ± SE of 6 animals per group. (**), Significantly ($P < 0.01$) greater than control values. (From[41] with permission, © The Endocrine Society.)

tissue to lumen. Whether all IgA in uterine secretions following estradiol and IFN-γ treatment is polymeric and the result of SC-mediated IgA transport, remains to be determined.

More recently, we examined the possibility that interleukin-6 (IL-6) may be involved in IgA movement into uterine secretions. Since IL-6 is synthesized by epithelial and stromal cells in the uterine endometrium,[44,50] we instilled IL-6 into the uteri of ovariectomized rats. Under these conditions we found that IL-6 had a pronounced stimulatory effect on both SC and IgA accumulation within the uterine lumen.[51] What remains to be established is whether IL-6 increased the movement of IgA from serum into uterine tissues as well as stimulated SC-mediated IgA transport, or whether IL-6 stimulated the differentiation of reproductive tract IgA-lymphoid cells into plasma cells which then synthesized polymeric IgA for transport form uterine tissue into secretions.

Influence of Hormones on Mitogen Responses in the Spleen

To investigate the role of the reproductive cycle on T- and B-lymphocyte responses to mitogens under in vivo conditions, animals were selected by daily vaginal smears after they had gone through at least one normal (4 day) estrous cycle. Spleen cells were incubated with concanavalin A (Con A) (1 μg/ml), phytohemagglutinin (PHA) (5 μg/ml), or lipopolysoccharide (LPS) (10 μg/ml) in 96-well microtiter plate for 3 days, and cell proliferation was evaluated by measuring the incorporation of ^{3}H-thymidine added to incubation wells for the last 24 h. As seen in Figure 4.11, spleen cell mitogenesis is influenced by the stage of the estrous cycle. Mitogenesis of lymphocytes from proestrous rats in response to Con A, PHA, and LPS was significantly greater (two- to threefold) than that seen with spleen cells from animals at either the estrous or diestrous stage of the cycle.

To determine whether the changes in mitogenesis observed during the estrous cycle are under the control of the female sex hormones,

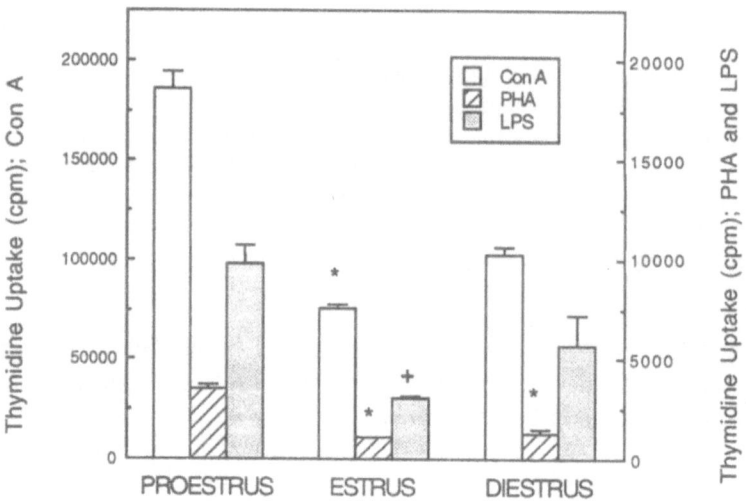

FIGURE 4.11. Mitogenic response of isolated spleen cells from intact female rats at various stages of the reproductive cycle. Animals were selected by routine vaginal smears, and spleens were recovered during proestrus, estrus, and diestrus (day 2). Splenocytes were prepared as described previously,[10] and incubated with ConA (1 μg/ml), PHA (5 μg/ml), and LPS (10 μg/ml) for 3 days. ^{3}H-Thymidine was added to culture wells for the last 24 h of each incubation. Each *bar* represents the mean ± SE minus background (counts/min per well in the absence of mitogen) of splenocytes pooled from 4–6 animals per group. (+), Significantly ($P < 0.05$) lower than proestrous values; (*), significantly ($P < 0.01$) lower than proestrous values. (From[54] with permission.)

TABLE 4.1. Effect of estradiol on the mitogenic response of spleen cells. (From[54] with permission.)

Groups	Thymidine incorporation (cpm)[a]		
	ConA	PHA	LPS
Control	36813 ± 3061	3037 ± 436	6430 ± 1218
Estradiol	61949 ± 10065*	11684 ± 869*	14738 ± 1936*

[a] Results represent mean and SEM of a pool of six animals.
* Significantly different ($P < 0.05$) than control.

ovariectomized animals were treated with estradiol ($2\,\mu g$/day) or saline ($0.1\,ml$) for 3 days prior to sacrifice $24\,h$ after the third injection. As shown in Table 1, spleen cell responses to both T- and B-cell mitogens were significantly higher in those animals that received estradiol, relative to saline controls. These findings suggest that increases in mitogenesis that occur at the proestrous stage of the estrous cycle are most likely due to the effect of estradiol, which is elevated in blood at this time.[52] Further studies are needed to determine whether the magnitude of lymphocyte responses measured in intact and hormonally-treated animals reflects either altered sensitivity of spleen cells to mitogen or the number of mitogen-responsive cells in the spleen.

Conclusions

Knowledge of the secretory immune system in the male and female reproductive tract has progressed slowly during the past decade. The recognition that the secretory immune system may be essential in controlling the spread of venereal diseases including HIV-1 has resulted in a growing awareness of the need to more fully identify the elements of the immune system in reproductive tract tissues and the factors that influence their presence.

Our studies using the rat as a model system have demonstrated that, depending on the site analyzed, androgens, estrogens, glucocorticoids, and selected cytokines exert regulatory influences on all aspects of mucosal immunity. In studies of the female reproductive tract, our goal was to define the origin(s) of antibodies, and the role of sex hormones in the expression of this response in uterine and cervico-vaginal secretions. Using sheep erythrocytes as our antigen, we found that PP, IP and UT immunization can lead to specific IgA- and IgG-antibody responses in the reproductive tract. These findings led us to conclude that some reproductive tract antibodies are derived from the gastrointestinal tract, whereas others are produced locally in the uterus following intrauterine immunization. Moreover, we found that the presence of antibodies in the reproductive tract is dependent on estradiol, which enhances oral- and IP-induced antibodies in uterine secretions and inhibits their presence in the vagina. We also found that intrauterine immunization stimulates antibody responses that are more pronounced than those seen after either PP or IP immunization. In addition, immunization within the uterus results in antibody sharing throughout the genital tract (contralateral nonimmunized horn, cervix/vagina), in serum, and at other mucosal sites such as the salivary gland.[29]

In an attempt to determine whether endocrine events comparable to those seen in the female occur in the male reproductive tract, studies were undertaken to determine whether androgens and estrogens influence the presence of immunoglobulins in the reproductive tract tissues and/or secretions. These studies extend the findings of Parr and Parr that demonstrated the presence of SC in epithelial cells at several sites, including the ejaculatory ducts, excretory ducts, and several glands of the rat reproductive tract.[9] We found that hormones exert a profound effect on the levels of SC, the IgA receptor, and to a lesser extent on IgA in specific tissues of the male reproductive tract. Further studies are needed to identify the origins of antibodies in the male reproductive tract, and the mechanisms through which androgens and estrogens exert their regulatory effects.

Our studies also demonstrate that glucocorticoids influence mucosal and systemic humoral immunity. When total IgA or mucosally-derived anti-SRBC IgA antibodies were measured, glucocorticoid treatment led to a redistribution of polymeric IgA from mucosal surfaces into blood. As discussed elsewhere,[35] these findings suggest that stress-induced elevations in serum glucocortcoids, possibly in response to systemic infection, may redistribute IgA from secretions to systemic sites to confer protection after mucosal immune defenses have been breached. What appears likely is that glucocorticoids increase polymeric IgA in blood by increasing serum SC levels, and SC binds IgA, retarding its clearance from blood into bile. Whether glucocorticoids redistribute immune cells as well as immunoglobulins from mucosal surfaces to central sites in the body, remains to be established.

In other studies, we found that IFN-γ placed in the uterine lumina of ovariectomized rats, stimulates the accumulation of SC in uterine secretions.[41,53] This finding, along with our recent observation that IL-6 increases both IgA and SC in uterine secretions,[51] extends our understanding of immune regulators in the reproductive tract beyond that of the female sex hormones estradiol and progesterone. Further, it suggests that endocrine events in the reproductive tract previously attributed to the direct action of sex hormones, may involve cytokines which could act as intermediaries of estradiol and progesterone during the reproductive cycle and throughout pregnancy.[36,37,47] We also found that IFN-γ placed in the uterine lumen increases the mitogenic response of isolated spleen cells.[41] When considered along with our observations that stage of the estrous cycle and treatment of ovariectomized rats with estradiol enhances spleen cell mitogenesis,[54] these findings suggest that reproductive tract mucosal immunity involves the interactions of lymphoid and reproductive tract tissues that are regulated by both sex hormones and selected cytokines. Further studies are needed to define the nature of these interactions.

Acknowledgments. This work was supported by research grants AI-13541 from NIH, and CA 23108 from NCI.

References

1. Heremans JF. Immunoglobulin A. In: Sela M, ed. The Anitgens. New York: Academic Press; 1974:365–522.
2. Mestecky J, McGhee JR. Immunoglobulin A (IgA): Molecular and cellular interactions involved in IgA biosynthesis and immune response. Adv Immunol 1987: 40:153–245.
3. Underdown BJ, Schiff JM. Immunoglobulin A: Strategic defense initiative at the mucosal surface. Annu Rev Immunol 1986; 4:389–417.
4. Williams RC, Gibbons RJ. Inhibition of bacterial adherence by secretory immunoglobulin A: A mechanism for antigen disposal. Science 1972; 177:697–699.
5. Fanger MW, Goldstine SN, Shen L. Cytofluorographic analysis of receptors for IgA on human polymorphonuclear cells and monocytes and the correlation of receptor expression with phagocytosis. Mol Immunol 1983; 20: 1019–1027.
6. Shen L, Fanger MW. Secretory IgA antibodies synergize with IgG in promoting ADCC by human polymorphonuclear cells, monocytes, and lymphocytes. Cell Immunol 1981; 59:75–81.
7. Anderson DJ, Hill JA. Immunological aspects of the reproductive organs and implications of intercourse. Curr Opin Immunol 1989; 1:1119–1124.
8. Anderson DJ, Wolff H, Zhang W, Pudney J. Immunology of the Male Reproductive Tract: Implications for the sexual transmission of human immunodeficiency virus. In: Voeller. B, ed. Fourth Kinsey Symposium on AIDs and Sex: Integrated biomedical and behavioral approach. Oxford University Press, New York 1990:311–333.
9. Parr MB, Parr EL. Immunohistochemical localization of secretory component and immunoglobulin A in the urogenital tract of the male rodent. J Reprod Fertil 1989; 85:115–124.
10. El-Demiry MIM, Hargreave, TB, Busuttil, A, James, K, Richie, AW, Chisholm GD. Lymphocyte subpopulations in the male genital tract. Br J Urol 1985; 57:769–774.
11. Koskimics AI, Kormano M, Lahti AA. Difference in the immunoglobulin content of seminiferous tubule fluid and rete testis fluid of the rat. J Reprod Fertil 1971; 27:463–465.
12. Rumke P. The origin of immunoglobulins in semen. Clin Exp Immunol 1974; 17:287–297.

13. Vaerman J-P, Férin J. Local immunological response in the vagina, cervix, and endometrium. Acta Endocrinol 1974; 194:281–301.
14. Ogra P, Yamanaka T, Losonsky GA. Local immunologic defenses in the genital tract. In: Reproductive Immunology New York: Alan R. Liss, Inc.; 1981:381–394.
15. Wira CR, Sandoe CP. Sex steroid hormone regulation of immunoglobin G (IgG) and A (IgA) in rat uterine secretions. Nature 1977; 268:534–536.
16. Schumacher GFB. Humoral immune factors in the female reproductive tract and their changes during the cycle. In: Dinsda D, Schumacher G, eds. Immunological Aspects of Infertility and Fertility Control. North Holland, NY: Elsevier; 1980:93–141.
17. Sullivan DA, Wira CR. Hormonal regulation of immunoglobulins in the rat uterus: Uterine response to multiple estradiol treatments. Endocrinology 1984; 114:650–658.
18. Wira CR, Stern J. Endocrine regulation of the mucosal immune system in the female reproductive tract: Control of IgA, IgG and secretory component during the reproductive cycle, at implantation and thoroughout pregnancy. In: Pasqualini JR, Scholler R, eds. Hormones and Fetal Pathophysiology. New York: Marcel Decker, Inc.; 1992:343–368.
19. Lippes J, Ogra S, Tomasi TBJ, Tourville DR. Immunohistochemical localization of γG, γA, γM, secretory piece, and lactoferrin in the human female genital tract. Contraception 1970; 1:163–183.
20. Rebello R, Green FHY, Fox HA. Study of the secretory immune system of the female genital tract. J Obstet Gynecol 1975; 82:812–816.
21. Kelly JK, Fox H. The local immunological defense system of the human endometrium. J Reprod Immunol 1979; 1:39–45.
22. Tourville DR, Ogra SS, Lippes J, Tomasi TBJ. The human female reproductive tract: Immunohistological localization of A, G, M, secretory piece, and lactoferrin. Am J Obstet Gynec 1970; 108:1102–1108.
23. Ogra PL, Ogra SS. Local antibody response to poliovaccine in the human female genital tract. J Immunol 1973; 110:1307–1311.
24. Kerr WR. Vaginal and uterine antibodies in cattle with particular reference to brucella abortus. Br Vet J 1955; 111:169–178.
25. Bell EB, Wolf B. Antibody synthesis in vitro by the rabbit vagina against diptheria toxoid. Nature 1967; 214:423–424.
26. Yang S, Schumacher GFB. Immune response after vaginal application of antigens in the rhesus monkey. Fertil Steril 1979; 32:588–598.
27. Parr EL, Parr MB, Thapar MA. Comparison of specific antibody responses in mouse vaginal fluid after immunization by several routes. J Reprod Immunol 1988; 14:165–176.
28. Wira CR, Sandoe CP. Specific IgA and IgG antibodies in the secretions of the female reproductive tract: Effects of immunization and estradiol on expression of this response in vivo. J Immunol 1987; 138:4159–4164.
29. Wira CR, Sandoe CP. Effect of uterine immunization and oestradiol on specific IgA and IgG antibodies in uterine, vaginal, and salivary secretions. Immunology 1989; 68:24–30.
30. Wira CR, Prabhala RH. The female reproductive tract is an inductive site for immune responses: Effect of estradiol and antigen on antibody and secretory component levels in uterine and cervico-vaginal secretions following various

routes of immunization. In: Griffin PD, Johnson PM, ed. Scientific Basis of Fertility Regulation: Local Immunity in Reproductive Tract Tissues. Oxford University Press NY; 1993:271–293.

31. Wira CR, Sandoe CP. Hormone regulation of immunoglobins: Influence of estradiol on IgA and IgG in the rat uterus. Endocrinology 1980; 106: 1020–1026.

32. Sullivan DA, Wira CR. Estradiol regulation of secretory component in the female reproductive tract. J Steroid Biochem 1981; 15:439–444.

33. Sullivan DA, Underdown BJ, Wira CR. Steroid hormone regulation of free secretory component in the rat uterus. Immunology 1983; 49:379–386.

34. Sullivan DA, Richardson GS, MacLaughlin DT, Wira CR. Variations in the levels of secretory component in human uterine fluid during the menstrual cycle. J Steroid Biochem 1984; 20:509–513.

35. Wira CR, Sandoe CP, Steele MG. Glucocorticoid regulation of the humoral immune system. I. In vivo effects of dexamethasone on IgA and IgG in serum and at mucosal surfaces. J Immunol 1990; 144:142–146.

36. McMaster MT, Newton RC, Dey SK, Andrews GK. Activation and distribution of inflammatory cells in the mouse uterus during the preimplantation period. J Immunol 1992; 148:1699–1705.

37. De M, Sanford TH, Wood GW. Detection of interleukin-1, interleukin-6, and tumor necrosis factor-alpha in the uterus during the second half of pregnancy in the mouse. Endocrinology 1992; 131:14–20.

38. Stern JE, Gardner S, Quirk D, Wira CR. Secretory immune system of the male reproductive tract: Effects of dihydrotesterone and estradiol on IgA and secretory component levels. J Reprod Immunol 1992; 22:73–85.

39. Wira CR, Sullivan DA. Estradiol and progesterone regulation of IgA, IgG, and secretory component in cervico-vaginal secretions of the rat. Biol Reprod 1985; 32:90–95.

40. Sullivan DA, Wira CR. Hormonal regulation of immunoglobulins in the rat uterus: Uterine response to a single estradiol treatment. Endocrinology 1983; 112:260–268.

41. Prabhala RH, Wira CR. Cytokine regulation of the mucosal immune system: In vivo stimulation by interferon-gamma of secretory component and immunoglobulin A in uterine secretions and proliferation of lymphocytes from spleen. Endocrinology 1991; 129:2915–2923.

42. Wira CR, Colby EM. Regulation of secretory component by glucocorticoids in primary cultures of rat hepatocytes. J Immunol 1985; 134:1744–1748.

43. Wira CR, Rossoll RM. Glucocorticoid regulation of the humoral immune system. Dexamethasone stimulation of secretory component in serum, saliva, and bile. Endocrinology 1991; 128:835–842.

44. Tabibzadeh SS, Santhanam U, Sehgal PB, May LT. Cytokine-induced production of IFN-beta 2/IL-6 by freshly explanted human endometrial stromal cells. Modulation by estradiol-17beta. J Immunol 1989; 142:3134–3139.

45. Tabibzadeh S. Ubiquitous expression of TNF-alpha/cachectin immunoreactivity in human endometrium. Am J Reprod Immunol 1991; 26:1–4.

46. Jacobs AL, Sehgal PB, Julian J, Carson DD. Secretion and hormonal regulation of interleukin-6 production by mouse uterine stromal and polarized epithelial cells cultured in vitro. Endocrinology 1992; 131:1037–1046.

47. Robertson SA, Mayrhofer G, Seamark RF. Uterine epithelial cells synthesize granulocyte-macrophage colony-stimulating factor and interleukin-6 in pregnant and nonpregnant mice. Biol Reprod 1992; 46:1069–1079.
48. Sollid LM, Kvale D, Brandtzaeg P, Markussen G, Thorsby E. Interferon-γ enhances expression of secretory component, the epithelial receptor for polymeric immunoglobulins. J Immunol 1987; 138:4303–4306.
49. Kvale D, Lovhaug D, Sollid LM, Brandtzaeg P. Tumor necrosis factor upregulates expression of secretory component, the epithelial receptor for polymeric Ig. J Immunol 1988; 140:3086–3089.
50. Jacobs AL, Sehgal PB, Julian J, Carson DD. Secretion and hormonal regulation of Interleukin-6 production by mouse uterine stromal and polarized epithelial cells cultured in vitro. Endocrinology 1992; 131:1037–1046.
51. Wira CR, O'Mara B, Richardson J, Prabhala R. The mucosal immune system in the female reproductive tract: Influence of sex hormones and cytokines on immune recognition and responses to antigen. Vaccine Res 1992; 1:151–167.
52. Shaikh AA. Estrone and estradiol levels in the ovarian venous blood from rats during the estrous cycle and pregnancy. Biol Reprod 1971; 5:297.
53. Wira CR, Bodwell JE, Prabhala RH. In vivo response of secretory component in the rat uterus to antigen, IFN-γ, and estradiol. J Immunol 1991; 146:1893–1899.
54. Prabhala RH, Wira CR. Influence of estrous cycle and estradiol on mitogenic responses of splenic T and B lymphocytes. 1993; In Press.

5

Suppressive and Permissive Actions of Glucocorticoids: A Way to Control Innate Immunity and to Facilitate Specificity of Adaptive Immunity?

ROEL DERIJK AND FRANK BERKENBOSCH*

The French physiologist Claude Bernard was the first to contribute to the concept of stress by proposing that in living organisms there must be a constancy in the 'milieu interieur,' and that the true understanding of the living process must be concerned with internal regulatory mechanisms for maintaining the internal environment. In the first half of this century, the extreme sensitivity of adrenal-deficient animals to stress from various sources (e.g., infections, exercise) was evident for many researchers.[1] The adrenocortical functions of conferring resistance to stress was eventually ascribed to the release and actions of glucocorticoids. Such a view was particularly stimulated by the introduction of Hans Selye's general adapatation syndrome (GAS) which he defined as the sum of nonspecific, systemic reactions of the body in response to exposure to stress.[2]

By defining GAS Selye focused attention on the stereotyped aspects of the response to stress elicited by any stimulus. The important elements, such as thymus involution and lymphopenia were considered to be due to actions of elevated plasma levels of glucocorticoids. GAS was ultimately connected to the concept of 'diseases of adaptation.' Selye predicted that such diseases, among which allergy, diffuse collagen disease, and rheumatic diseases were listed, were due to overactivity of the adrenal cortex. The demonstration of relief of rheumatoid arthritis following treatment with cortisone were therefore unexpected,[3] introducing the

---

*Frank Berkenbosch's sudden death on April 3, 1993, took away a teacher, a mentor, and a good friend. He introduced me to science and always supported me whenever I needed him. In addition, he was a special person, who approached others in an honest and positive way. His death is a great loss to us all, but the seeds of his ideas live on. EDITOR.

concept of pharmacological effects in glucocorticoid physiology. The overall outcome was a loss of interest in the area of glucocorticoids and stress. However, the discovery of glucocorticoid receptors and the basic molecular mechanisms of their action, together with the discovery of their broad distribution in almost every nucleated cell in the body, has recently generated renewed interest in this area. In fact, the apparent lack of evidence collected over the years that glucocorticoids enhance the body's normal defense mechanisms, led Munck and colleagues[4] to introduce a novel hypothesis concerning how glucocorticoids confer protection during stress.

These workers evaluated the evidence and proposed that: (1) the physiological function of stress-induced increases in glucocorticoids levels is to protect not against the source of stress itself (as put forward by Selye), but against the normal defense reactions that are activated by stress; and (2) glucocorticoids accomplish this function by suppressing those defense reactions, thus preventing them from overshooting and threatening homeostasis. The basis of this unifying conceptual framework, designed to accommodate apparently unrelated physiological and pharmacological effects of glucocorticoids, has mostly been derived from the wealth of information that glucocorticoids generally suppress immune and inflammatory reactions. However, the concept that glucocorticoids only suppress the primary defense reactions to stress has, paradoxically, been challenged by recent data demonstrating that some important aspects of the immune response are actually facilitated or enhanced by glucocorticoids.

In this paper, the immune system will be considered as divided in two functional divisions, namely the innate immune system and the adaptive immune system. Innate immunity acts as first line of defense against infectious agents, has no memory, and consists of acute phase proteins, complement and eicosanoids as soluble mediators, and phagocytes as cellular constituents. However, the adaptive immune system produces specific reactions to each individual infectious agent, and the effector elements are T and B cells that display memory for a particular antigen.

We propose the hypothesis that glucocorticoids exert a dual action on the immune system and are selectively *immune suppressive* and *permissive enhancing*, controlling the consequences of the innate immune system, while at the same time boosting essential components of the adaptive immune system, leading to increased specificity of the immune reaction. In this way we integrate and unify the general, and seemingly paradoxical, views of the enhancing and suppressing effects of glucocorticoids.

Evidence That Plasma Glucocorticoid Concentrations Increase During Inflammation and Immune Responses

Inflammatory Stimuli

Several studies have demonstrated that plasma corticosterone levels in animals rapidly increase after administrations of viral or bacterial products.[5] Intraperitoneal administration of NewCastle disease virus (NDV, nonvirulent in rodents) in mice has frequently been demonstrated to induce a fast and long-lasting (several hours) increase in both plasma adrenocorticotropin hormone (ACTH) and corticosterone concentrations.[6,7] In addition, in a variety of studies it has been consistently demonstrated that administration of low doses of lipopolysaccharide (LPS), an inflammatory extract of bacterial membranes, induces a fast and long-lasting increase (up to 4 hours) of plasma ACTH and corticosterone levels.[8-11] We reported that the response is independent of the behavioral and febrile effects of LPS.[9,12] Moreover, the lack of effects on blood levels of prolactin, the gonadotropins, and of adrenaline and noradrenaline has demonstrated that the effects of non-pyrogenic doses of LPS are very selective and clearly differ from stimuli generating a more general stress response.[9,12]

Production and release of glucocorticoids by the adrenal glands is primarily under control of ACTH released from the anterior pituitary gland. In turn, the release of ACTH is regulated by a variety of neurohypophysial peptides produced by hypothalamic neurons. Two of the main regulating peptides are corticotropin-releasing factor (CRF) and arginine vasopressin (AVP), both produced in the paraventricular nucleus.[13] This system is known as the hypothalamus-pituitary-adrenal axis. LPS and NDV have been shown to stimulate the production of small quantities of an ACTH-like substance from lymphocytes.[14,15] Based on findings that only a small fraction of total lymphocytes produce this ACTH-like substance and related peptides,[14,15] it can be anticipated that ACTH released from lymphocytes may play a paracrine rather than an endocrine role. Nevertheless, Blalock and Smith[14] hypothesized that ACTH produced by lymphocytes is sufficient to trigger CORT release by the adrenal cortex. In support of their hypothesis, they showed that hypophysectomized mice injected with NDV exhibited an increase in circulating corticosterone.[16] However, in a series of experiments on mice tested for the completeness of the hypophysectomy, Dunn and collegues[7] failed to replicate the evidence for the existence of the so-called 'lymphoid-adrenal axis.' In fact, the ACTH depletion of the pituitary gland in response to administration of NDV appears to be the only nonconflicting observation demonstrating the involvement of the pituitary gland in NDV-induced adrenocortical response.[5]

The requirement of the hypothalamus and the pituitary gland for the corticosterone response to LPS has found more solid experimental evidence. Early studies in rats involving hypothalamic lesions and/or pharmacological blockade of CRF secretion have clearly shown that ACTH or corticosterone released in response to LPS predominantly originates from the pituitary gland and involves a central mechanism.[10,11] Recently, we have demonstrated the validity of these observations, showing that passive immunoneutralization of CRF completely prevents the ACTH response to subpyrogenic doses of LPS (Schotanus et al. submitted).[17]

TABLE 5.1. Criteria for cytokines as mediators for pituitary-adrenal responses to inflammation and infection.

Criterion 1
The putative cytokine released should have some quantitative and temporal relationship to the magnitude and time course of the pituitary-adrenal response, respectively.

Criterion 2
Injection of the putative cytokine must result in pituitary-adrenal activation.

Criterion 3
Substances that block the production and/or action of the putative cytokine should prevent the pituitary-adrenal response.

It can be anticipated that neuroendocrine regulation can not be conceived without afferent signals originating from the immune system. Recently, we demonstrated that selective elimination of peripheral macrophages in the rat by means of the liposome-mediated macrophages suicide technique[9,12] completely blocks both the increase in plasma ACTH and corticosterone after administration of nonpyrogenic doses of LPS. These results led us to hypothesize that soluble mediators released from peripheral macrophages may mediate the pituitary-adrenal response. Among the many soluble madiators released by stimulated macrophages in vitro are growth factors, proteases, protease inhibitors, colony-stimulating factors, complement components, and cytokines.[18] Various criteria, listed in Table 5.1, must be fulfilled a substance to be classified as a mediator. At this stage, various arguments point to a complementary role for the cytokines interleukin (IL) -1, TNF, and IL-6 in LPS-induced pituitary-adrenal activation. Administration of the 3 cytokines to rats or mice has been shown to increase plasma levels of ACTH and corticosterone via mechanisms involving CRF release.[19-22] Moreover, injection of LPS in doses that lead to pituitary-adrenal activation result in a parallel induction of the above-mentioned cytokines in the circulation.[11,23-28]

It should be emphasized that the observations described here are only suggestive and, do not prove that these cytokines actually participate in the response. Passive immunization studies or experiments involving selective receptor antagonists should give further insight into the relative roles of each of these cytokines. In part, this criterium has been met for the role of IL-1. First, supernatants from in vitro-stimulated macrophages have been shown to increase plasma corticosterone concentrations in mice, and this response was prevented by preincubation of the supernatants with an antiserum raised against IL-1.[6] Second, IL-1 receptor blockade with antisera raised to the IL-1 alpha receptor has been shown to attenuate the LPS-induced increase in plasma ACTH, although no data were provided concerning the plasma corticosterone response.[29]

Third, we have recently demonstrated that injection of an endogenous, human IL-1 receptor antagonist markedly attenuates the ACTH response to injection of subpyrogenic doses of LPS (Schotanus and Berkenbosch, submitted).[30]

Antigenic Stimuli

In rats and mice,[5] increased glucocorticoid blood levels occurring at the same time as the peak of the humoral immune response have also been observed after antigenic challenge with different antigens. This response is thought to be mediated by the release of glucocorticoid-inducing factor (GIF) from stimulated T cells. The characteristics of GIF differ from any of the known cytokines released from T cells. Preliminary experiments demonstrate that purified GIF preparations are able to stimulate the release of ACTH from primary anterior pituitary cultures in vitro. These observations suggest that, unlike IL-1, GIF my act at the level of the pituitary gland (Berkenbosch and Besedovsky, unpublished observations).

Summary

In summary, the administration of antigens or inflammatory stimuli induce increased plasma corticosterone concentrations. Differences in the time course of the corticosterone response suggests that antigenic and inflammatory stimuli may act through other mediators to increase plasma corticosterone levels. The increase in plasma corticosterone after injection of a low dose of LPS is selective, macrophage dependent, and is likely to involve IL-1 as an important signal. The increase in plasma corticosterone concentrations during the peak of the humoral response to antigenic challenge is likely to be dependent on the induction of a noncharacterized T-cell factor, designated GIF.

Corticosteroid Receptor Diversity and Specificity-Conferring Mechanisms Involving Glucocorticoid-Binding Protein

Corticosteroid Receptors in the Immune System

Two separate, high-affinity, cytosolic receptors for glucocorticoids, type I and type II, have been characterized by receptor binding studies,[31] and cDNA clones corresponding to the two receptor types have recently been isolated.[32,33] Type I receptors are also referred to as mineralocorticoid receptors (MRs), whereas type II receptors are commonly refered to as glucocorticoid receptors (GRs). The MRs have high affinity for aldosterone (ALDO), a mineralocorticoid, and for cortisol and corticosterone (Kd approximately 1 nM), both glucocorticoids whereas they have a two- to five-fold lower affinity for dexamethasone (DEX), a synthetic glucocorticoid. In contrast, GRs have high affinity for dexamethasone (Kd = 0.4–1 nM), whereas they have a three- to five-fold lower affinity for corticosterone, and a 10- to 20-fold lower affinity for the mineralocorticoid ALDO.[31] Due to their higher affinity for corticosterone or cortisol, MRs have a much larger fractional occupation by endogenous glucocorticoids than GRs, even when circulating glucocorticoid levels are at basal morning values. GRs become progressively occupied during the rise of circulating glucocorticoids after stress and during the circadian rhytmicity.[34] The MRs are most concentrated in the hippocampus. Many fewer have been detected in peripheral tissues, including the spleen, and no MRs have been detected in the thymus.[32,35] Moreover, MRs have been detected in peripheral blood lymphocytes of humans[36,37] but not of rats.[38] Recently, it has been shown that ALDO-selectivity of MRs is conferred by the enzyme 11β-hydroxysteroid dehydrogenease (11β-OHSD) which converts glucocorticoids to an inactive metabolite, and which allows binding of ALDO to MRs.[39] Whether the MRs detected in the spleen and blood lymphocytes are ALDO- or glucocorticoid-preferring sites has not been established.

The GRs are evenly distributed throughout the brain and peripheral tissue and are found in high concentrations in the spleen and thymus,[35,38] and on human peripheral blood cells.[36–37] In vitro studies have demonstrated that the number of GRs on individual human lymphocytes is increased by mitogenic stimulation.[40] Moreover, this increase in GRs seems to be cell-stage dependent, as receptor number correlates with the proliferative stage of the cell cycle.

Recent molecular genetic studies using cells transfected with MR or GR gene expression vectors has demonstrated that, if coexpressed, the two receptors are capable of interacting with closely overlapping gene networks.[41] In this way, MRs and GRs are proposed to function as a binary hormone response system in which low concentrations of glucocorticoids will act through MRs while higher concentrations would expand the range of gene control via activation of the GRs. Although MRs and GRs are coexpressed in hippocampal neurons, too little is known of MR- and GR-mediated gene control in hippocampal neurons to test the elegant hypothesis of coordinate genomic control exerted by these receptors. However, in support of the hypothesis of coordinated control, it has recently been demonstrated that MRs and GRs control the cellular excitability of hippocampal neurons in a coordinate antagonistic mode, depending on the concentration of corticosterone added to the hippocampal slices.[42,43] A coordinated control exerted by coexpression of MRs and GRs on lymphoid tissue may also be an attractive explanation for the observed dual effects of glucocorticoids on adaptive immune responses, as will be discussed later. However, data on coexpression of MRs and GRs are lacking, and dual effects of glucocorticoids can also be explained by assuming that GR-mediated genomic regulation is controlled by additional factors such as the timing of the cell cycle, or the absence or presence of cytokines.

Glucocorticoid-Binding Protein (CBG)

Changes in the numbers of measurable binding sites are considered to be a sensitive idex for receptor activation; the greater the receptor activation, the lower the number of measurable bindings sites, and vice versa.[44-46] Recently, it has been demonstrated that acute restraint stress for 1 hour, leading to peak levels of circulating corticosterone in rats, reduces GR binding in the hippocampus but does not affect GR binding in the lymphoid tissue; whereas injection of the synthetic glucocorticoid was shown to reduce GR binding at both sites.[44] These far-reaching observations have been explained by the fact that circulating glucocorticoids, but not DEX, are protein-bound to CBG. CBG, a protein of 383 amino acids, is found in the periphery but not in the brain,[47] and has been thought to buffer peripheral tissue from corticosterone during rest and after stress. CBG-bound glucocorticoid is considered to be the biologically inactive form of glucocorticoids in plasma.[48] In keeping with the biological activity of only the free fraction of glucocorticoids, Dallman and collegues[48] have estimated that, at resting plasma levels of corticosterone (10–50 nM), the non-CBG-bound fraction of corticosterone in the circulation is sufficient to saturate MRs but not the GRs. Moreover, at approximate concentrations over 100 nM, free corticosterone in plasma is logarithmically related to total corticosterone concentrations and is sufficient to occupy the low-affinity GRs. Thus, the lack of effect of stress-induced acute elevations of glucocorticoids to activate GRs in the spleen is not likely to be due to the buffering capacity of CBG in the circulation. Various peripheral tissues have been shown to contain high concentrations of CBG. The CBG binding capacity of the spleen is relatively high,[44] which might be due to the ability of macrophages to produce CBG.[47] Therefore, the acute elevation of plasma glucocorticoid is likely to be adsorbed by the local high concentrations of CBG in the spleen, and this may account for the minimal changes in GR binding in stressed animals. A similar mechanism to diminish GR activation has been described for the pituitary gland.[49,50] Such local production of CBG may be an efficient specificity-conferring mechanism causing differential effects of endogenous glucocorticoids in the different compartements of the immune system. Specificity-conferring mechanisms have also been shown to be active in local inflammation. In this regard, it is worth noting that CBG acts as a substrate for neutrophil elastase, which cleaves CBG and thus may promote the local delivery of glucocorticoids during inflammation.[47]

Summary

In summary, high numbers of GRs and relatively low numbers of MRs have been detected in the spleen and on cells of the immune system. Whether MRs are glucocorticoid or aldosterone-preferring sites has not been established. Although coordinate control of gene networks by MRs and GRs is an interesting possible explanation for the dual actions of glucocorticoids on the immune system, the basis for it (i.e., coexpression of MRs and GRs on single cells) is lacking. Efficient specificity-conferring mechanisms mediated by glucocorticoid-binding proteins, such as CBG or proteases that specifically degrade binding-proteins, may be involved in compartmentalization of the actions of glucocorticoids on immune cells.

Glucocorticosteroid Actions on Innate Immunity

Innate Immunity

Innate immunity acts as a first line of defense against infectious agents, and most potential pathogens are controlled before they can accomplish overt infection. Acute-phase proteins, complement factors, and eicosanoids are the main soluble factors that play a role in innate immunity. These factors are responsible for recruitment and activation of phagocytes, the main cellular constituents of innate immunity. It is well established that innate and adaptive immune systems do not act in isolation. For instance, antibodies produced by the cooperative activities of T and B cells help phagocytes to recognize the infectious agent. Moreover, cytokines released by cells of the adaptive immune system enhance the activity of phagocytes to destroy the infectious agent more effectively. In turn, macrophages are able to process and present antigen, and their activity is a requisite for clonal activation of antigen-committed T cells.

Acute Phase Proteins

Regardless of the cause of inflammation (physical or chemical tissue injury; bacterial, viral, or parasitic infections; neoplastic growth), a common systemic consequence is a change in plasma concentrations of a group of proteins collectively designated as acute-phase proteins. The bulk of these proteins are of hepatic origin, but some of them are also produced at extrahepatic sites. Although the true physiological role of a number of the acute-phase proteins remains unclear, various activities suggest a homeostatic role in inflammation.[51] Among these functions are direct immobilization and scavenging of foreign particles and immune complexes, functions in the clotting cascade, activation of several kinds of lymphoid cells, and protection in endotoxin shock. In addition, a large part of the acute-phase proteins is formed by various proteinase inhibitors (e.g., α_2-macroglobulin, cysteine proteinase inhibitor, α^1-proteinase inhibitor, and α_1-antichymotrypsin in the rat). It is generally accepted that these protease inhibitors protect the tissue against damage that could be inflicted by the enhanced production of proteases at the inflammatory site. Remarkably, the broad nature of inhibition against various proteinases is maintained across the different species, including man. This emphasizes the importance of proteinase inhibitory activity during the acute-phase response. Among the regulatory signals for the production of the acute-phase proteins are the cytokines IL-1, IL-6, tumor necrosis factor (TNF), and glucocorticoids, of which IL-6 is now believed to be the most important.[48,51] Glucocorticoids do not directly induce production of acute-phase proteins by hepatic cells, but rather facilitate the action of IL-6, probably by the induction of the IL-6 receptor on hepatic cells.[48,51-53]

Complement

The complement system is composed of circulating proteins of which a number could be classified as acute-phase proteins, since during infection their concentrations increase several-fold in the circulation. During an immune response the complement system is responsible for a number of important events including opsonization of pathogens, chemotaxis, vasodilatation, and a direct cytotoxic effect exerted by the membrane attack complex.[54] Because this very reactive and broad acting system is located in the peripheral circulation, it can affect all body cells. It is thus essential that this system is carefully regulated to prevent damage. In vitro, DEX down-regulates the release of C_3 the key regulatory component from both human endothelial cells and monocytes.[55-57] In addition, expression of factor B, which can stabilize the reactive form of C3 (i.e., C3b), is also inhibited, while in contrast, factor H expression is induced on human endothelial cells.[55,57] Factor H is an intrinsic inhibitory component of the complement system and is able to interrupt the cascade induced by C3b. This indicates that glucocorticoids are regulating the proinflammatory actions of the complement system not only by inhibiting the production of the proinflammatory parts of the system, but also by selectively inducing an inhibitor of the system. In this context it is worth noting that the cytokine IL-1 has exactly the opposing effect as glucocorticoids, because IL-1 induces the production of C3 and factor B, while factor H expression is inhibited.[57]

Eicosanoids

In addition to systemic changes, local inflammatory substances such as the eicosanoids are produced and found in nearly every tissue of the body. Generally, eicosanoids are considered to be proinflammatory substances having local activities.[58] It has been stated for quite some time that glucocorticoids inhibit the formation of arachidonic acid, the precursor molecule of both the lipo-oxygenase (leukotrienes and hydroxy eicosatetraenoic acids) and the cyclo-oxygenase derivates (thromboxanes and prostaglandins). In addition, it has been suggested that this effect of glucocorticoids is mediated via the induction of a second messenger protein, called lipocortin, inhibiting the action of phospholipase A_2, the key enzyme generating arachidonic acid from membrane derived phospholipids.[59] However, these findings have recently been questioned.[60] First, although in vitro data mainly show inhibition of eicosanoid production by glucocorticoids, in vivo experiments are less consistent showing increasing or decreasing eicosanoid production after glucocorticoid treatment. Second, the induction of lipocortins by glucocorticoids has been questioned.[61,62] Third, the mode of action of lipocortins is unclear. Furthermore, it has been proposed that not the amount but the availability of arachidonic acid is the rate limiting step in eicosanoid synsthesis. As an alternative, glucocorticoids can affect eicosanoid synthesis at different levels.[60] Glucocorticoids are main regulators of the lipid metabolisms and of other mediators (e.g., cytokines, Ca^{2+}, G-proteins) which possibly have regulatory effects on the action of phospholipase A_2. Taken together, substantial evidence indicates that glucocorticoids influence eicosanoid production and release, but this can be accomplished by several means and the exact mechanism remains to be elucidated.

Antibody-Dependent Cellular Cytotoxicity (ADCC)

A powerful cellular effector mechanism which can be considered as an interplay of innate and adaptive immunity is ADCC, the process of direct cellular killing of pathogens that are opsonized by specific antibodies. The effector cells, for example granulocytes, large granular lymphocytes, or monocytes/macrophages, bind antibodies with Fc receptors and phagocytose the opsonized particles. It can be anticipated that antibody specificity, antibody titers, and the level of expression of Fc receptors will greatly determine the efficacy of the ADCC. Interestingly, the addition of DEX alone down-regulates the expression of Fc receptors on the human granulocytic cell line HL-60.[63] In contrast, glucocorticoids augment Fc expression by interferon γ (IFN-γ), as has been shown for cultured human monocytes.[64] Furthermore, antibody responses are improved when cytokines and glucocorticoids are both present, as will be discussed below. Finally, addition of DEX causes a functional enhancement of the in vitro

ADCC of cultured monocytes in the presence of IFNγ.[65] Taken together, both Fc expression and the end point in the process of ADCC can be facilitated or inhibited by glucocorticoids, and the final outcome appears to be dependent on the presence of cofactors such as cytokines.

Glucocorticoid Actions on Adaptive Immunity

Adaptive Immunity: Importance of Specific and Nonspecific Signals

Clonal expansion of antigen-committed cells is an issue of critical importance for the adaptive immune response. It is now well established that the central role of antigen-presenting cells in the initiation of clonal expansion of immune cells is dependent on the capacity to generate specific and nonspecific signals recognized by immune cells. The specific signal is formed by a complex of processed antigen bound to self major histocompatibility complex (MHC) displayed on the surface of antigen-presenting cells; the complex is then recognized by a clonally restricted T-cell receptor complex.[66]

Evidence is growing that recognition of the MHC–antigen complex alone is insufficient to activate committed T cells. Costimulatory molecules are essential for activation and multiplication; the lack of costimulatory molecules has even been demonstrated to result in T-cell tolerance.[66] In general, cytokines have now been recognized as critically important costimulatory signals. For instance, it is clear from studies in several laboratories that IL-1 is a requisite costimulator for the clonal expansion of restricted T cells.[67] Glucocorticoids have been demonstrated to affect the steps leading to antigen presentation as well as critically regulate the costimulator signals. Although the effects are certainly very complex, and the consequences for immunity difficult to understand on basis of the current knowledge, it can be recognized that timing of glucocorticoid exposure as well as the concentrations of the glucocorticoid used are critical variables in the outcome of the effects of these steroids. Some of the basic principles, largely derived from in vitro studies, will be discussed briefly below.

Glucocorticoid Modulation of Cell Proliferation

Effects of glucocorticoids on proliferation of a wide variety of cells including those of the immune system have long been studied.[68] Most of the studies have been performed in vitro and both stimulatory and inhibitory effects have been described. It has been recognized that the specific cell type, concentration of the hormone, and stage of the growth cycle when the hormone is added are of critical importance whether glucocorticoids act as inhibitory or stimulatory agents.[68] The inhibitory effects of glucocorticoids on clonal expansion of immune cells have been overwhelmingly demonstrated, which has led to the generally accepted and dogmatic view that glucocorticoids are profound physiological inhibitors of lymphocyte proliferation.[4] Admittedly, only a few studies have been published demonstrating permissive effects of glucocorticoids on lymphocyte proliferation. For instance, without discussing the observations, Neifeld et al.[69] have demonstrated that T-cell proliferation in response to a mitogen is augmented by low concentrations of DEX and hydrocortisone. Higher pharmacological concentrations were found to inhibit T-cell proliferation. Moreover, even earlier studies show that T-cell growth becomes resistant to the inhibitory effects of glucocorticoids, depending on the time at which cells are exposed to glucocorticoids: T-cell proliferation in response to the T-cell mitogen phytohemagglutinin (PHA) is not affected when glucocorticoids are added 10 min or longer after the addition of PHA.[70] This illustrates the cell-cycle dependency of glucocorticoid actions on cell growth. Furthermore, Almawi et al.[71] showed that DEX-mediated inhibition of T-cell proliferation is completely abrogated by the synergistic action of the cytokines IL-1, IL-6, and IFN-γ. These data indicate that the effect of glucocorticoids on cell proliferation depends on the life cycle of the cell, which in turn is critically regulated by the actions of cytokines.

Major Histocompatibility Complex

Since regulation of clonal expansion of T and B cells involves expression of antigen bound to MHC molecules, it seems obvious to ask if MHC expression is regulated by glucocorticoids. In this respect, it is worth noting that the relevance of glucocorticoid regulation of MHC expression must be demonstrated, since MHC expression is not necessarily associated with antigen presentation.[72,73] Effects of glucocorticoids on MHC expression are complex. Snyder and Uanue[74] have shown that hydrocortisone or prednisolone suppresses MHC-class II expression on cultured murine monocytes. By contrast, class II expression on human monocytes can be enhanced by hydrocortisone or DEX.[73] Moreover, DEX has been shown to markedly potentiate IFN-γ-induced MHC-class I and -class II expression on human monocytes.[65] These results strongly suggest that the effect of glucocorticoids on MHC expression (one of the important requisites for clonal expansion of T cells) may depend on the species studied, on the activation stage of the cell, and/or the presence of cytokines.

Costimulatory Cytokines

There is a general consensus that glucocorticoids are profound inhibitors of the production and release of most of the known cytokines, both in vivo and in vitro. It is worth noting that the molecular mechanisms governing the biosynthesis and secretion of the cytokines are poorly understood at the present time. This is in spite of their enormous importance to the control of adaptive immunity. Consequently, only a limited amount of data are available on the molecular mechanisms of the cytokine regulation by glucocorticoids. In early experiments, it was shown that DEX could inhibit the production and release of T-cell growth factor (TCGF) a supernatant produced by activated peripheral blood cells and probably composed of a mixture of the cytokines IL-2, IL-1 and IL-6.[75] After cloning and characterization of the different cytokines, it has been consistently demonstrated that DEX, prednisolone, hydrocortisone, or cortisol can decrease expression of IL-1, IL-2, IL-6, IFN-γ, and TNF mRNA and protein of in vitro stimulated immune cells[76–82] However, an important question which has been poorly addressed concerns the timing of effects of glucocorticoids on cytokine production and release. In vivo, plasma glucocorticoids start to rise during antigen presentation, which is a time when cytokines are already induced. Furthermore, it has been reported that once the TNF mRNA is initiated, DEX is incapable of preventing TNF protein production and secretion.[77] Moreover, resistence of IL-1 production to hydocortisone occurs when monocytes are primed with IFN-γ.[79] It is not known if these mechanisms also function in the regulation of other cytokines.

Glucocorticoids can also differentially regulate cytokine production. In vivo treatment of mice with slow release corticosterone pellets has been shown to shift the in vitro cytokine production in previously isolated lymphoid cells from predominantly IL-2 to IL-4;[83] IL-2 production was decreased while IL-4 production was enhanced. While IL-2 is involved in regulatory clonal expansion of T cells, the cytokine IL-4 is involved in control and modulation of antibody responses.[83,84] Additionally, it serves as a costimulant not only in antigen driven activation and enhancement of MHC-molecule expression,[84] but also in B-cell differentiation. Here, IL-4 is believed to promote immunoglobulin switching of B cells from IgM to IgG$_1$ and IgE, and to inhibit IFN-γ-induced switching to IgG$_{2a}$.[84,85] It is tempting to speculate that such cytokine switching in response to glucocorticoids is related to the requirement of glucocorticoids for optimal and specific B-cell responses in vitro,[86] resulting in the increase in titers of the specific antibodies generated.[87]

Cytokine Receptors

Intriguing observations show that DEX or prednisolone: (1) up-regulates the expression of high-affinity IL-6 receptors on human epithelial cells, and on a human hepatoma cell line[88,89] (2) up-regulates the IL-1 receptor binding and expression on a glioblastoma cell line and human blood lymphocytes,[90,91] and (3) enhances the number of IFN-γ binding sites on cultured human monocytes.[92] In contrast, DEX has no effect or may slightly decrease the number and expression of IL-2 receptors on T cells.[78,93] Assuming the absence of spare receptors and, therefore, that cytokine receptor number is related to the magnitude of the biological effects, it seems obvious to suggest that the increased expression of cytokine receptors induced by glucocorticoids may allow glucocorticoids to promote clonal expansion of antigen-committed T cells. Interestingly, Munck et al.[94] recently proposed, using a mathematical model, that the dual regulatory actions of glucocorticoids (e.g., stimulatory on cytokine receptor expression and inhibitory on cytokine production and release) can combine to stimulate activity of a homeostatic mechanism. Admittedly, for this assumption to work, a critical factor is the temporal relationship between glucocorticoids, cytokine production and/or switching, and the corresponding receptors. At the present time, this relationship is difficult to reconstruct since no studies are available in which both parameters are assessed during the same experimental paradigm. Increased receptor expression can also be considered as a specificity-conferring mechanism of the adaptive immune response. It can be anticipated that T cells with the highest affinity for the MHC-antigen complex will express the highest number of receptors for costimulatory cytokines. Glucocorticoids may additionally augment cytokine receptor expression induced by the restricted T-cell receptor with the best fit for the presented MHC-antigen complex. The reality of this possibility is reinforced by data of Gilles et al.[75] demonstrating that committed T cells with low affinity for an antigen are down-regulated by glucocorticoids, whereas committed T cells with a high affinity for the antigen are favored to proliferate in the presence glucocorticoids. Also, Sorkin and collegues[95-97] have presented evidence that the physiological function of the glucocorticoid response to infection may be to preserve the antigenic specificity of the response preventing lymphocytes with little affinity for the antigen from unrestricted proliferation. In the absence of such regulation, enhanced risk for autoimmunity may be envisioned.

Tolerance to Self Antigens

The idea that glucocorticoids are involved in regulation of tolerance to self-antigens is based on the findings that glucocorticoids can relieve the clinical signs of rheumatoid arthritis in humans.[3] Recently, we have reviewed in detail the evidence that glucocorticoids play a role in regulation of self-recognition[98] and, therefore, here we will only briefly discuss the evidence. Most of the evidence for a critical role of glucocorticoids in recognition between self and nonself is based on studies with experimental animals. For instance, the fact that experimental autoimmune encephalomyelitis (EAE), an animal model for multiple sclerosis, can be induced only in susceptible Lewis rats appears to depend on defective activation and function of the pituitary-adrenal system in this rat strain.[99,100] More importantly, histocompatable Fisher rats, which are normally resistant for the induction of EAE, become susceptible to EAE after treatement with the GR antagonist RU-486.[100] In obese strain chickens (representing a spontaneous model of thyroid autoimmunity), both an impaired function of the pituitary-adrenal system and a two-fold increase in plasma CBG levels has been noted.[101,102] Correction of the pituitary-adrenal impairment in these chickens results in a complete remission of autoimmunity. Moreover, biobreeding (BB) rats, who develop pancreatic and thyroid autoimmunity, show a reduced binding of corticosterone to CBG as compared to histocompatible Wistar rats. This impairment has been attributed to a single point mutation in CBG.[98] In addition to an impaired regulation of plasma glucocorticoids, BB rats display a diminished capacity to secrete cytokines such as IL-1.[98] Similar defects including a diminished capacity to secrete TNF have been reported in nonobese (NOD) mice (a mouse model for pancreatic autoimmunity).[104] These data taken together strongly favor the view that dysfunctions in specificity-conferring mechanisms, such as altered functions of CBG or the diminished capacity to increase plasma glucocorticoids levels due to dysfunctions in the hypothalamic-pituitary-adrenal system, are (co)factors that play a critical role in controlling recognition of self antigens. Although currently there is a lack of knowledge at the molecular level with respect to the role of glucocorticoids, it can be anticipated that self-tolerance is maintained by glucocorticoids through active control and down-regulation of uncontrolled antigen presentation, and production of costimulatory signals. As we have discussed previously, both are essential for T-cell activation and multiplication.

The Glucocorticoid Paradox: Do Glucocorticoids Enhance the Body's Defence Reaction, or Do They Prevent Defence Reactions from Overschooting?

Viewing the discussed data, we can conclude that glucocorticoids are important determinants in controlling the extent of activation of innate immunity. The receptors that contribute to this control are mainly GRs. A role for MRs has not been studied. As briefly discussed, the complement system which can be potentially lethal as illustrated during septic shock,[105] appears to be under strict control by glucocorticoids. Furthermore, glucocorticoids may direct and down-regulate local inflammation by inducing the production of acute-phase proteins, including proteinase inhibitors, while glucocorticoids probably also can modulate the formation of proinflammatory arachidonic-acid derivatives. Moreover, specificity-conferring mechanisms, such as CBG cleavage by enzymes released by neutrophils, are likely to promote the delivery of glucocorticoids at the sites of the inflammation. Although most of the components of innate immunity are effectively down-regulated by glucocorticoids, some powerful effector mechanisms of innate immunity such as ADCC are facilitated by glucocorticoids. The enhancement of these functions appears to be caused mainly by permissive effects of glucocorticoids on some aspects of adaptive immunity that are involved in the regulation of these innate effector mechanisms.

By contrast, the evidence collected by various workers over the last few years favors the concept that glucocorticoids can facilitate adaptive immunity. These effects are likely to be mediated via GRs. Although MRs are present on immune cells, their role in regulation of adaptive immunity has been poorly addressed. Glucocorticoids can facilitate clonal expansion of antigen-committed immune cells. Moreover, the specificity of the adaptive immune response can be facilitated by glucocorticoids. The molecular basis of the promotion of clonal expansion, which is critical for adaptive immunity, appears to be mediated via complex effects of glucocorticoids on antigen presentation, production and release of costimulatory cytokines, and the expression of cytokine receptors. The enhancing role of glucocorticoids on the specificity of adaptive immunity is exemplified by the observations that committed cells with high affinities for antigens are favored to proliferate and that a normal glucocorticoid physiology is an important factor in controlling tolerance to self-antigens.

Last but not least, it should be emphasized that facilitation of growth and selectivity of adaptive immunity may depend largely on the temporal sequence of cytokine and glucocorticoid secretion. Under conditions of inflammation and infection, cytokine secretion is likely to precede glucocorticoid secretion. Various arguments favor the view that this temporal sequence of signaling to immune cells is a requisite for the permissive effects of glucocorticoids on growth of committed cells, and possibly on the selectivity of adaptive immune response. Glucocorticoid exposure of immune cells prior to their activation has been demonstrated to down-regulate virtually all molecular events recognized to be necessary for the development of the adaptive immune response. The general immune suppression that occurs when higher organisms are exposed to psychological stress, resulting in chronically elevated plasma glucocortcoid levels, further illustrates the notion of the importance of the temporal sequence of events for the outcome of adaptive immune responses.[106]

In summary, the data reviewed in this paper clearly illustrate that glucocorticoids can influence the immune system in a complex way. Glucocorticoid concentrations, the species studied, specificity-conferring mechanisms, different receptor subtypes which can act in a coordinate agonistic and antagonistic fashion, temporal sequence of integration of the actions of cytokines and glucocorticoids at the level of immune cells, and the diversity of the immunological regulatory compartments and the interaction of these compartments (e.g., innate and adaptive immunity), all define the outcome of the physiological action of glucocorticoids on immunity in general. In one perspective, glucocorticoid action on the immune system can be described as permissive and enhancing. This action of glucocorticoids can be considered to fit with the traditional view that glucocorticoids enhance defense systems and are involved in protection against the source of stress itself as proposed by Hans Selye.[2] From another perspective, glucocorticoid action on the immune system can be described as suppressive. This action of glucocorticoids meets with the more recent view that glucocorticoids do not protect against the source of stress itself but rather against the body's normal reaction to stress, as recently proposed by Munck and collegues.[4] Our point of view is based on the synthesis of both seemingly paradoxical perspectives, and we suggest that glucocorticoids increase resistance to stress through complex and dual interactions involving integrated permissive and suppressive effects on defense reactions to stress. Such integration of permissive and suppressive actions of glucocorticoids have also recently be described for the actions of these hormones on brain neurochemistry and behavior.[107]

References

1. Gaunt R. History of the adrenal cortex. In: Blaschko H, Sayers G, Smith AD, eds. Handbook of Physiology Washington, D.C.: American Physiological Society; 1974:1–12.
2. Selye H. Stress. Montreal: Acta Inc. Medical Publisher 1950.
3. Hench PS, Kendall EC, Slocumb CH, Polley HF. The effect of a hormone of the adrenal cortex (17-hydroxy-11-dehydrocorticosterone: compound E) and of pituitary adrenocorticotropic hormone on rheumatoid arthritis. Proc Staff Meet Mayo Clin Rochester 1949; 24:181–197.
4. Munck A, Guyer PM, Holbrook NY. Physiological functions of glucocorticoids in stress and their relation to pharmacological actions. Endocr Rev, 1984 5:25–44.
5. Besedovsky HO, Del Rey A, Sorkin E. Immune-neuroendocrine interactions. J Immunol 1985; 135:750s–754s.
6. Besedovsky HO, Del Rey A, Sorkin E, Dinarello CA. Immunoregulatory feedback between interleukin-1 and glucocorticoid hormones. Science 1986; 233:652–654.
7. Dunn AJ, Powell ML, Gaskin JM. Virus-induced increases in plasma corticosterone: A technical comment on Smith, Meyer, and Blalock. Science 1987; 238:1423–1423.
8. Berkenbosch F, DeRijk R, Del Rey A, Besedovsky HO. Neuroendocrinology of interleukin-1. In: Porter JC, Jezova D, eds. Circulating regulatory factors and neuroendocrine function. New York: Plenum Press; 1990: 303–314.
9. DeRijk RH, Van Rooijen N, Tilders FJH, Besedovsky HO, Del Rey A, Berkenbosch F. Selective depletion of macrophages prevents pituitary-adrenal activation in response to subpyrogenic, but not to pyrogenic, doses of bacterial endotoxin. Endocrinology, 1991; 129:330–338.

10. Moberg GP. Site of action of endotoxin on hypothalamic-pituitary-adrenal axis. Am J Physiol 1971; 220:397–400.
11. Yasuda N, Greer MA. Evidence that the hypothalamus mediates the endotoxin stimulation of adrenocorticotropic hormone secretion. Endocrinology 1987; 102:947–953.
12. DeRijk RH, Van Rooijen N, Berkenbosch F. The role of macrophages in the pituitaryadrenal activation in response to endotoxin (LPS). Res Immunol 1991; 143:224–229.
13. Tilders FJH, Berkenbosch F, Smelik PG. Control of secretion of peptides related to adrenocorticotropin, melanocytes stimulating hormone and endorphin. Front Horm Res 1985; 14:161–196.
14. Kavelaars A, Berkenbosch F, Croiset G, Ballieux RE, Heijnen CJ. Induction of beta-endorphin secretion by lymphocytes after subcutaneous administration of CRF. Endocrinology 1990; 126:759–764.
15. Blalock J, Smith EM. A complete regulatory loop between the immune system and neuroendocrine systems. Fed Proc 1985; 44:108–111.
16. Smith EM, Meyer JW, Blalock JE. Virus induced corticosterone in hypophysectomized mice: A possible lymphoid-adrenal axis. Science 1982; 218:1311–1312.
17. Schotanus K, Makara GB, Tilders FJH, Berkenbosch F. ACTH response to bacterial endotoxin in rats is mediated by corticotropin-releasing hormone (CRH). 1993; submitted.
18. Nathan C. Secretory products of macrophages. J Clin Invest 1987; 79: 319–326.
19. Sapolsky RM, Rivier C, Yamamoto P, Plotsky P, Vale W. Interleukin-1 stimulates the secretion of hypothalamic corticotropin releasing factor. Science 1987; 238:522–524.
20. Sharp B, Matta SG, Peterson RN, Chao C, McAllen K. Tumor necrosis factor-alpha is a potent ACTH secretagogue: Comparison to interleukin-1 beta. Endocrinology 1989; 124:3131–3133.
21. Naitoh Y, Fukuta J, Tominaga T, Nakai Y, Tamai S, Mori K, Imura H. Interleukin-6 stimulates the secretion of adrenocorticotropin hormone in conscious, freely moving rats. Biochem Biophys Res Commun 1988; 155: 1459–1463.
22. Berkenbosch F, van Oers JWAM, Del Rey A, Tilders FJH, Besedovsky HO. Corticotropin releasing factor-producing neurons in the rat activated by interleukin-1. Science 1987; 238:524–526.
23. DeRijk RH, Berkenbosch F. Development and application of a radioimmunoassay to detect interleukin-1 in rat peripheral circulation. Am J Physiol 1992; 263:E1092–E1098.
24. Bristow AF, Mosley K, Poole S. Interleukin-1 beta production in vivo and in vitro in rats and mice measured using specific immunoradiometric assays. J Mol Endocrinol 1991; 7:1–7.
25. Butler LD, Layman NK, Riedl PE, Cain RL, Shellhaas J, Evans GF, Zuckerman SH. Neuroendocrine regulation of in vivo cytokine production and effects: I in vivo regulatory networks involving the neuroendocrine system, interleukin-1 and tumor necrosis factor-a. J Neuroimmunol 1989; 24:143–153.

26. Fong Y, et al. Antibodies to cachectin/tumor necrosis factor reduce interleukin-1 and interleukin-6 appearance during lethal shock. J Exp Med 1989; 170:1627–1633.

27. Hogquist KA, Nett MA, Sheehan CF, Pendleton KD, Schreiber RD, Chaplin DD. Generation of monoclonal antibodies to murine IL-1beta and demonstration of IL-1 in vivo. J Immunol 1991; 146:1534–1540.

28. Moldawer LL, Gelin J, Schersten T, Lundholm KG. Circulating interleukin 1 and tumor necrosis factor during inflammation. Am J Physiol 1987; 253:R922–R928.

29. Rivier C, Chizzonite R, Vale W. In the mouse, the activation of the hypothalamic-pituitaryadrenal axis by a lypopolysaccharide (endotoxin) is mediated through interleukin-1. Endocrinology 1989; 125:2800–2805.

30. Schotanus K, Berkenbosch F, Tilders FJH. Human recombinant interleukin-1 receptor antagonist prevents ACTH but not interleukin-6 responses to low doses of bacterial endotoxin in rats. Endocrinology 1993; in press.

31. Reul JMHM, Kloet ER. Two receptor systems for corticosteronein rat brain: microdistribution and differential occupation. Endocrinology 1985; 117:2505–2511.

32. Arizza JL, Weinberger C, Cerelli G, Glaser TM, Handelin BL, Housman EE, Evans RM. Cloning of human mineralocorticoid receptor complementary DNA: Structural and functional relationship with the glucocorticoid receptor. Science 1987; 237:268–275.

33. Hollenberg SM, Weinberger C, Ong ES, Cerelli G, Oro A, Lebo R, Thompson EB, Rosenfeld MG, Evans RM. Primary expression of a functional human glucocorticoid receptor cDNA. Nature 1985; 318:635–641.

34. Reul JMHW, Van den Bosch FR, De Kloet ER. Differential response of Type I and Type II corticosteroid receptors in rat brain following stress and dexamethasone treatment: Functional implications. Neuroendocrinology 1987; 45:407–412.

35. Spencer L, Miller AH, Stein M, McEwen BS. Coricosterone regulation of Type I and II adrenal steroid receptors in brain, pituitary and immune tissue. Brain Res 1991; 549:236–246.

36. Armanini D, Strasser T, Weber PC. Characterization of aldosterone binding sites in circulating human mononuclear lymphocytes. Am J Physiol 1985; 248:E388–E390.

37. Armanini D, Witzgall H, Strasser T, Weber PC. Mineralocorticoid and glucocorticoid receptors in circulating mononuclear leukocytes of patients with primary hyperaldosteronism. Cardiol 1985; 72:99–101.

38. Lowy MT. Quantification of type I and II adrenal steroid receptors in neuronal, lymphoid and pituitary tissues. Brain Res 1989; 503:191–197.

39. Funder JW, Pearce PT, Smith R, Smith AI. Mineralocorticoid action: Target tissue specificity is enzyme, not receptor, mediated. Science 1988; 242:583–585.

40. Smith KA, Crabtree GR, Kennedy SJ, Munck AU. Glucocorticoid receptors and glucocorticoid sensitivity of mitogen stimulated and unstimulated human lymphocytes. Nature 1977; 267:523–526.

41. Evans RM, Arriza JL. A molecular Framework for the action of glucocorticoid hormones in the nervous system. Neuron 1989; 2:1105–1112.

42. Joels M, De Kloet ER. Effects of glucocorticoids and norepinephrine on the excitability in the hippocampus. Science 1989; 245:1503–1505.

43. Joels M, De Kloet ER. Mineralo-glucocorticoid receptor-mediated effects on membrane properties of the rat CA1 pyramidal neurons in vitro. Proc Natl Acad Sci 1990; 87:4495–4498.

44. Miller AH, Spencer RL, Stein M, McEwin BS. Adrenal steroid receptor binding in spleen and thymus after stress and dexamethasone. Am J Physiol 1990; 22:E405–E412.

45. Miller AH, Spencer RL, Trestman RL, Kim C, McEwen BS, Stein M. Adrenal steroid receptor activation in vivo and immune function. Am J Physiol 1991; 261:E126–E131.

46. Spencer RL, Young EA, Choo PH, McEwen BS. Adrenal steroid type I and type II receptor binding: Estimates of in vivo receptor number, occupancy and activation with varying level of steroid. Brain Res 1990; 514:37–48.

47. Hammond GL. Molecular properties of corticosteroid binding globulin and the sex-steroid binding proteins. Endocr Rev 1990; 11:65–79.

48. Dallman MF, Akana SF, Cascio CS, Darlington DN, Jacobson L, Levin N. Regulation of ACTH secretion: Variations on a theme of B. Recent Prog Horm Res 1987; 43:113–173.

49. De Kloet ER, Voorhuis TAM, Leunissen JLM, Koch B. Intracellular CBG-like molecules in the rat pituitary. J Steroid Biochem 1984; 20: 367–371.

50. Kuhn RW, Green AL, Raymore WL, Siiteri PK. Immunocytochemical localization of corticosteroid-binding globulin in rat tissue. J Endocr 1986; 108:31–36.

51. Richards C, Gauldie J, Baumann H. Cytokine control of acute phase protein expression. In: Bienvenu J, Fradelizi D, eds. Cytokines and Inflammation. Paris: John Libbey Eurotext; 1991:29–50.

52. Koj A, Gauldie J, Regoeczi E, Sauder DN, Sweeney GD. The acute phase response of cultured rat hepatocytes. Biochem J 1984; 224:505–514.

53. Baumann H, Richards C, Gauldie J. Interaction amoung hepatocyte-stimulating factors, interleukin 1 and glucocorticoids for regulation of acute phase plasma proteins in human hepatoma (HepG2) cells. J Immunol 1987; 139:4122–4128.

54. Roitt I. Immunology. London, New York: Gower Medical publishing; 1985.

55. Lemercier C, Julen N, Coulpier M, Dauchel H, Ozanne D, Fontaine M, Ripoche J. Differential modulation by glucocorticoids of alternative complement protein secretion in cells of the monocyte/macrophage lineage. Eur J Immunol 1992; 22:909–915.

56. Lappin DF, Whaley K. Modulation of complement gene expression by glucocorticoids. Biochem J 1991; 280:117–123.

57. Dauchel H, Julen N, Lemercier C, Daveau M, Ozanne D, Fontaine M, Ripoche J. Expression of complement alternative pathway proteins by endothelial cells. Differential regulation by interleukin-1 and glucocorticoids. Eur J Immunol 1990; 20:1669–1675.

58. Salman AJ, Higgs CA. The eicosanoids. In: Dale MM, Foreman JC, eds. Textbook of Immunopharmacology. London: Blackwell Scientific Publishers; 1989:129–141.

59. Flower RJ. Lipocortin and the mechanisms of action on glucocorticoids. Br J Pharmacol 1988; 65:987–1015.

60. Duval D, Freyss-Beguin M. Glucocorticoids and prostaglandin synthesis: We cannot see the wood for the trees. Prost Leuk Essential Fatty Acids 1992; 45:86–112.
61. Bronnegard M, Andersson O, Edwall D, Lund J, Norstedt G, Caristedt-Duke J. Human calpactin II (lipocortin I) Messenger ribonucleic acid is not induced by glucocorticoids. Mol Endocrinol 1988; 2:732–739.
62. Bienkowski MJ, Petro MA, Robinson LJ. Inhibition of thromboxane a synthesis in U937 cells by glucocorticoids. 1989; 264(11):6536–6544
63. Crabtree GR, Munck A, Smith KA. Glucocorticoids inhibit expression of Fc receptors on the human granulocytic cell line HL-60. Nature 1979; 279:338–339.
64. Girard MT, Hjaltadottir S, Fejes-Toth AN, Guyre PM. Glucocorticoids enhance the gamma-interferon augmentation of human monocyte immunoglobin G Fc receptor expression. J Immunol 1987; 138:3235–3241.
65. Shen L, Guyre PM, Ball ED, Fanger MW. Glucocorticoids enhances gamma interferon effects on human monocyte antigen expression and ADCC. Clin Exp Immunol 1986; 65:387–395.
66. Weaver CT, Unanua ER. The costimulatory function of antigen presenting cells. Immunol Today 1990; 11:49–55.
67. Rotteveel FTM, Verhoef MHAM, DeRijk RH, van den Berg H, Wolvers DAW, Berkenbosch F. Both interleukin-1 alpha and interleukin-1 beta are involved as accessory molecules in primary antigen (Tetanus Toxoid) induced human T-cell activation. Cell Immunol 1991; 138:245–250.
68. Cristofalo VJ, Rosner BA. Glucocorticoid modulation of cell proliferation. In: Baserga R, ed. Tissue Growth Factors. Berlin: Springer Verlag; 1981: 209–228.
69. Neifeld JP, Lippman ME, Tormey DC. Steroid hormone receptors in normal human lymphocytes. J Biol Chem 1977; 252:2972–2977.
70. Elves MW, Gough J, Israels MCG. The place of the lymphocyte in the reticuloendothelial system: A study of the in vitro effects of prednisolone on lymphocytes. Acta Haematol 1964; 32:100–107.
71. Almawi WY, Lipman ML, Stevens AC, Zanker B, Hadro ET, Strom TB. Abrogation of glucocorticoid-mediated inhibition of T-cell proliferation by the synergistic action of IL-1, IL-6 and IFNgamma. J Immunol 1991; 146:3523–3527.
72. Gerrard TL, Cupps TR, Jurgensen CH, Fauchi AS. Hydrocortisone-mediated inhibition of monocyte antigen presentation: Dissociation of inhibitory effect and expression of DR antigens. Cell Immunol 1984; 85:330–339.
73. Rhodes J, Ivanayi J, Cozens P. Antigen presentation by monocytes: Effect of modifying major histocompatibility complex class II antigen expression and interleukin 1 production by using interferons and corticosteroids. Eur J Immunol 1986; 16:370–375.
74. Snyder DS, Unanue ER. Corticosteroids inhibit murine macrophage Ia expression and interleukin-1 production. J Immunol 1982; 129(5):1803–1805.
75. Gilles S, Crabtree GC, Smith KA. Glucocorticoid-induced inhibition of T cell growth factor production. J Immunol 1979; 123:1624–1631.
76. Arya SK, Wong-Staal F, Gallo RC. Dexamethasone-mediated inhibition of human T-cell growth factor and gamma-interferon messenger RNA. J Immunol 1984; 133:273–276.

77. Beutler B, Krochin N, Milsark IW, Luedka C, Cerami A. Control of cathectin (Tumor Necrosis Factor) synthesis: Mechanisms of endotoxin resistance. Science 1986; 232:977–979.
78. Grabstein K, Dower S, Gilles S, Urdal D, Larsen A. Expression of inter-leukin 2, interferon-gamma, and the IL 2 receptor by human peripheral blood lymphocytes. J Immonol 1986; 136:4503–4508.
79. Lee SW, Tsou A, Chan H, Thomas J, Petrie K, Eugui EM, Allison AC. Glucocorticoids selectively inhibit the transcription of the interleukin 1beta gene and decrease the stability of interleukin 1beta mRNA. Proc Natl Acad Sci 1988; 85:1204–1208.
80. Lew W, Oppenheim JJ, Matsushima K. Analysis of the suppression of IL-1alpha and IL-1beta production in human peripheral blood mononuclear adherent cells by a glucocorticoid hormone. J Immunol 1988; 140:1895–1902.
81. Uehara A, Kohda H, Sekiya C, Takasugi Y, Namika M. Inhibition of interleukine-1 beta release from cultured human peripheral blood mononu-clear cells by prednisolone. Experienta 1988; 45:166–167.
82. Zanker B, Walz F, Wieder KJ, Strom TB. Evidence that glucocorticoids block the expression of the human interleukin-6 gene by accessory cells. Transpl 1990; 49:183–185.
83. Daynes RA, Araneo BA, Dowell TA, Huang K, Dudley D. Regulation of murine lymphokine production in vivo. J Exp Med 1990; 171:979–996.
84. Paul WE. Interleukin 4/B cell stimulatory factor 1: One lymphokine, many functions. FASEB J 1987; 1:456–461.
85. Jabara HH, Ahern DJ, Vercelli D, Geha RS. Hydrocorticosterone and IL-4 induce IgE isotype switching in human B cells. J Immunol 1991; 147:1557–1560.
86. Emilie D, Crevon M, Auffredou MT, Galanaud P. Glucocorticosteroid-dependent synergy between interleukin-1 and interleukin-6 for human B lymphocyte differentiation. Eur J Immunol 1988; 18:2043–2047.
87. Tuchinda M, Newcomb RW, De Vald BL. Effects of prednisolone on the human immune response to keyhole limpet hemocyanin. Int Arch Allergy 1972; 42:533–544.
88. Snyders L, Wit L, Content J. Glucocorticoid upregulation of high affinity interleukin 6 receptors on human epithelial cells. Proc Natl Acad Sci 1990; 87:2838–2842.
89. Rose-John S, Schooltink H, Lenz DR, Hipp E, Schmitz H, Schiel X, Hirano T, Kishimoto T, Heinrich PC. Studies on the structure and regulation of the human hepatic interleukin-6 receptor. Eur J Biochem 1990; 190:79–83.
90. Akahoshi T, Oppenheim JJ, Matsushima K. Induction of high affinity interleukin-1 receptors on human peripheral blood lymphocytes. J Exp Med 1988; 167:924–936.
91. Gottschall PE, Koves K, Mizuno K, Tatsuno I, Arimura A. Glucocorticoid upregulation of interleukin-1 receptor expression in a glioblastoma cell line. Am J Physiol 1991; 261:E362–E368.
92. Strickland RW, Wahl LM, Finbloom DS. Corticosteroids enhance the binding of gamma-interferon to cultered human monocytes. J Immunol 1986; 137:1577–1580.
93. Redondo JM, Fresno M, Lopez-Rivas A. Inhibition of interleukin 2-induced proliferation of cloned murine T-cells by glucocorticoids. Possible involve-ment of an inhibitory protein. Eur J Immunol 1988; 18:1555–1559.

94. Munck A, Naray-Fejes-Toth A. The ups and downs of glucocorticoid physiology: Permissive and suppressive effects revisited. Mol Cel Endocrinology 1992; 90:C1–C4.
95. Besedovsky HO, Sorkin E. Network of immune-neuroendocrine interactions. Clin Exp Immunol 1977; 27:1–12.
96. Besedovsky HO, Del Rey A, Sorkin E. Antigenic competion between horse and sheep red blood cells as a hormone dependent phenomenon. Clin Exp Immunol 1979; 37:106–113.
97. Besedovsky HO, Del Rey A, Sorkin E. Lymphokine containing supernatant from Con A-stimulated cells increase corticosteroid levels. J Immunol 1981; 126:385–392.
98. DeRijk, RH, Berkenbosch F. The immune-hypothalamo-pituitary adrenal axis and autoimmunity. Int J Neurosci 1991; 59:91–100.
99. MacPhee IAM, Antoni FA, Mason DW. Spontaneous recovery of rats from experimental allergic encephalomyelitis is dependent on regulation of the immune system by exogenous adrenal corticosteroids. J Exp Med 1989; 169:431–445.
100. Sternberg EM, Young III WS, Bernardini R, Calogero AE, Chrousos GP, Gold PW, Wilder RL. A central nervous system defect in biosynthesis of corticotropin-releasin hormone is associated with susceptibility to streptococcal cell wall arthritis in Lewis rats. Proc Natl Acad Sci (USA), 1989 J; 86:4771–4775.
101. Schauenstein K, Fassler R, Dietrich H, Schwarz S, Kromer G, Wick G. Disturbed immune-endocrine communication in autoimmune disease. J Immunol 1987; 6:1830–1833.
102. Fassler R, Schauenstein K, Kromer G, Schwarz S, Wick G. Elevation of corticosteroid-binding globulin in obese strain (OS) chickens: Possible implications for the disturbed immunoregulation and the development of spontaneous autoimmune thyroiditis. J Immunol 1986; 136:3657–3661.
103. Smith CL, Hammond GL. An amino acid substitution in BioBreeding rat corticosteroid binding globulin results in reduced steroid binding affinity. J Biol Chem 1991; 266:18555–18559.
104. Jacob CO, Sadakazu A, Michie SA, McDevitt HO, Acha-Orbea H. Prevention of diabetes in nonobese diabetic mice by tumor necrosis factor (TNF): Similarities between TNF and Interleukin-1. Proc Natl Acad Sci 1990; 87:968–972.
105. Hack CE, Thijs LG. The orchestra of mediators in the pathogenesis of septic shock: A review. In: Vincent JL, ed. Update in intensive care and emergency medicine. Heidelberg, Springer-Verlag; 1990:232–246.
106. Khansari DN, Murgo AJ, Faith RE. Effect of stress on the immune system. Immunol Today 1990; 11:170–175.
107. de Kloet ER. Brain corticosteroid receptor balance and homeostatic control. Front Neuroendocrinology 1991; 12:95–164.

6
Hormonal Interactions Between the Pituitary and Immune Systems

Istvan Berczi

The first observations that neurohormonal factors influence lymphoid organs were made by pathologists at the beginning of the twentieth century. It was noted that the thymus frequently involutes under the influence of environmental or emotional factors and that hormonal changes such as castration, Graves' disease, Addison's disease, and acromegaly may be associated with thymic hyperplasia.[1] In 1930, Smith first demonstrated experimentally the role of the pituitary gland in thymic growth.[2] He observed that in hypophysectomized rats the thymus regressed in weight to less than half that of control animals, whereas the thymus of partially hypophysectomized animals did not show accelerated involution. The profound influence of steroid hormones on lymphoid tissue was first shown by Selye in 1936.[3] He found that in rats a variety of noxious stimuli that produce a so-called alarm reaction also cause an acute involution of the thymus and other lymphoid organs in intact, but not in adrenalectomized animals. Furthermore, thymic atrophy could readily be induced in rats by adrenocortical extracts.[4] Selye also established that steroid hormones had a similar influence on the bursa of Fabricius in birds.[5] These initial observations inspired numerous studies on the effect of hormones on lymphoid tissue. However, the findings were so controversial that Dougherty[6] was not able to reach any definitive conclusions after reviewing the literature. Similarly, it was recognized in the 1950s that hypophysectomized animals become anemic and that, in humans, hypopituitarism is also associated with anemia. However, after surveying the literature, Crafts and Meinecke[7] concluded that pituitary, thyroid, and adrenocortical hormones do not affect bone marrow function directly, but rather, a secondary metabolic effect exists. Therefore, the idea of neuroendocrine regulation of lymphoid tissue fell into disrepute and was not considered seriously until recently.

During the past decade, interest in the interaction of neuroendocrine and immune systems has been rejuvenated, and antigens, soluble mediators, and receptors shared by both systems have been identified in increasing numbers. The innervation of lymphoid organs provides the morphological basis for interaction. By now, a substantial body of evidence, summarized in several recent volumes and in numerous reviews, indicates that there is indeed a close functional and regulatory relationship between the neuroendocrine and immune systems.[8-21] Moreover, there are compelling indications that the malfunction of this regulatory interaction may lead to disease and even to death. Owing to space limitations, only a brief overview can be provided here, and the reader is referred to the cited literature for more detailed information. Those areas that are discussed in detail elsewhere in this volume will only be considered generally in this chapter.

Pituitary Hormones and Immune Function

The pituitary gland plays a key role in immunoregulation. Homeostasis of the immune system is maintained by a proper balance between immunostimulatory (prolactin and growth hormone) and immunosuppressive (adrenocortical) hormones. Other pituitary hormones also influence immune function.[22,14]

The Role of Growth and Lactogenic Hormones

Growth Hormone

Although it has long been proposed on the basis of animal experiments that growth hormone (GH) plays a role in the maintenance of immune function, these observations were seriously compromised by the fact that human pituitary dwarfs do not show major symptoms of immunodeficiency.[23] This long-standing controversy has been solved by studies in hypophysectomized (Hypox) rats. It was found that the profound immunodeficiency of such rats could be fully restored by treatment with either GH or prolactin (PRL).[24-30] As it turned out, human pituitary dwarfs have normal levels of PRL,[31] which explains their immunocompetence. In contrast, the dwarf mice studied immunologically are deficient in both PRL and GH.[32,33] GH treatment restores the immune function of deficient dwarf animals.[22]

Hypophysectomized rats exhibit general immunodeficiency, anemia, an involution of the thymus and lymphoid organs, and severe impairment of nucleic acid synthesis in lymphoid tissue and bone marrow. All these hematological and immunological abnormalities can be restored by treatment with GH. GH is also effective in restoring the immunocompetence of rats suppressed by bromocriptine (BRC) or adrenocorticotropic hormone (ACTH) treatment. Natural killer (NK) cell function is also stimulated by GH. Some lymphoid cell lines express well-defined receptors for GH, although the presence of GH receptors on normal lymphocytes is not easily demonstrable. On the other hand, human monocytes express clearly detectable GH receptors. Under proper experimental conditions, a direct mitogenic effect of GH on lymphocytes and augmentation of interleuking (IL)-2 production can also be demonstrated. GH stimulates the production of IL-1 as well as superoxide anions, and also potentiates the induction of tumor necrosis factor-α (TNF-α) by bacterial lipopolysaccharide (LPS) in mononuclear phagocytes.[34–45] Neutrophilic leukocytes are also affected by GH. For example, stimulation of lysosomal enzyme production and oxidative metabolism, stimulation of adhesiveness and inhibition of chemotaxis, and priming for superoxide production have been reported.[45–50]

The effect of GH treatment on the immune system of GH-deficient children has been studied by several investigators. Shifts in helper/suppressor (CD4$^+$/CD8$^+$) T-cell ratios, changes in the proportion of peripheral B lymphocytes, greater spontaneous proliferation and alteration of lymphocyte response to mitogens, changes in immunoglobulin secretion in vitro, and an increase in NK-cell activity were observed. Most investigators emphasized that there were no obvious immune abnormalities in these children. It was also shown that these changes are transient and that normalization of altered parameters takes place upon long term treatment, although others did not observe any alteration after GH treatment.[51–59] Two children with renal allografts had acute rejection episodes after GH treatment.[60] In 14 girls with Turner syndrome the CD4$^+$/CD8$^+$ T-cell ratio was decreased, and the number of NK cells (CD16$^+$) increased, compared to controls. Treatment with GH induced a slight reduction in the percentage of B cells (CD20$^+$), and the number of CD16$^+$ NK cells returned to normal. The number of children with thyroid antibodies increased from 2 before treatment to 5 after 1 year.[61] Women with impaired GH secretion and healthy adults, both treated with GH, had significantly increased target cell lysis by NK cells.[62,63]

Receptors have been found on thymocytes and activated lymphocytes for somatomedins (or insulin-like growth factors [IGF]).[64–66] IGF-1 enhanced the mitogenic response of human peripheral blood lymphocytes to phytohemagglutinin (PHA), whereas insulin had no effect.[67] However, the proliferation and antibody formation of murine spleen cells induced by IL-2 was suppressed in vitro by physiological concentrations of IGF-1. Pharmacological concentrations of insulin had a similar effect.[68] Primary X-ray-induced thymic lymphomas had the phenotypic characteristics of pre-T cells, and showed no response to interleukins, but proliferated in response to IGF-1 and to an autocrine peptide termed lymphoma growth factor.[69] Treatment of rats with GH or IGF-1 accelerated thymic regeneration after injury induced by cyclosporine A (CSA).[70] The weight of the thymus in diabetic rats was restored by insulin and also by IGF-1. IGF-1 was effective despite persisting hyperglycemia and adrenal hyperplasia. Insulin and IGF-1 treatment of diabetic rats increased [^{3}H]thymidine incorporation and restored the expression of the Thy-1 antigen and the number of double-positive (CD4$^+$, CD8$^+$) thymocytes. The antibody response was normal in diabetic rats.[71] Treatment of GH deficient children with GH significantly increased the serum level of thymulin for at least 48 h. In addition, positive correlation was found between the serum level of IGF-1, but not of GH, and thymulin activity.[72] IGF-1 was also shown to enhance erythropoiesis and granulopoiesis, and it was suggested that the hematopoietic effects of GH are mediated by IGF-1. Furthermore, macrophages have the capacity to produce IGF-1.[73-76] Normal human B lymphocytes transformed with Epstein-Barr virus (EBV) respond to stimulation by GH with the production of significant amounts of IGF-1 and enhanced proliferation. EBV-transformed B cells derived from pygmies produced significantly less IGF-1 after exposure to GH.[77] Human T-cell lines derived from normal individuals by transformation with the human T-lymphocyte virus-I or -II responded to stimulation by GH with proliferation and the production of low levels of IGF-1. IGF-1 also stimulated colony formation in such cultures. This increased cloning efficiency in response to GH or IGF-1 was almost completely eliminated by the preincubation of cells with antibodies to either IGF-1 or the type I IGF receptor. Similar T-cell lines derived from individuals with Laron-type dwarfism did not respond to stimulation by GH with proliferation or IGF-1 production.[78] Murine spleen cells also produced IGF-1 which was stimulated by GH.[79]

Monocytes express high-affinity insulin receptors, and insulin has an influence on the expression of Fc receptors and on phagocytosis, fibrinolysis, and antibody-dependent cytotoxic reactions. Activated T and B lymphocytes also express insulin receptors. Insulin has a stimulatory effect on lymphocytes and was reported to induce nonspecific cytotoxic T cells, to increase the number of antibody forming cells, and to potentiate anaphylactic shock. Physiologic concentrations of insulin enhanced the cytotoxic effect of rat lymphocytes. Lymphocytes of rats, rabbits, pigs, cows, and from human tonsils elaborated a proinflammatory factor, termed anaphylactoid inflammation promoting factor, after exposure to insulin. A chemotactic activity of porcine insulin was observed for human T lymphocytes in vitro. Insulin reduced the sensitivity of human platelets to aggregating agents. Glucagon and somatostatin antagonized insulin action on lymphoid tissue.[10,14,80,81]

Prolactin

The immunoregulatory role of PRL was revealed by the observation that syngeneic pituitary grafts placed under the kidney capsule of Hypox rats restored their immunocompetence. Such grafts are known to secrete only PRL in significant amounts. Similar restoration could be achieved if hypophysectomized rats were treated with daily injections of PRL. Moreover, the immunosuppressive effect of dopaminergic agents (BRC, pergolide), which inhibit PRL secretion, could also be restored by PRL treatment. Subsequent experiments revealed that the anemia, involution of lymphoid organs, and impaired nucleic acid synthesis in lymphoid tissue of Hypox rats could also be normalized by syngeneic pituitary graft or treatment with PRL.[24–27,29,30,34,82–84] Many of these original findings have been confirmed and further developed by other investigators.[44,45,85–88]

Receptors for PRL have been identified on lymphocytes and monocytes, and a direct mitogenic effect of this hormone on lymphoid cells was demonstrated in vitro. Moreover, it has been found in three different laboratories that the potent immunosuppresive agent CSA interferes with the binding of PRL to lymphoid cells. CSA was proposed to be a PRL receptor antagonist agent, or, alternatively, a regulator of receptor expression.[89–92] However, Varma and Ebner[93] found that CSA has no effect on PRL binding by Nb2 rat lymphoma cells. The Nb2 pre-T rat lymphoma expresses a novel short form of PRL receptor consisting of 393 amino acids, which has a higher affinity for PRL ($Ka = 29.1 \times 10^9 \, M^{-1}$) compared to the long receptor ($Ka = 8.8 \times 10^9 \, M^{-1}$).[94] Thymic epithelial cells also express functional PRL receptors. PRL stimulates the expression of cytokeratin, secretion of thymulin, and proliferation of thymic epithelial cells.[95] Prolactin stimulates thymus growth and has a direct mitogenic effect on thymocytes.[96,97]

Prolactin was shown to stimulate the antibody response in various species.[84,98–100] Prolactin is necessary for the mixed lymphocyte reaction. Dopamine agonist agents (e.g., BRC, CPP 201–403) acted synergistically with CSA in the inhibition of graft rejection.[101,102] BRC treatment of mice prevented the T cell-dependent induction of macrophage tumoricidal activity which could be reversed by additional treatment with PRL. The production of interferon (IFN)-γ by T lymphocytes, and lymphocyte proliferation in response to mitogens were also depressed in spleen cells of BRC-treated mice, and were reversed after co-administration of PRL. Moreover, the number of deaths resulting from the inoculation of mice with Listeria was increased after BRC treatment and could be reversed by exogenous PRL.[103]

In most patients with cardiac allografts, serum PRL levels were increased prior to the primary rejection episode. Such increase was not always observed, however, during recurrent rejections.[104–106]

NK-cell activity of spleen lymphocytes from pituitary grafted male and female Ames dwarf mice was greatly enhanced.[107] There are contrasting observations with regard to the effect of hyperprolactinemia on NK-cell activity in humans.[108–110] Matera et al.[111] showed that PRL stimulates the proliferation and cytotoxic activity of purified NK cells, but it has no effect on NK activity of unseparated peripheral blood lymphocytes. The different susceptibility of purified NK cells and peripheral blood lymphocytes to PRL was due to the presence in the unseparated cell population of PRL-sensitive T cells capable of suppressing NK activity.

PRL enhanced the recovery of the sheep red blood cell (SRBC) receptor on human T lymphocytes after treatment with trypsin. Elevated serum PRL levels induced in males by chlorpromazine and in females by lactation raised the number of large granular lymphocytes in the peripheral blood that exert NK activity. Moreover, human sera containing elevated PRL levels stimulated the metabolic activity of peripheral neutrophilic leukocytes.[112]

Prolactin also plays a role in the immune function of the mammary gland and seems to promote the migration of lymphocytes to hormonally activated mammary tissue and initiate immunoglobulin secretion into the colostrum and milk.[113] The production of an immunosuppressive cytokine by the submandibular gland was deficient in Hypox male rats. Treatment with PRL, testosterone, and triiodothyronine (T_3) produced the most effective restoration, although PRL alone showed significant activity.[114]

Placental Lactogen

We have observed that all the hematological and immunological abnormalities of Hypox rats could be restored by daily treatment with human placental lactogen. These findings are in full agreement with some preliminary observations reported earlier—namely, that placental lactogen is capable of raising the weight of the thymus and spleen in dwarf mice and that it may exert an erythropoietic effect.[34,115]

The ACTH-Adrenal Axis

Adrenocorticotropic Hormone, Alpha-Malanocyte-Stimulating Hormone, and Opioid Peptides

ACTH was shown to exert an immunosuppressive effect in various experimental systems, and it antagonizes the restoration of immunocompetence in Hypox or BRC-treated rats by treatment with GH or PRL.[22] Pigs treated with porcine ACTH (1 IU/kg body wt) i.v. exerted a dramatic increase in NK and IL-2-stimulated NK cytotoxicity. Physiological concentrations of ACTH had no direct effect on NK cells in vitro.[116] Recent studies revealed that ACTH has a direct effect on lymphoid cell proliferation.[117,118]

Alpha-melanocyte-stimulating hormone (α-MSH) has been found to antagonize several effects of IL-1, including pyrogenicity, thymocyte proliferation, neutrophilia, the induction of acute-phase proteins, depression of TNF and contact sensitivity, and induction of prostaglandin E in fibroblasts. These effects are not mediated by classical α-MSH receptors. Intracerebro-ventricular infusion of IL-1β to rats rapidly decreased NK-cell activity. PHA reactivity, and IL-2 production by peripheral blood and spleen lymphocytes. All these effects of IL-1 could be blocked by simultaneous infusion of α-MSH.[119-124] Intravenous α-MSH reduced only the first phase of the biphasic febrile response of rabbits to the i.v. injection of *Staphylococcus aureus* cell walls. Intracerebro-ventricular α-MSH had no effect. Intravenous α-MSH had no effect on the fever or the serum iron response caused by muramyl dipeptide (MDP). It was concluded that the first phase of the thermal response to *S. aureus* is mediated by an endogenous pyrogen, and the second phase by a different mechanism, possibly by MDP.[125]

Lymphoid cells and monocyte macrophages have receptors for opioid peptides, some of which can be inhibited by the morphine receptor antagonist drug naloxone, but others are not inhibited. Although it is certain that immune function is influenced by endogenous opioid peptides, thus far the findings are controversial and do not permit definite conclusions. Antibody production, natural killer activity lymphokine activated killer activity, cytotoxic T-cell activity, the mixed lymphocyte reaction, IL-1, IL-2, prostaglandin, and interferon synthesis, the degranulation of mast cells, and chemotaxis of neutrophilic leukocytes were all affected by opioid peptides. Opiates are capable of immunomodulation by acting indirectly through the brain.[20,126-131]

Glucocorticoids

All the lymphoid organs and leukocytes possess glucocorticoid receptors, thymic epithelial cells and bone marrow cells having the highest concentration. The number of receptors is increased in stimulated lymphocytes. The circadian rhythm of leukocyte recirculation inversely correlates with the daily variation of endogenous cortisol. The thymus undergoes a profound involution under the influence of glucocorticoids. In highly sensitive species such as the rat and mouse, glucocorticoids activate in thymocytes and spleen cells an endogenous nuclease that cleaves nuclear DNA and causes cell death (apoptosis). This DNA fragmentation is a calcium-dependent process. Cortical epithelial reticular cells of the mouse thymus become spherical under the influence of dexamethasone and lose their major histocompatibility (MHC) antigens, whereas medullary epithelial cells remain unaffected under the same conditions. The production of prostaglandins by the thymic reticulum is also decreased by glucocorticoids. Thymic hormones and genes of the MHC complex influence the glucocorticoid sensitivity of thymocytes.[10,132-134]

Virtually all the functions of the monocyte macropahge cell series are inhibited by glucocorticoids. These include cell metabolism, chemotaxis, phagocytosis, and cytotoxic reactions, as well as the capacity to present antigen, secrete cytokines, and produce enzymes and other factors. On human monocytes, glucocorticoids increased the expression of human leukocyte D-related (HLA-DR) antigens, and IFN-γ and Fc-γ receptors.

The helper, suppressor, and killer function of T lymphocytes and the production of interleukins by them are also inhibited by glucocorticoids. This inhibitory effect can be abrogated by IL-2 and by insulin. IL-2 also protects murine-cytotoxic lymphocytes from glucocorticoid-induced DNA apoptosis. Glucocorticoids have a marked suppressive effect on the early stages of B-lymphocyte activation but do not seem to affect the proliferative response of activated B cells. In glucocorticoid-treated animals, the number of B lymphocytes in the spleen and lymph nodes is decreased, whereas those in the bone marrow are unaffected. Glucocorticoids enhance immunoglobulin secretion by human B cells in vitro, which was attributed to the selective inhibition of suppressor T-cell function in the system. Glucocorticoids potentiated the synergistic stimulatory effect of IL-1 and IL-6 on immunoglobulin production by activated B cells. Thymic hormones, IL-1, IL-2, and interferons all antagonize the inhibitory effects of glucocorticoids on lymphoid tissue.[10,14,132,135–137]

The inhibitory effect of glucorticoid on NK cells has been observed repeatedly. This inhibition is calcium dependent and can be abrogated by IFN-β.[138,139] Killer cells mediating antibody-dependent cellular cytotoxicity are also inhibited by glucocorticoids, which is potentiated by prostaglandin E_2 and abrogated by interferon or IL-2. Lymphokine-activated killer (LAK) cells, which destroy target cells similarly to NK cells, are suppressed by cortisone. Glucocorticoid treatment reduces the number of mast cells in both humans and animals. Immunologically triggered mediator release from mast cells and basophilic leukocytes is also inhibited. In mouse bone marrow mast cells dexamethasone down-regulated Fc-ε receptors and the IgE-dependent release of leukotrienes, whereas the release of prostaglandin D_2 was increased significantly. The chemotactic response of human eosinophils was also inhibited by glucocorticoids. Fc receptors, complement receptors, and chemotactic receptors were rendered nonfunctional, and β-adrenergic receptors in neutrophils were found to be uncoupled from adenylate cyclase by glucocorticoids.[10,14]

Systemic treatment with glucocorticoids is immunosuppressive in a variety of species including humans, mice, rats, guinea pigs, rabbits, chickens, lizards, and frogs. Immunoglobulin levels and humoral and cell-mediated immune reactions are depressed by chronic treatment. Immunological memory and the cells responsible for the induction of graft-versus-host reaction were not affected.[10]

The Pituitary-Gonadal Axis

Gonadotropins

Until recently it was believed that gonadotropins could modify immune reactions only through their effect on sex hormone production. However, it was found that luteinizing hormone (LH) significantly increases the proliferative response of murine lymphocytes to some mitogens and also stimulates the production of IL-1 and IL-2. Moreover, LH enhanced significantly the primary and secondary antibody response in BALB/c mice.[140] This finding opens the possibility that tropic pituitary hormones may have a direct modulatory effect on the immune system. It is also indicated by the direct effect of ACTH on lymphoid cells.

Treatment of mice with human chorionic gonadotropin (hCG) suppressed delayed-type hypersensitivity reactions and enhanced NK-cell activity, which were dependent on the presence of the gonads. In vitro treatment of murine lymphocytes led to the induction of suppressor cells. Several attempts in rats to modulate various immune reactions by treatment with hCG yielded negative results. Treatment of guinea pigs with 4000 IU of hCG i.p. 1–7 days prior to skin testing inhibited the development of delayed-type hypersensitivity skin responses for 3 weeks. Lymphocytes of hCG-treated guinea pigs showed depressed responses to PHA and purified protein derivative (PPD).[10]

Several investigators reported that the response of human peripheral blood lymphocytes to various mitogens was depressed by hCG, due to the generation of suppressor cells. The mixed lymphocyte reaction was also suppressed by hCG. A number of investigators pointed out, however, that commercial hCG preparations contain impurities that are responsible for these in vitro effects.[10] Therefore, the direct effect of hCG on lymphoid cells needs to be reexamined.

Sex Hormones

Estrogen and androgen receptors of high affinity and low capacity are present in the thymus and also in the bursa of Fabricius. Sex hormone receptors in mature lymphocytes are not detectable, with the exception of $CD8^+$ T cells that express well-defined receptors. Progesterone seems to affect immune function through glucocorticoid receptors, although the existence of specific receptors for this hormone in lymphoid tissue has also been proposed. Estrogens and androgens also have the capacity to combine with glucocorticoid receptors of lymphocytes and, at high concentrations, may affect their function through such receptors.[14,141–144]

Estradiol (E2) causes bone marrow deficiency and thymic involution, and inhibits various T-lymphocyte functions that include regulatory (helper and suppressor) and effector (killer and delayed hypersensitivity) T-cell mechanisms. NK cells, neutrophils, and mast cell degranulation are also inhibited by E2. However, phagocytosis, humoral immune reactions, and certain autoimmune diseases are enhanced in laboratory animals by E2.[141,143,145,146]

The development of the bursa of Fabricius can be prevented in chicken embryos by testosterone treatment. In general, androgens have a suppressive or moderating effect on immune reactions, and antagonize the enhancing effect of estrogens in a variety of animal autoimmune disease models. The hematopoietic effect of androgens is well established.[141,146,147]

Testosterone promotes the secretion of IgA and the synthesis of secretory component in the lacrimal gland. Estradiol, progesterone, and PRL stimulate the mammary gland for lactation, which leads to the migration of lymphoid cells to mammary tissue and the enhanced synthesis and secretion of IgA. Testosterone inhibits mammary immune function. Estradiol stimulates the secretion of immunoglobulin in the uterus. Progesterone antagonizes this function of E2 but promotes cervical and vaginal IgA secretion, in the latter case synergistically with E2.[148,113]

The mechanism by which sex hormones modulate the immune system is not clear. Grossman[142] suggested that sex hormones act on the thymus, possibly by the alteration of the thymic hormones, which in turn would influence lymphocyte reactivity. Testosterone was suggested to favor the maturation of suppressor T lymphocytes in the thymus.[146] Modification of bone marrow function[149] and direct action on lymphoid cells have also been proposed.[150] However, the stimulatory effect of estradiol on mononuclear phagocytes is well demonstrated, which allows direct influence on immune reactions through antigen-presenting cells.[151] Because these antigen-presenting cells secrete powerful soluble mediators such as IL-1 and TNF, the regulation of these cytokines by sex hormones would be expected to have important consequences. One may note in this context that E2 stimulates the release of PRL from the pituitary gland, which opens yet another pathway by which the immune system could be influenced by estrogens.

The Pituitary-Thyroid Axis

Thyroid Stimulating Hormone (TSH)

Human monocytes and NK cells express cell surface receptors for TSH, whereas similar receptors are barely detectable in human T and B lymphocytes. On the other hand, activated B lymphocytes and established human B-cell lines possess easily detectable receptors. The binding of TSH to T cells was not affected by activation. TSH did not have a stimulatory effect on lymphocytes, but increased moderately immunoglobulin secretion by activated B lymphocytes.[152,153] Human thyroid epithelial cells (thymocytes) express HLA class II molecules after exposure to IFN-γ, which is enhanced by TSH in vitro. Moreover, a proportion of thymocytes expressed MHC-II following treatment with TSH or dibutryl cyclic adenosine monophosphate (dibutryl CAMP) in the absence of IFN-γ, provided that some preexisting class II expression was present.[154]

Thyroid Hormones (Thyroxine or T_4; Triiodo-thyronine or T_3)

Nuclear receptors for T_3 have been detected in the IM-9 human B-cell lymphoma line, and for both T_3 and T_4 in human mononuclear blood cells.[155,156] Human peripheral blood lymphocytes have the ability to convert T_4 to T_3 which is the active form of the hormone. T_3 was reported to influence sodium exchange and glucose uptake by lymphoid cells. T_3 has a stimulatory effect on thymus growth and hormone production and was reported to promote erythroid burst forming colonies and B-cell maturation. The effect of thyroid hormones on lymphoproliferation and immune function remains controversial. Enhancement, suppression, or no effect was reported in various species in relation to mitogen-induced lymphoproliferation, antibody formation to a number of antigens, and for various forms of cell-mediated immunity that include graft rejection, delayed-type hypersensitivity reaction, and NK activity. In a number of experiments in which thyroid hormone deficiency was artificially created, immunodeficiency was also observed, which could be restored by treatment with T_3. On the other hand, supplemental treatment of normal animals often yielded negative results.[10,157-169]

Other Pituitary Hormones

Arginine Vasopressin (AVP)

Receptors for AVP of the V_1 type have been identified on human peripheral blood mononuclear cells and on mouse splenic lymphocytes. AVP stimulated the production of prostaglandin E_2 by human mononuclear phagocytes and enhanced proliferation in the autologous mixed lymphocyte culture. Recently, AVP was reported to stimulate the production of β-endorphin by human peripheral blood mononuclear cells. AVP is able to attenuate fever after central administration and thus may function as an antipyretic hormone.[10,170-175]

Other Hormones and Factors

An antiproliferative hormone called *suppressin* was isolated by LeBoeuf and coworkers[176,177] from bovine pituitaries. This polypeptide hormone had a molecular weight of 63 kd and inhibited mitogen-induced and IL-2-dependent lymphocyte proliferation. A pituitary factor isolated from bovine glands induced thymic epithelial cell proliferation in vitro. GH, PRL, ACTH, FSH, LH, TSH, AVP, and oxytocin were ineffective alone when used to stimulate thymic cell proliferation.[178]

Neurohormonal Immunoregulatory Mechanisms

Growth Control

We have proposed earlier that growth control is the principal mechanism by which the pituitary gland regulates immune function.[34] This theory was prompted by the profound immunodeficiency, rapid involution of the thymus and spleen, and grossly impaired DNA synthesis in the lymphoid tissues of rats after hypophysectomy, and by the remarkable ability of GH and PRL to restore immunocompetence and nucleic acid synthesis, and to stimulate growth in these organs. The following facts support this hypothesis: (1) The pituitary gland controls the growth of the entire organism and there is no immune response without lymphocyte growth;[178,180] (2) Normal immune reactivity in rats requires the presence of either GH or PRL; (3) The GH_3 pituitary tumor, which secretes GH and PRL, was shown to reverse age-related thymic involution and to increase immunocompetence in old rats;[181] (4) A proportion of myeloid and lymphoid tumors are pituitary dependent,[182,183] whereas in others the c-*myc* proto-oncogene is deregulated through translocation to the vicinity of promoters that are normally active in the cell type from which the tumor has originated.[184,185] The expression of the c-*myc* gene in the thymus and spleen is regulated by GH and PRL.[186] Therefore, one may argue that c-*myc* deregulation allows the tumor to escape from pituitary growth control; and (5) Transgenic mice, which possess deregulated c-*myc*, are characterized by general and uncontrolled proliferation of lymphoid cells in bone marrow, thymus, spleen, and lymph nodes, and by frequent occurrence of lymphoid malignancy.[187,188]

The above listed facts fit the *competence progression* model of cell proliferation. This theory states that a minumum of two hormones, one inducing competence in the cell but not mitogenic on its own, and the second stimulating growth, are required for the initiation of DNA synthesis and cell proliferation.[189] It was also suggested that competence hormones activate c-*myc*.[190,191] The competence hormone has the power of limiting the ability of the cell to respond to growth factors and to proliferate. Indeed, the proliferation rate of the Nb2 lymphoma is directly proportional to the concentration of lactogenic hormones present in the medium.[192] Moreover, these cells are able to respond to additional growth factors present in serum, but only in the presence of lactogenic hormones.[193,194]

Primary Lymphoid Tissue

The immune system may be divided into primary lymphoid organs (including the bone marrow, the bursa of Fabricius in birds, and the thymus), which produce the cells of the immune system, and secondary lymphoid organs (spleen, lymph nodes, tonsils, Peyer's patches), which are concerned with specific immune reactions. In mammals, the bone marrow produces all the formed elements of the blood (erythrocytes, platelets, neutrophilic, eosinophilic, and basophilic granulocytes, monocytes, and B lymphocytes) with the exception of T cells. T-lymphocyte precursors, which are also generated in the bone marrow, have to home to the thymus in order to finish their maturation into functional T cells. Similarly in birds, T-cell precursors migrate into the thymus, and B-cell precursors home to the bursa of Fabricius where they differentiate into functional B lymphocytes.[195]

The primary lymphoid organs are characterized by continuous cell proliferation, which is easily demonstrated in vitro by overnight pulsing with radioactive nucleotide precursors.[34,38] Cell proliferation in the bone marrow is regulated by the sequential action of hormones, granulocyte-macrophage colony-stimulating factor (GM-CSF), and IL-3-stimulating stem cells and immature precursors, whereas erythropoietin, granulocyte colony-stimulating factor (G-CSF), and macrophage colony-stimulating factor (M-CSF) act on committed precursor cells and on mature leukocytes. The thymus and bursa also have hormonal factors that regulate cell proliferation and maturation.[196-200] Recent studies revealed that in the thymus the recognition of MHC class I and class II self-antigens by antigen receptors of maturing thymocytes provides a major proliferative stimulus. Apparently, cells that react strongly to MHC self-antigen components are eliminated in situ through apoptosis. Current findings also suggest that T-cell precursors that are not stimulated in the thymus by MHC self-antigens will never mature. Therefore, T-cell precursors that are stimulated moderately by MHC self-antigens ('self-recognition') will reach a stage of full differentiation in the thymus and will be released to the periphery.[201,202]

During hematopoiesis, there is a hierarchy of growth factors that act sequentially during the proliferation, commitment, and differentiation of hematopoietic stem cells into various effector cells.[197,199,200] The existence of synergistic or permissive growth factors has also been indicated.[203] Such synergistic factors are believed to be nonmitogenic on their own, but capable of potentiating the effect of other growth factors during cell division.

The observation that cell proliferation in bone marrow and thymus is dependent on growth and lactogenic hormones suggests that PRL and GH may function directly, as *competence hormones* on primary lymphoid tissue. Alternatively, it is possible that these hormones indirectly control the production of growth factors (i.e., colony-stimulating factors and thymic hormones) that are necessary for proliferation, or both mechanisms may be operative, which would be analogous to current ideas of GH action. GH is now believed to act on its targets directly and indirectly through IGF-1. PRL also generates intermediate hormones called synlactins. Both PRL and GH have already been shown to induce thymic hormones.[204-207] Some thymic factors stimulate LH, PRL, and GH release from pituitary cells in vitro,[208] whereas others inhibit the release of TSH and GH.[209] G-CSF has been demonstrated to release ACTH from human pituitary corticotroph adenomas.[210] These findings indicate the existence of feedback interaction between primary lymphoid tissue and the pituitary gland (Table 6.1).

Secondary Lymphoid Tissue

The function of the secondary lymphoid organs is to mount specific immune reactions. This is often referred to in the literature as antigen-driven differentiation, in contrast to *antigen-independent differentiation* in the primary lymphoid organs. According to current understanding, partially digested (processed) antigen associated with surface MHC molecules is presented by cells of the monocyte macrophage series or by some related cell types (antigen-presenting cells) to antigen-sensitive clones of T lymphocytes of the helper subset. In addition, B-cells may also present antigen fragments to T-cells. Antigen-presenting cells also secrete IL-1, which is necessary to trigger helper cells to secrete IL-2 and other varieties of interleukins. Immature precursors of T and B lymphocytes that express surface receptors capable of recognizing the antigen (antigen-specific clones) are then driven into the proliferation process by the combined action of MHC-antigen complex and interleukins that act as growth factors. At some point, this antigen-driven clonal proliferation of lymphoid cells is terminated by differentiation into effector cells, which results in the production of killer, delayed-type hypersenstive, and regulatory (e.g., helper or suppressor) T lymphocytes. B lymphocytes mature into cells secreting IgM initially and may switch to the production of other immunoglobulin classes in the later stage of development.[195,211,212]

That lymphocytes require at least two signals for activation was proposed first by Bretscher and Cohn.[213] In essence, this theory is analogous to the competence-progression model of cell proliferation. One may suggest that, here, antigen acts as a competence factor, preparing the cells for proliferation, as well as inducing the production of growth factors. Current evidence indicates that PRL and GH are necessary for primary immune reaction and that the ACTH-adrenal axis exerts a powerful suppressive influence. However, the secondary immune response is less dependent on pituitary hormones.[24] Several mechanisms may be envisaged with regard to the influence of pituitary hormones on antigen-driven differentiation. First, it is possible that GH and PRL affect antigen presentation, since both hormones influence macrophage function. Alternatively, it is possible that PRL and GH govern lymphocyte proliferation up to a certain stage during the primary response, which leads to the production of antigen-sensitive memory cells. Such memory cells

TABLE 6.1. Lymphoid and inflammatory feedback signals toward the pituitary gland.

Species	Mediator	Target	Biological effect	Reference
Rat	Thymosin	HYP	Stimulation of GnRH and LH release	311
Rat	Thymopoietin Thymopentin	PIT	ACTH, β-END release	312
Rat	Thymosin-α1	HYP	Inhibition of ACTH, TSH, PRL release	313
		PIT	Release of TSH, ACTH, LH	
Rat	MB-35	PIT	GH, PRL release	314
Human	Thymosin-5	PITA	ACTH release	210
Human	G-CSF	PITA	ACTH release	210
Rat	IL-1α,β	HYP	ACTH, GnRH and IL-6 release; inhibition of LH release	217, 220, 315–319 241, 320
Rat	IL-1α,β	PIT	ACTH, GH, LH, TSH release; inhibition of PRL release; IL-6 induction	321 322
Mouse	IL-1α,β	PITA	ACTH and β-END release	249, 323, 324
Human	IL-1β	PITA	ACTH release	210
Rat, mouse	IL-2	PIT	Inhibition of GH, LH, FSH release; PRL, ACTH, TSH release	325, 326
Human	IL-2	?	ACTH, β-END, GH, PRL release	327, 328
Mouse	IL-6	PITA	ACTH and β-END release	249, 323
Rat	IL-6	HYP	ACTH release; inhibition of TSH release	329, 330
		PIT	Inhibition of ACTH release	
Rat	IFN-γ	HYP	ACTH release; inhibition of GH, TSH release	330–333
		PIT	Inhibition of ACTH, PRL, GH release;	330–333
			Increased release of ACTH, LH, FSH, GH, PRL; inhibition of ACTH production	334, 335
Human	IFN-α	?	ACTH, GH release	336, 337
Human	IFN-γ	PITA	ACTH release	210
Rat	TNF-α	HYP	ACTH, GnRH, IL-6 release	247, 315, 319, 338
Calf	TNF-α	PIT	Blocking of GH release	341
Rat	TGF-β1	PIT	Inhibition of basal PRL secretion and TSH mediated PRL release; stimulation of basal GH secretion	339
Rat	TGF-β	PITA	Inhibition of PRL gene expression	340
Rat	PAF	HYP	ACTH release; β-END release	342–344
		PIT	GH, PRL release	
Rat	PDGF	PITA	Decrease of PRL production	345
Rat	Bradykinin	PIT	PRL release	346, 347
Rat	histamine	HYP	ACTH, β-END, PRL release	348, 349
Rat	H₂-histamine agonists	Brain	PRL release	350

ACTH, adrenocorticotropic hormone; END, endorphin; G-CSF, granulocyte colony-stimulating factor; GH, growth hormone; GnRH, gonadotropin-releasing hormone; HYP, hypothalamus; IFN, interferon; IL, interleukin; LH, luteinizing hormone; PAF, platelet-activating factor; PDGF, platelet-derived growth factor; PIT, pituitary; PITA, pituitary adenoma; PRL, prolactin; TNF, tumor necrosis factor; TSH, thyroid-stimulating hormone.

are able to respond to antigen as a competence signal by proliferation through the autocrine secretion of IL-2,[214] and may not respond to GH or PRL. Memory cells are also glucocorticoid resistant. On exposure of memory cells to antigen, IL production is initiated, which in turn stimulates the proliferation of immature antigen-sensitive cells (PRL- or GH-dependent) as well as the proliferation of the memory cells. The observation that cytotoxic T lymphocytes can be maintained in the state of continuous proliferation either in vitro or in vivo for long periods of time by stimulation with IL-2, if activated first by antigen, fully supports this assumption.[212,215]

There is indication that immune reactions are capable of stimulating PRL release from the pituitary gland, whereas excessive immune inflammatory events are known to lead to growth retardation. It is well established that the level of glucocorticoids rises gradually during immune reactions, due to the stimulation of ACTH release by IL-1 and possibly by some other cytokines[10,216–220] (Table 6.1). These observations indicate that both the stimulatory (PRL and GH) and inhibitory (ACTH-adrenal axis) pituitary regulatory pathways interact dynamically with the immune system. This regulation is superimposed on the elaborate internal regulatory circuits of the immune system.[195] The function of the pituitary gland may be viewed as one of setting upper and lower thresholds for immune activity within which the immune system is allowed to operate in a compatible manner to maintain the homeostasis and harmony of the organism.

Regulation of Effector Immune Mechanisms

Effector T lymphocytes recirculate, migrate to the sites of antigen deposits, initiate inflammation (delayed hypersensitivity), and exert cytotoxicity. Antibodies can also initiate inflammation by complexing with the antigen, which in turn activates the complement system and triggers polymorphonuclear and mononuclear phagocytes for phagocytosis or cell-mediated cytotoxicity. IgE antibodies mediate the degranulation of basophilic leukocytes and mast cells. Some of these reactions, especially those that involve basophil and mast cell degranulation, may develop rapidly into allergic reactions and lead to life-threatening situations.[195]

Current evidence suggests that adrenergic, cholinergic, and sensory nerves are all involved in the regulation of allergic reactions. This regulatory mechanism permits fast local intervention, which is required in such situations. Glucocorticoids, which are potent antiinflammatory agents, also play a role in the regulation of these reactions.[132]

The influence of GH and PRL on mature antigen-presenting cells (superoxide production, IL-1, and TNF-α induction) and on mature T cells (IL-2 and IFN-γ production) suggests that these hormones also play a role in the function of effector cells. It is unknown whether these effects coincide with a proliferative stimulus. Similar observations were made with regard to some of the hematopoietic growth factors (G-CSF, M-CSF, GM-CSF), which support the maturation and also the function of phagocytic cells. Thus, GM-CSF 'primes' neutrophils so that they will be hyperresponsive to a second stimulus, such as chemotactic agents, complement split products, or arachidonate metabolites. Such primed neutrophils respond with enhanced oxidative burst, membrane depolarization, and phagocytosis, which prepares them for maximum antibacterial response. GM-CSF also enhances the cytotoxic, phagocytic, and bactericidal activity of monocytes and macrophages, promotes the proliferation of tissue macrophages, potentiates the production of IL-1, TNF-α, and prostaglandin E_2 when a costimulator is used, and enhances antigen presentation. Epidermal Langerhans' cells mature into dendritic cells in the presence of GM-CSF, which is enhanced by IL-1.[221]

The Role of Shared Mediators

A number of mediators, which include ACTH, bombesin, corticotropin-releasing factor (CRF), endorphins, methionine enkephalin, chorionic gonadotropin, GH, growth hormone releasing hormone (GHRH), IL-1, IL-3, LH, luteinizing hormone-releasing hormone (LHRH), neurophysins, oxytocin, PRL, somatostatin (SRIH), substance P, TSH, vasoactive intestinal peptide (VIP), and AVP, have been found to be common to the nervous and immune systems by immunoassay, high-performance liquid chromatography, electrophoresis, or bioassay. The homology of mRNA and/or amino acid sequence identity has also been established for ACTH, β-endorphin, GH, and VIP.[14,222-228]

These findings have been cited as evidence for regulatory interaction between the nervous and immune systems.[229] However, other organs and tissues also share at least some of these mediators; IL-1 has been detected in the skin and in blood vessels, for instance.[230,231] For this reason, substances earlier named interleukins or lymphokines are now preferentially called cytokines, indicating that they are not restricted to the immune system.[211] Hematopoietic growth factors, interferons, leukotrienes, and prostaglandins are all mediators of the immune system and are shared with other tissues. Moreover, the production of some 28 neuropeptides has been described to date in the anterior pituitary gland, and specific receptors could also be identified for many within the gland. Because these peptides are synthesized in small quantities, they are also called 'minority' peptides, and an autocrine/paracrine role has been suggested for them.[232] Apparently interleukins are no exception, as the production of IL-6 by the pituitary gland has also been described.[233,234] The brain also produces several interleukins, and neurotransmitter function has been suggested for the locally produced cytokines.[235] A number of neuropeptides and their specific receptors also exist within the thymus.[236]

The observation that CRF, which could be produced within the immune system, stimulates the release of lymphocyte-derived ACTH and β-endorphin[237] supports the assumption that a significant proportion of the shared mediators are in fact involved in local regulation in both the neuroendocrine and immune systems. Others may have both local and intersystem regulatory functions, as was shown already for IL-1 and for a number of other cytokines, as well as for ACTH, LH, and TSH. The shared substances with local function may simply represent gene economy, by which the same mediator is utilized to transmit regulatory signals in various organs and tissues that are not necessarily identical.[238]

In certain situations, such as pregnancy, wound healing, tissue regeneration, etc., there is an urgent need for local enhancement of growth that may be mediated, at least in part, by locally generated and shared growth regulatory hormones. Immune reactions represent an analogous situation. Placental hormones, many of which are identical or similar to pituitary hormones, growth factors released at the site of injury by platelets and macrophages, and the rapid generation of growth regulatory substances within the immune system fulfill this need.[75,239] In addition, there is evidence to indicate a role for lymphocyte-derived growth factors in the development of the mammalian embryo, in tissue regeneration in general, and even in the stimulation of tumor growth.[240] Nevertheless, there is strong evidence to indicate that both the initiation of pregnancy and immunocompetence are dependent on pituitary function in spite of the ectopic hormone production. Much remains to be done for the elucidation of the exact role(s) of shared mediators.

The Systemic Immunoregulatory Network

By now it is clear that immune-derived mediators interact with all tissues and organs in the body. Thus, IL-1 induces fever, releases ACTH and possibly other pituitary hormones, antagonizes opioid receptors in the brain, promotes slow-wave sleep, decreases appetite, stimulates acute-phase proteins in the liver, promotes proteolysis in muscle, inhibits thyroglobulin gene expression, stimulates thyroid growth, stimulates insulin release (though in high doses the effect is inhibitory), inhibits steroid synthesis by the gonads and the adrenals, and stimulates bone resorption.[14,230,241,242] IL-1 infused into the lateral cerebral ventricle of rats led to the rapid suppression, within 15 minutes, of natural killer cytotoxicity and the response to PHA and IL-2 production by blood and spleen lymphocytes. This suppression was also present in adrenalectomized animals and could be antagonized by the local administration of α-MSH.[122] The intracerebro-ventricular administration of IL-1β to mice inhibited the production of IL-1 by splenic macrophages. This suppressive effect could be eliminated either by adrenalectomy or splenic denervation, which suggests that both the hypothalamic-pituitary-adrenal axis and the sympathetic nervous system are involved in the IL-1-induced immunosuppression.[243]

TNF (cachectin) has many overlapping functions with IL-1, including pyrogenicity, promotion of slow-wave sleep, a strong catabolic effect, release of ACTH, T- and B-cell activation, and stimulation of bone resorption. Neutrophils, eosinophils, and macrophages are also activated by TNF. In addition, TNF is cytotoxic for certain tumors and other targets by the activation of the suicide pathway, and causes inflammation, hemorrhage, and shock if produced in excess. TNF plays a major role in the multiple endocrine and metabolic changes associated with trauma and sepsis. IL-1 and TNF inhibit the β-adrenergic responsiveness of cardiac myocytes.[244-247]

IL-6 (hepatocyte-stimulating factor) is emerging as a proinflammatory cytokine, and it plays a major role in the initiation of the acute-phase response. In addition, IL-6 also released ACTH from mouse pituitary tumor cells.[248,249] Other substances of importance are the interferons produced in the immune system (INF-γ) and in many other tissues and organs (INF-α and INF-β). Interferons are known for their antiviral, antiproliferative, and immunoregulatory actions, but they also affect cell metabolism, stimulate adrenal steroidogenesis, and inhibit steroidogenesis in Leydig cells, as well as influence insulin and thyroid hormone secretion.[250-256]

Evidence of the influence on the immune system of nearly all the classical hormones, endocrine organs, and some other tissues and cells exists and has been reviewed elsewhere.[257] The neurohormonal system receives signals that are initiated both within as wells as from outside the body, and which lead to adaptive responses in hormonal secretions. By now it is clear that the endocrine changes associated with stressful stimuli do, in fact, modulate the immune system.[258] The presence of receptors on lymphocytes for numerous hormones and neurotransmitters indicates that the immune system is capable of receiving signals from many organs and tissues in the body. Shared mediators facilitate this multidirectional interaction, and therefore, one may suggest that immune function is the result of a network of signals that acts simultaneously on the immune system. Order is maintained by the hierarchy and sequential nature of signals, which may be classified as primary, secondary, or tertiary regulators. Any signal that is capable of inducing competence for lymphocyte proliferation (e.g., GH, PRL, antigen) is categorized as a *primary regulator*. The factors that govern cell proliferation and differentiation are *secondary regulators* that can act only after the delivery of the primary signal. Many of these factors show some target specificity (e.g., G-CSF, M-CSF, interleukins). Primary and secondary regulators govern the function of genes that are involved in cell proliferation and differentiation. Finally, the function of fully differentiated immune effector cells is ruled by *tertiary regulators*. These functions include secretion, locomotion (chemotaxis), phagocytosis, cytotoxicity, and the like. Neurotransmitters appear to be potent regulators of these processes.

Possible Relevance to Disease

Autoimmunity

In healthy individuals, autoantibodies are commonly demonstrated and autoimmune disease can readily be induced in various laboratory animal models by deliberate immunization. This indicates the presence of potentially autoreactive lymphocyte clones in healthy hosts. That disease does not develop is the result of various immunosuppressive regulatory mechanisms that are able to keep these clones in a dormant state.[259] As already discussed, self-tolerance of T lymphocytes is established in the thymus, but whether a similar selection of B lymphocytes is taking place in the bone marrow is unknown. It is also clear from the evidence presented in this review that GH and PRL are thymotropic whereas glucocorticoids are thymolytic. Furthermore, sex hormones also affect thymus function. On the basis of this information, one may predict that endocrine alterations may lead to disturbance of thymus function. Because these hormones also influence mature lymphoid tissue, immunoregulatory cells and mechanisms may be affected by them during autoaggression.

A severe autoimmune condition called autologous graft-versus-host disease can be induced in rats by lethal irradiation, syngenic or autologous bone marrow reconstitution, and CSA treatment. Apparently, during regeneration CSA interferes with thymocyte selection so that clones with strong autoreactivity are released to the periphery rather than committed to the suicide pathway. Once these clones are relieved of drug inhibition, a serious autoimmune condition evolves.[260] Although the exact mechanism of erroneous T-cell maturation has not been elucidated, one may suggest that these T cells could mature in the thymus because their autoreactivity was moderate (e.g., self-recognition) under the influence of CSA. As pointed out earlier, CSA interferes with PRL binding to lymphoid cells. Therefore, it is conceivable that PRL deficiency could also lead to autoimmune disease according to a similar mechanism. Indeed, we found that patients with rheumatoid arthritis are deficient in circulating PRL.[193] This is the first disease to be associated with PRL deficiency. GH and IGF-1 deficiency has also been observed in juvenile rheumatoid arthritis.[261,262] Hyperprolactinemia has been detected in association with several autoimmune conditions in humans, including autoimmune hypophysitis,[263] autoimmune thyroid disease,[264] Addison's disease,[265] endogenous iridocyclitis,[266] and systemic lupus erythematosus (SLE) in men.[267]

A malfunction of the ACTH-adrenal axis can also lead to autoimmune disease. This possibility is illustrated by the finding that the obese strain of chickens, which develop spontaneous autoimmune thyroid disease, do not respond to immunization with elevated levels of glucocorticoid.[268] Additionally, in adrenalectomized rats, the development of severe experimental autoimmune encephalomyelitis may lead to death.[10,269] Inbred Lewis rats had a markedly impaired ACTH and glucocorticoid response to group A streptococcal cell wall peptidoglycan polysaccharide, and they developed arthritis which was similar to rheumatoid arthritis. Histocompatible Fisher rats exhibited normal ACTH and glucocorticoid responses to the same stimulus and did not develop arthritis. Accordingly defective corticotropin-releasing hormone production by hypothalamic neurons was found to be the underlying abnormality responsible for the development of disease in Lewis rats.[270,271]

Women are more prone to autoimmune disease than are men, and the male–female ratio for SLE is approximately 1:10, which makes SLE a predominantly female disease. Observations on inbred strains of mice that are prone to develop an SLE-like syndrome also show that this condition develops earlier and the course of the disease is more serious in female animals. Oophorectomy inhibits the development of auto-immunity, which can be reversed by estradiol treatment. Moreover, estradiol accelerates the development of SLE syndrome in castrated male animals, while treatment with testosterone antagonizes the disease-promoting effect of estradiol. Prolactin also has an influence on the SLE-like disease of mice. Several observations on patients of both sexes with SLE showed that this condition is associated with androgen deficiency and elevated PRL serum levels, especially in males.[145,146,267,272–277] Auto-immune reactions against neuroendocrine organs and the central nervous system are also fairly common. Here, one can envisage a vicious circle in which the initial abnormality (neuroendocrine or immunological) may cause additional abnormalities (endocrine or immunological) that can greatly aggravate the disease process.[278–281]

Allergy and Asthma

Although recently the immunological etiology of allergy and asthma has been receiving much attention, it is clear that identical symptoms can be elicited by chemical or physical stimuli.[282] A β-adrenergic theory of allergy and bronchial asthma has been developed by Szentivanyi,[283] who proposed that asthma is not an immunological disease but, rather, a unique pattern of bronchial hypersensitivity to a broad spectrum of stimuli that include immune reactions, cyclic infections, and chemical and physical irritations. The development of disease is due to the reduced function of the β-adrenergic system. Neurogenic and myogenic theories and, more recently, the inflammatory augmentation of airway reactivity have been proposed for the pathogenesis of asthma.[282] Given the recent evidence that substance P and other neuropeptides are potent regulators of inflammation and that these peptides are also involved in allergic reactions,[284] one may now propose that neurogenic inflammatory mechanisms play an important role in the etiology of allergy and asthma. A role for neurogenic inflammation has also been suggested in the pathogenesis of symmetrical arthritis.[285] Nevertheless, the efficiency of glucocorticoid therapy points to the role of hormonal regulatory factors in these diseases.

Infection

Trauma and sepsis are typically associated with fever, changes in serum hormone levels (ACTH, endorphins, glucocorticoids, catecholamines, PRL, GH, AVP, insulin, glucagon, and thyroid hormones), insulin resistance, and the synthesis of acute-phase proteins by the liver.[248,286–289] Many of these changes are induced by immune-derived mediators, primarily IL-1, IL-6, and TNF, as outlined earlier. The effect of hormones on host resistance to infectious agents has been reviewed.[257] Although it is clear that hormones affect host resistance, the exact pathophysiological significance of the massive neuroendocrine and metabolic changes during infection remains to be elucidated.

Many pathogenic microorganisms have the capacity to activate lymphocytes polyclonally.[290] A massive activation of the immune system poses dangers because of the autoimmune dormant reaction by clones, and the toxicity of lymphokines produced in large amounts.[291–293] Excess production of TNF is responsible for many of the pathological changes in endotoxin (LPS) shock and murine cerebral malaria.[244,294] However, it is clear that TNF, at lower concentrations, has beneficial effects on endotoxin shock and infections.[295,296]

The sensitivity of adrenalectomized mice to LPS was increased 3–400 times. We observed that 2 h after toxin treatment, serum TNF levels were 40–60 times higher in adrenalectomized mice than in controls. There was a glucocorticoid response to LPS injection in intact animals, and the development of high TNF levels could be inhibited by glucocorticoid treatment in adrenalectomized mice, also protecting them from the lethal effect of LPS. The sensitivity to LPS of mice treated with metyrapone, which inhibits glucocorticoid biosynthesis in the adrenal glands, was also greatly increased. In addition, plasma PRL was increased significantly 1 h after LPS injection but returned promptly to basal levels in both intact and adrenalectomized mice.[297] Finally, similar observations have also been made by other investigators.[298,299] There is evidence to indicate that under the influence of glucocorticoids, T lymphocytes and macrophages secrete factors permitting lymphocyte activation, as outlined earlier. This may be an important mechanism to counteract the immunosuppressive effect of polyclonal lymphocyte activators or any other stimuli that activate the ACTH-adrenal axis.

It is intriguing to note that trauma elicits a neuroendocrine and metabolic response that is very similar to that of infection.[286] A possible mechanism for the induction of this endocrine response is that under traumatic conditions LPS absorbs from the intestinal tract[300] and stimulates the release of TNF and other immune-derived mediators, which in turn initiate the response. However, it is also possible that the response is initiated by substances released from damaged tissues. Platelet-activating factor, platelet-derived growth factor, bradykinin, and histamine, which are commonly associated with trauma and inflammation, are all capable of influencing pituitary hormone secretion (Table 6.1). Neurogenic or stress-induced hormonal alterations are likely to contribute to the development of systemic reaction to trauma.

Anemia

There are anemias of unknown etiology that are refractory to any treatment, and the anemia associated with chronic disease belongs to this group. Recently we studied serum PRL levels in rheumatoid arthritis patients with anemia and found that PRL bioactivity was higher in anemic patients who also had reticulocytosis, whereas in anemic patients without reticulocytosis there was a significantly lower level of PRL when compared to nonanemic rheumatoid patients. Thus, there was a direct correlation between reticulocytosis and PRL bioactivity.[301] This is fully compatible with our findings in animals that bone marrow function is pituitary dependent and that GH or PRL is required for maintenance of hematopoiesis.[38]

Cancer

A number of tumors secrete hormones and growth factors that could influence immune function. Tumors are also known to express embryonic antigens and, according to recent findings in reproduction biology, such antigens can stimulate the production of lymphocyte-derived growth factors that would facilitate tumor growth.[240] Cancer patients frequently develop severe cachexia, which is caused by the excess production of cachectin or TNF.[302] Just why such a massive amount of TNF is produced in cancer patients in at present not understood. Certainly, immunological induction is a possible mechanism[303] while infection could be another explanation. Breakdown products released from necrotizing tumor masses and perhaps also from other tissues damaged by tumor growth may also be involved, since this might act to stimulate macrophages to release TNF.

Reproduction

The mammalian conceptus is the equivalent of an allograft, since paternal histocompatibility antigens are expressed by fetal tissues. Nonetheless, the fetus is not rejected. On the contrary, genetic disparity between parents has long been recognized as a desirable situation for reproduction (hybrid vigor). Recent observations suggest that immune-derived growth factors may, in fact, be necessary for optimal mammalian reproduction.[240,304]

Discussion

There is a dynamic regulatory interaction between the neuroendocrine and immune systems that elicits functional consequences for both. The major immunoregulatory hormones and feedback regulatory signals are illustrated in Figure 6.1, and a list of possible feedback signals has been provided in Table 6.1. These would suggest that PRL and GH maintain both the primary and secondary lymphoid tissues, and thus may be designated as the *hormones of immunocompetence*. Because a complete deficiency of GH and PRL has never been fully documented, this would suggest that such mutations are lethal. However, the lymphoid organs develop normally in utero in the absence of the hypophysis or, indeed, in the absence of much of the central nervous system.[305] Apparently, placental hormones fulfill the role of regulating lymphoid development at this stage. After birth, the pituitary gland takes over the role of placental hormones. GH is assumed to be more prevalent in growing animals and children, whereas PRL would be expected to have increasing lymphoregulatory power in adults and at the later stages of life. The function of the ACTH-adrenal axis is to suppress lymphoid tissue and to antagonize excess stimulation. It is now believed that the pituitary gland maintains lymphoid homeostasis thorugh its stimulatory (GH, PRL) and suppressor (ACTH-adrenal axis) hormones. Certainly, if defects occur in this primary regulatory circuit, this may lead to serious consequences for the individual and result in premature death. Sex hormones are regarded as immunomodulators, mainly because they are not essential for the maintenance of immune function. One may suggest that many of the effects attributable to sex hormones would be to act on immune function and this, in turn, promote successful reproduction.

The competence progression model for cell proliferation is suggested as a likely mechanism for the regulation of lymphoid tissue by pituitary hormones. It is envisioned that growth and lactogenic hormones induce competence for cell division in lymphoid cells. In addition, these hormones also stimulate a variety of growth factors that are necessary for cell proliferation. Some, such as insulin-like growth factor, act on a wide

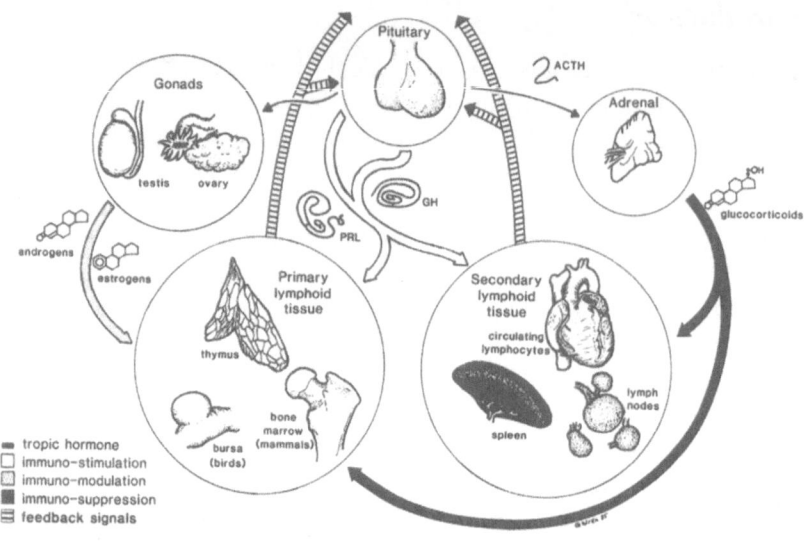

FIGURE 6.1. Immunoregulation by pituitary hormones. Prolactin (PRL) and growth hormone (GH) stimulate lymphoproliferation in both primary and secondary lymphoid organs and maintain immunocompetence. The ACTH-adrenal axis has an inhibitory effect on both kinds of lymphoid tissue. Feedback regulatory signals (Table 6.1) are emitted by both the primary and secondary lymphoid tissues toward the pituitary gland and the hypothalamus, which in turn influence pituitary hormone release and some other functions of the central nervous system. This regulatory circuit is vital for the maintenance of immune homeostasis. The profound endocrine and metabolic changes characteristic of infection, inflammation, and trauma are due, at least in part, to the effect of immune-derived mediators on the neuroendocrine system and on some other ogans and tissues. Sex hormones are designated as immunomodulators, since they are not indispensable for immune function, although sex hormones have a significant influence on immunity, mainly in the interest of reproduction. In addition to the hormones shown in the figure, numerous other hormones, neurotransmitters, and growth and differentiation factors participate in the regulation of the immune system. A hierarchy and sequential order of these regulatory signals exists, and according to their importance and order of action, the signals may be classified as primary, secondary, or tertiary regulators, as explained in the text. (From Berczi, 'Neurohormonal immunoregulation.' *Endocrine Pathology, Volume 1, Number 4*. December 1990, p. 210. Reprinted by permission of Blackwell Scientific Publications, Inc.)

variety of target cells, whereas others that may be induced, such as colony-stimulating factors, interleukins, and the like, act more specifically on cells at various stages of development. The hierarchy and sequential action of growth regulatory hormones is an important mechanism for the regulation of cell proliferation and differentiation within lymphoid tissues.

The levels of these factors may set the rate of cell growth, as exemplified by the Nb2 lymphoma proliferation assay for lactogenic hormones. Apparently, cells will die in the absence of growth-promoting stimuli, as revealed by studies on hematopoiesis in vitro.[200] In this context, it is interesting to note that the activation of the suicide pathway in lymphoid cells by glucocorticoids can successfully be antagonized by growth factors.[10,137] Hence, it is possible that an important feature of thymic selection is the precise regulation of the availability of growth factors. If this is altered (by CSA, for instance), autoimmune disease may result.

For the activation of mature lymphoid cells, two pathways are envisioned: one is neuroendocrine and the other immunological. It is suggested that during antigen-driven differentiation, the cell may gradually gain independence from hormonal regulation and come under the influence of antigen as a primary regulator (memory cells). The exact relationship between these two pathways remains to be elucidated. However, current views imply that normally mature lymphocytes are in a state of inhibition, and thus remain dormant.[306] Our observation that there is spontaneous DNA synthesis in the spleen of normal rats would suggest that continuous cell division is taking place in secondary lymphoid tissue, and this process is under the control of GH or PRL. Hence, GH and PRL are likely to maintain mature lymphoid cells in the absence of antigenic stimulation.

The observation that single molecules such as plant lectins or hematopoietic growth factors are capable of inducing cell proliferation, in some cases even when chemically defined medium is used, seems to contradict the competence progression model. Since lymphoid cells are heterogeneous, it is possible that the growth factors necessary for cell proliferation are induced by the lectin from mature cells, which in turn could exert an autocrine or paracrine function. Stimulation of more than one receptor by the same lectin is also conceivable. Alternatively, growth factors may be available from the medium if serum is applied, or some of the cells investigated may have undergone neoplastic changes and thus would not require as many growth factors as normal cells. Finally, it is possible that the cells have already acquired competence prior to experimentation or, indeed, they are able to respond to a single factor with proliferation. These possibilities should be investigated.

The regulation of inflammation by hormones and neuropeptides is firmly established, and abnormalities of this regulatory system may lead to disease. The variable effect of a number of hormones, neurotransmitters, and neuropeptides on immune reactions may be due to the fact that these agents have the ability to modulate the second messenger pathways of various lymphocyte signals. For instance, catecholamines regulate cAMP and intracellular calcium.[307,308] In lymphocytes, these pathways are influenced by numerous other signals that are hormone- or antigen-initiated and thus, ultimately, the status quo (e.g., cAMP or calcium level) of the cell will determine whether a particular neurotransmitter will have an effect and in which direction. Receptor heterogeneity and the fact that various lymphocyte-activating signals may travel on different second messenger pathways add further opporunities for variation of the responses.[309,310] Nevertheless, this signal-amplifying or signal-inhibiting function of certain hormones and neurotransmitters may fulfill important regulatory functions.

Finally, the reader must be reminded that most, if not all, hormones and neurotransmitters that influence the immune system can do so in more than one way. Thus, the primary lymphoid tissues and mature lymphoid cells and their subsets may be affected by the same mediator. Some hormones induce secondary factors, which in turn affect lymphoid function. This may be one reason why the effect of GH and PRL on lymphocyte reactions is difficult to demonstrate in vitro, whereas the in vivo effect is very reproducible. Some hormones and neuropeptides may act on the endocrine system or on the central nervous system, which in turn alters immune function. On the other hand, the immune system affects the function of the neuroendocrine system, and through neuroendocrine alterations (but also by direct action) interacts with other tissues and organs. In addition to defending the body against infectious and other noxious agents, the immune system may fulfill a number of other important functions that may include promotion of embryonic growth, regeneration, would healing, and bone remodeling. Thus, immunocytes may be regarded as mobile endocrine cells promoting growth, regeneration, and the like, locally whenever needed. In pathological situations (e.g., severe infection, inflammation, trauma), a systemic endocrine and metabolic response is initiated by various mediators, many of which are derived from the immune system, during which novel proteins appear in the serum and catabolism prevails. This may lead to cachexia and growth retardation if the illness is prolonged. The details and the pathophysiological significance of these changes are to be elucidated.

During the short history of this field, which Ader[8] called *psychoneuroimmunology*, many exciting new findings and concepts have emerged. One can be sure that this is only the beginning and that much more is to come. These truly multidisciplinary observations not only have advanced our knowledge and understanding, but also have given a new perspective to biomedical sciences (i.e., to view phenomena in relation to the complexity óf the organism).

Conclusions

The immune system may be divided into primary lymphoid organs (bone marrow, bursa of Fabricius, and thymus), which produce mature leukocytes, and secondary organs (spleen, lymph nodes, tonsils, Peyer's patches, etc.), which are concerned with specific immune responses. In the primary organs, stem cells proliferate and differentiate into various subsets of polymorphonuclear and mononuclear cells. Evidence is increasing that cell proliferation in the primary lymphoid organs is dependent on pituitary growth hormone (GH) and prolactin (PRL), which control the expression of growth regulatory genes (protooncogenes) such as c-*myc*, and also induce essential growth factors (insulin-like growth factor, thymic and bursal hormones, etc.) and, possibly, their receptors. The adrenocorticotropic hormone-adrenal axis serves as an inhibitory pathway, antagonizing the action of PRL and GH on primary lymphoid tissue. The effect of glucocorticoids is especially forceful on thymocytes through the activation of the genetically programmed suicide pathway. Sex hormones also regulate the primary lymphoid organs, but their mechanism of action remains to be clarified. Thymus-derived feedback signals toward the pituitary gland have already been described. The pituitary gland exerts a similar regulatory influence on mature lymphocytes during their antigen-driven differentiation. PRL or GH is required for primary immune reactions; however, the secondary immune response may be less dependent on these hormones. Once the immune system is primed, antigen itself becomes a primary regulator. Exposure of memory cells to antigen leads to the production of growth factors (interleukins) and to the expression of their receptors. Therefore, at this stage antigen appears to fulfill a role that is originally played by GH or PRL in the primary lymphoid organs and, to some extent, also during antigen-driven differentiation. During immune reactions, interleukin-1 and tumor necrosis factor activate the adrenocorticotropic hormone-adrenal axis, which plays an important role in setting upper limits to and terminating responses. Lymphocytes have receptors for, and react to, numerous hormones, neurotransmitters, and mediators derived from a number of organs and tissues. Therefore, ultimately, the reaction of a lymphocyte will be the vector of all positive and negative signals received. A hierarchy and sequential system of signals exists. *Primary regulatory signals* (competence signals) represent the most powerful regulators (e.g., PRL, GH, or antigen) of lymphoid cells. The delivery of a competence signal is the prerequisite for subsequent lymphoproliferation, which is regulated by growth factors that are specific for a certain developmental stage of the lymphoid cell, and which also act sequentially. Hormonal factors that promote growth and differentiation deliver the *secondary regulatory signals*. Competence factors, and growth and differentiation hormones regulate gene expression in lymphocytes. The *tertiary regulatory signals* modulates the function of mature effector cells (e.g., locomotion, secretion, phagocytosis, cytotoxicity). Neurotransmitters appear to function as secondary signal modulators and tertiary functional regulators.

Acknowledgments. The work discussed in this chapter has been supported in part by grants from the Arthritis Society of Canada, the Medical Research Council of Canada, and the Manitoba Health Research Council. The author is indebted to Mrs. Jean Sylwester for her devoted work on this manuscript.

References

1. Hammar JA. The new views as to the morphology of the thymus gland and their bearing on the problem of the function of the thymus. Endocrinology 1921; 5:543–573
2. Smith PE. Effect of hypophysectomy upon the involution of the thymus in the rat. Anat Rec 1930; 47:119–129.
3. Selye H. Thymus and adrenals in the response of the organism to injuries and intoxications. Br J Exp Pathol 1936; 17:234–248.
4. Selye H. A syndrome produced by diverse nocuous agents. Nature 1936; 183:32.
5. Selye H. The pharmacology of steroid hormones and their derivatives. Rev Can Biol 1942; 1:577–632.
6. Dougherty TF. Effect of hormones on lymphatic tissue. Physiol Rev 1952; 32:379–407.
7. Crafts RC, Meinecke HA. The anemia of hypophysectomized animals. Ann NY Acad Sci 1959; 77:501–517.
8. Ader R, ed. Psychoneuroimmunology. New York: Academic; 1981.
9. Ader R, Felten D, Cohen N, eds. Psychoneuroimmunology II. New York: Academic; 1990.
10. Berczi I. The influence of pituitary-adrenal axis on the immune system. In: Berczi I, ed. Pituitary Function and Immunity. Boca Raton, Florida: CRC Press; 1986:49–132.
11. Berczi I, Kovacs K, eds. Hormones and Immunity. Lancaster, UL: MTP Press; 1987.
12. Berczi I. The influence of pituitary hormones and neurotransmitters on the immune system. EOS Riv Immun Immunofarm 1988; 8:186–194.
13. Berczi I. Immunoregulation by neuroendocrine factors. Dev Comp Immunol 1989; 13:329–341.
14. Berczi I. Neurohormonal–immune interactions. In: Kovacs K, Asa S, eds. Functional Endocrine Pathology. Boston: Blackwell Scientific; 1990: 990–1004.
15. Berczi I, Nagy E. Effects of hypophysectomy on immune function. In: Ader R, Felten DL, Cohen N, eds. Psychoneuroimmunology II. New York: Academic; 1990.
16. Goetzl EJ, ed. Proceedings of a Conference on Neuromodulation of Immunity and Hypersensitivity. J Immunol (Suppl) 1985; 135(2).
17. Goetzl EJ, Spector NH, eds. Neuroimmune Networks: Physiology and Diseases. New York: Alan R. Liss; 1989.
18. Guillemin R, Cohn M, Melnechuk T, eds. Neural Modulation of Immunity. New York: Raven; 1985.

19. Jankovic BD. Neuroimmunomodulation: Facts and dilemmas. Immunol Lett 1989; 21:101–118.
20. Plotnikoff NP, Faith RE, Murgo AJ, Good RA, eds. Enkephalins and Endorphins: Stress and the Immune System. New York: Plenum; 1986.
21. Wolstenholme GE, Knight J, eds. Hormones and the Immune Response (Ciba Study Group, No. 36). London: Churchill Livingston; 1970.
22. Berczi I. The effects of growth hormone and related hormones on the immune system. In: Berczi I, ed. Pituitary Function and Immunity. Boca Raton, Florida: CRC Press; 1986:133–159.
23. Ramos-Zepeda R, Kretschmer R, Lopez-Osuna M, Parra-Covarrubias A, Perez-Pasten E. Evaluación de la función immunologica en el hipopituitarismo humano. Arch Invest Med (Mex) 1973; 4:197–206.
24. Berczi I, Nagy E, Kovacs K, Horvath E. Regulation of humoral immunity in rats by pituitary hormones. Acta Endocrinol (Copenh) 1981; 98:506–513.
25. Berczi I, Nagy E. A posible role of prolactin in adjuvant arthritis. Arthritis Rheum 1982; 25:591–594.
26. Berczi I, Nagy E, Asa SL, Kovacs K. Pituitary hormones and contact sensitivity in rats. Allergy 1983; 38:325–330.
27. Berczi I, Nagy E, Asa SL, Kovacs K. The influence of pituitary hormones on adjuvant arthritis. Arthritis Rheum 1984; 27:682–688.
28. Nagy E, Berczi I. Immunodeficiency in hypophysectomized rats. Acta Endocrinol (Copenh) 1978; 89:530–537.
29. Nagy E, Berczi I, Friesen HG. Regulation of immunity in rats by lactogenic and growth hormones. Acta Endocrinol (Copen) 1983; 102:351–357.
30. Nagy E, Berczi I, Wren GE, Asa SL, Kovacs K. Immunomodulation by bromocriptine. Immunopharmacology 1983; 6:231–243.
31. Kaplan SL, Grumbach MM, Friesen HG, Costom BH. Thyrotropin-releasing factor (TRF) effect on secretion of human pituitary prolactin and thyrotropin in children and in idiopathic hypopituitary dwarfism: Further evidence for hypophysiotropic hormone deficiencies. J Clin Endocrinol Metab 1972; 35:825–830.
32. Barkley MS, Bartke A, Gross DS, Sinha YN. Prolactin status of hereditary dwarf mice. Endocrinology 1981; 110:2088–2096.
33. Bartke A. Prolactin deficiency in genetically sterile dwarf mice. Mem Soc Endocrinol 1966; 15:193–197.
34. Berczi I, Nagy E. The effect of prolactin and growth hormone on hemolymphopoietic tissue and immune function. In: Berczi I, Kovacs K, eds. Hormones and Immunity. Lancaster, UK: MTP Press; 1987:145–171.
35. Edwards CK III, Lorence RM, Dunham DM, Yunger LM, Kelley KW. Peritoneal macrophages from hypophysectomized rats treated in vivo with interferon-gamma or growth hormone are primed to release tumor necrosis factor-alpha (abstract No. 93-20:618). In: Proceedings of the Seventh International Congress on Immunology. Berlin: Gustav Fischer Verlag; 1989.
36. Kelley KW. Growth homone, lymphocytes and macrophages. Biochem Pharmacol 1989; 38:705–713.
37. Kelley KW. Growth hormone in immunobiology. In: Ader R, Felten D, Cohen N, eds. Psychoneuroimmunology II. New York: Academic; 1990: 377–402.

38. Nagy E, Berczi I. Pituitary dependence of bone marrow function. Br J Haematol 1989; 71:457–462.
39. Exon JH, Bussiere JL, Williams JR. Hypophysectomy and growth hormone replacement effects on multiple immune responses in rats. Brain Behav Immun 1990; 4:118–128.
40. Khansari DN, Gustad T. Effects of long-term, low-dose growth hormone therapy on immune function and life expectancy of mice. Mech Ageing Dev 1991; 57:87–100.
41. Schimpff RM, Repellin AM. In vitro effect of human growth hormone on lymphocyte transformation and lymphocyte growth factors secretion. Acta Endocrinol 1989; 120:745–752.
42. Schimpff RM, Repellin AM. Production of intereleukin-1-alpha and inter-leukin-2 by mononuclear cells in healthy adults in relation to different experimental conditions and to the presence of growth hormone. Horm Res 1990; 33:171–176.
43. Bozzola M, Valtorta A, Moretta A, Montagna D, Maccario R, Burgio GR. Modulating effect of growth hormone (GH) on PHA-induced lymphocyte proliferation. Thymus 1988; 12:157–165.
44. Jafari P, Khansari DN. Detection of somatotropin receptors on human monocytes. Immunol Lett 1990; 24:199–202.
45. Murphy WJ, Durum SK, Anver MR, Longo DL. Immunologic and hema-tologic effects of neuroendocrine hormones. J Immunol 1992; 148:3799–3805.
46. Rovensky J, Ferencikova J, Vigas M, Lukac P. Effect of growth hormone on the activity of some lysosomal enzymes in neutrophilic polymorphonuclear leukocytes of hypopituitary dwarfs. Int J Tissue React 1985; 7:153–159.
47. Spadoni GL, Spagnoli A, Cianfarani S, Del Principe D, Menichelli A, DiGiulio S, Boscherini B. Enhancement by growth hormone of phorbol diester-stimulated respiratory burst in human polymorphonuclear leukocytes. Acta Endocrinol 1991; 124:589–594.
48. Fu YK, Arkins S, Wang BS, Kelley KW. A noval role of growth hormone and insulin-lke growth factor-1. Priming neutrophils for superoxide anion secretion. J Immunol 1991; 146:1602–1608.
49. Wiedermann CJ, Niedermuhlbichler M, Beimpold H, Braunsteiner H. In vitro activation of neutrophils of the aged by recombinant human growth hormone. J Infect Dis 1991; 164:1017–1020.
50. Wiedermann CJ, Niedermuhlbicher M, Geissler D, Beimpold H, Braun-steiner H. Priming of normal human neutrophils by recombinant human growth hormone. Br J Haematol 1991; 78:19–22.
51. Rapaport R, Oleske J, Ahdieh H, Solomon S, Delfaus C, Denny T. Sup-pression of immune function in growth hormone deficient children during treatment with human growth hormone. J Pediatr 1986; 109:434–439.
52. Rapaport R, Oleske J, Ahdieh H, Skuza K, Holland BK, Passannante MR, Denny T. Effects of human growth hormone on immune functions: In vitro studies on cells of normal and growth hormone-deficient children. Life Sci 1987; 41:2319–2324.
53. Kiess, Weiland, Doerr H, Butenandt O, Belohradsky BH. Lymphocyte subsets and natural-killer activity in growth hormone deficiency. N Engl J Med 1986; 314:321.

54. Church JA, Costin G, Brooks J. Immune functions in children treated with biosynthetic growth hormone. J Pediatr 1989; 115:420–423.
55. Bozzola M, Maccario R, Cisternino M, DeAmici M, Valtorta A. Moretta A, Biscaldi I, Schimpff RM. Immunological and endocrinological response to growth hormone in short children. Acta Paediatr Scand 1988; 77:675–680.
56. Bozzola M, Cisternino M, Valtorta A, Moretta A, Biscaldi I, Maghnie M, DeAmici M, Schimpff RM. Effect of biosynthetic methionyl growth hormone (GH) therapy on the immune function in GH-deficient children. Horm Res 1989; 31:153–156.
57. Bozzola M, Valtorta A, Moretta A, Cisternino M, Biscaldi I, Schimpff RM. In vitro and in vivo effect of growth hormone on cytotoxic activity. J Pediatr 1990; 117:596–599.
58. Etzioni A, Pollack S, Hochberg Z. Immune function in growth hormone-deficient children treated with biosynthetic growth hormone. Acta Paediatr Scand 1988; 77:169–170.
59. Spadoni GL, Rossi P, Ragno W, Galli E, Cianfarani S, Galasso C, Boscherini B. Immune function in growth hormone-deficient children treated with biosynthetic growth hormone. Acta Paediatr Scand 1991; 80:75–79.
60. Tyden G, Berg U, Reinholt F. Acute renal graft rejection after treatment with human growth hormone. Lancet 1990; 336:1455–1456.
61. Rongen-Westerlaken C, Rijkers GT, Scholtens EJ, van Es A, Wit JM, van den Brande JL, Zegers BJ. Immunologic studies in Turner syndrome before and during treatment with growth hormone. J Pediatr 1991; 119:268–272.
62. Crist DM, Peake GT, Mackinnon LT, Sibbitt WL Jr, Kraner JC. Exogenous growth hormone treatment alters body composition and increases natural killer cell activity in women with impaired endogenous growth hormone secretion. Metabolism 1987; 36:1115–1117.
63. Crist DM, Kraner JC. Supplemental growth hormone increases the tumor cytotoxic activity of natural killer cells in healthy adults with normal growth hormone secretion. Metabolism 1990; 39:1320–1324.
64. Kozak RW, Haskell JF, Greenstein LA, Rechler MM, Waldmann TA, Nissley SP. Type I and II insulin-like growth factor receptors on human phytohemagglutinin-activated T lymphocytes. Cell Immunol 1987; 109:318–331.
65. Verland S, Gammeltoft S. Functional receptors for insulin-like growth factors I and II in rat thymocytes and mouse thymoma cells. Mol Cell Endocrinol 1989; 67:207–216.
66. Johnson EW, Jones LA, Kozak RW. Expression and function of insulin-like growth factor receptors on anti-CD3-activated human T lymphocytes. J Immunol 1992; 148:63–71.
67. Roldan A, Charreau E, Schillaci R, Eugui EM, Allison AC. Insulin-like growth factor-1 increases the mitogenic response of human peripheral blood lymphocytes to phytohemagglutinin. Immunol Lett 1989; 20:5–8.
68. Hunt P, Eardley DD. Suppressive effects of insulin and insulin-like growth factor-1 (IGF-1) on immune response. J Immunol 1986; 136:3994–3999.
69. Gjerset RA, Yeargin J, Volkman SK, Vila V, Arya J, Haas M. Insulin-like growth factor-1 supports proliferation of autocrine thymic lymphoma cells with a pre-T cell phenotype. J Immunol 1990; 145:3497–3501.

70. Beschorner WE, Divic J, Pulido H, Yao X, Kenworthy P, Bruce G. Enhancement of thymic recovery after cyclosporine by recombinant human growth hormone and insulin-like growth factor-1. Transplantation 1991; 52:879–884.

71. Binz K, Joller P, Froesch P, Binz H, Zapf J, Froesch ER. Repopulation of the atrophied thymus in diabetic rats by insulin-like growth factor 1. Proc Natl Acad Sci USA 1990; 87:3690–3694.

72. Mocchegiani E, Paolucci P, Balsamo A, Cacciari E, Fabris N. Influence of growth hormone on thymic endocrine activity in humans. Horm Res 1990; 33:248–255.

73. Merchav S, Tatarsky I, Hochberg Z. Enhancement of erythropoiesis in vitro by human growth hormone is mediated by insulin-like growth factor-1. Br J Haematol 1988; 70:267–271.

74. Merchav S, Tatarsky I, Hochberg Z. Enhancement of human granulopoiesis in vitro by biosynthetic insulin-like growth factor 1/somatomedin C and human growth hormone. J Clin Invest 1988; 81:791–797.

75. Rappolee DA, Mark D, Banda MJ, Werb Z. Wound macrophages express TGF-alpha and other growth factors in vivo: Analysis by mRNA phenotyping. Science 1988; 241:708–712.

76. Rom WN, Basset P, Fells GA, Nukiwa T, Trapnell BC, Crysal RG. Alveolar macrophages release an insulin-like growth factor-1 type molecule. J Clin Invest 1988; 82:1685–1693.

77. Merimee TJ, Grant MB, Broder CM, Cavalli-Sforza LL. Insulin-like growth factor secretion by human B lymphocytes: A comparison of cells from normal and pygmy subjects. J Clin Endocrinol Metab 1989; 69:978–984.

78. Geffner ME, Bersch N, Lippe BM, Rosenfeld RG, Hintz RL, Golde DW. Growth hormone mediates the growth to T-lymphoblast cell lines via locally generated insulin-like growth factor-1. J Clin Endocrinol Metab 1990; 71: 464–469.

79. Baxter JB, Blalock JE, Weigent DA. Characterization of immunoreactive insulin-like growth factor-1 from leukocytes and its regulation by growth hormone. Endocrinology 1991; 129:1727–1734.

80. Berman JS, Center DM. Chemotactic activity of porcine insulin for human T lymphocytes in vitro. J Immunol 1987; 138:2100–2103.

81. Trovati M, Anfossi G, Cavalot F, Massucco P, Mularoni E, Emanuelli G. Insulin directly reduces platelet sensitivity to aggregating agents: Studies in vitro and in vivo. Diabetes 1988; 37:780–786.

82. Nagy E, Berczi I. Prolactin and contact sensitivity. Allergy 1981; 36: 429–431.

83. Nagy E, Berczi I. Immunomodulation by tamoxifen and pergolide. Immunopharmacology 1986; 12:145–153.

84. Cross RJ, Roszman TL. Neuroendocrine modulation of immune function: The role of prolactin. Prog Neuroendocrinimmunol 1989; 2:17–20.

85. Holaday JW, Bryant HU, Kenner JR, Bernton EW. Pharmacologic manipulation of the endocrine-immune axis. Prog Neuroendocrinimmunol 1988; 1:6–8.

86. Gala RR. Prolactin and growth hormone in the regulation of the immune system. Proc Soc Exp Biol Med 1991; 198:513–527.

87. Bernton E, Dave J. Prolactin, growth hormone, and immune homeostasis. In: Meltzer MS, Mantovani A, eds. Cellular and Cytokine Networks in Tissue Immunity. (Progress in Leukocyte Biology, Vol. 11.) New York: Wiley-Liss Inc.; 1991:69.

88. Berczi I. The immunology of prolactin. In: McCoshen JA, ed. Seminars in Reproductive Endocrinology, Special Issue on 'Prolactin in Women.' Thieme Medical Publ. Inc., New-York, Stuttgart 1992; 10:196–219.

89. Hiestand PC, Melker P, Nordmann R, Grieder A, Permmongkol C. Prolactin as a modulator of lymphocyte responsiveness provides a possible mechanism of action for cyclosporine. Proc Natl Acad Sci USA 1986; 83:2599–2603.

90. Matera L, Muccioli G, Cesano A, Bellussi G, Genazzani E. Prolactin receptors on large granular lymphocytes: Dual regulation by cyclosporin A. Brain Behav Immun 1988; 2:1–10.

91. Russel DH, Kibler R, Martrisian L, Larson DF, Poulos B, Magun BE. Prolactin receptors on human T and B lymphocytes: Antagonism of prolactin binding by cyclosporin. J Immunol 1985; 134:3027–3031.

92. O'Neal KD, Schwarz LA, Yu-Lee LY. Prolactin receptor gene expression in lymphoid cells. Mol Cell Endocrinol 1991; 82:127–135.

93. Varma S, Ebner KE. The effect of cyclosporin A on the growth and prolactin binding to Nb-2 rat lymphoma cells. Biochem Biophys Res Commun 1988; 156:223–239.

94. Ali S, Pellegrini I, Kelly PA. A prolactin-dependent immune cell line (Nb2) expresses a mutant form of prolactin receptor. J Biol Chem 1991; 266: 20110–20117.

95. Dardenne M, Kelly PA, Bach JF, Savino W. Identification and functional activity of prolactin receptors in thymic epithelial cells. Proc Natl Acad Sci USA 1991; 88:9700–9704.

96. Skwarlo-Sonta K. Mitogenic effect of prolactin on chicken lymphocytes in vitro. Immunol Lett 1990; 24:171–178.

97. Berczi I, Nagy E, de Toledo SM, Matusik RJ, Friesen HG. Pituitary hormones regulate c-*myc* and DNA synthesis in lymphoid tissue. J Immunol 1991; 146:2201–2206.

98. Spangelo BL, Judd AM, Ross PC, Login IS, Jarvis WD, Badamchian M, Goldstein AL, MacLeod RM. Thymosin fraction 5 stimulates prolactin and growth hormone release from anterior pituitary cells in vitro. Endocrinology 1987; 121:2035–2043.

99. Sotowska-Brochocka J, Rosolowska-Huszcz D, Skwarlo-Sonta K, Gajewska A. Effect of exogenous prolactin on immunity in chickens. Res Vet Sci 1984; 37:123–125.

100. Skwarlo-Sonta K, Sotowska-Brochocka J, Rosolowska-Huszca D, Pawlowska-Wojewodka E, Gajewska A, Stepien D, Kochman K. Effect of prolactin on the diurnal changes in immune parameters and plasma corticosterone in white leghorn chickens. Acta Endocrinol 1987; 116:172–178.

101. Hiestand PC, Gale JM, Mekler P. Soft immunosuppression by inhibition of prolactin release: Synergism with cyclosporine in kidney allograft survival and in the localized graft-versus-host reaction. Transplant Proc 1986; 18: 870–872.

102. Wilner ML, Ettenger RB, Koyle MA, Rosenthal JT. The effect of hypopro-lactinemia alone and in combination with cyclosporine on allograft rejection. Transplantation 1990; 49:264–267.
103. Bernton EW, Meltzer MT, Holaday JW. Suppression of macrophage acti-vation and T-lymphocyte function in hypoprolactinemic mice. Science 1988; 239:401–404.
104. Larson DF, Copeland JG, Rossel DH. Prolactin predicts cardiac allograft rejection in cyclosporin immunosuppressed patients. Lancet 1985; II:53.
105. Carrier M, Emery RW, Wild-Mobley J, Perrotta NJ, Russell DH, Copeland JG. Prolactin as a marker of rejection in human heart transplantation. Transplant Proc 1987; 19:3442–3443.
106. Cosson C, Myara I, Guillemain R, Amrein C, Dreyfus G, Moatti N. Serum prolactin as a rejection marker in heart transplantation. Clin Chem 1989; 35:492–493.
107. Esquifino AI, Villanua MA, Szary A, Yau J, Bartke A. Ectopic pituitary transplants restore immunocompetence in Ames dwarf mice. Acta Endo-crinol 1991; 125:67–72.
108. Gerli R, Rambotti P, Nicoletti I, Orlandi S, Migliorati G, Riccardi C. Reduced number of natural killer cells in patients with pathological hyper-prolactinemia. Clin Exp Immunol 1986; 64:399–406.
109. Matera L, Ciccarelli E, Cesano A, Veglia F, Miola C, Camanni F. Natural killer activity in hyperprolactinemic patients. Immunopharmacology 1989; 18:143–146.
110. Vidaller A, Guadarrama F, Llorente L, Mendez JB, Larrea F, Villa AR, Alarcon-Segovia D. Hyperprolactinemia inhibits natural killer (NK) cell function in vivo and its bromocriptine treatment not only corrects it but makes it more efficient. J Clin Immunol 1992; 12:210–215.
111. Matera L, Cesano A, Muccioli G, Veglia F. Modulatory effect of prolactin on the DNA synthesis rate and NK activity of large granular lymphocytes. Int J Neurosci 1990; 51:265–267.
112. Rovensky J, Vigas M, Marek J, Blazickova S, Korcakova L, Vyletelkova L, Takac A. Evidence for immunomodulatory properties of prolactin in selected invitro and in vivo situations. Int J Immunopharmacol 1991; 13: 267–272.
113. Weisz-Carrington P. Secretory immunobiology of the mammary gland. In: Berczi I, Kovacs K, eds. Hormones and Immunity. Lancaster, UK: MTP Press; 1987:172–202.
114. Nagy E, Berczi I, Sabbadini E. Endocrine control of the immunosuppressive activity of the submandibular gland. Brain Behav Immun 1992; 6:418–428.
115. Berczi I, Nagy E. Pituitary dependence of bone marrow function (abstract no. 93-10:616). In: Proceedings of the Seventh International Congress on Immunology Berlin: Gustav Fischer Verlag; 1989.
116. McGlone JJ, Lumpkin EA, Norman RL. Adrenocorticotorpin stimulates natural killer cell activity. Endocrinology 1991; 129:1653–1658.
117. Heijnen CJ, Zijlstra J, Kavelaars A, Croiset G, Ballieux RE. Modulation of the immune response by POMC-derived peptides. I. Influence on prolifera-tion of human lymphocytes. Brain Behav Immun 1987; 1:284–291.
118. Kavelaars A, Ballieux RE, Heijnen C. Modulation of the immune response by proopiomelanocortin derived peptides. II. Influence of adrenocortico-

tropin hormone on the rise in intracellular free calcium concentration after T-cell activation. Brain Behav Immun 1988; 2:57–66.

119. Cannon JG, Tatro JB, Reichlin S, Dinarello CA. Alpha melanocyte stimulating hormone inhibits immunostimulatory and inflammatory actions of interleukin 1. J Immunol 1986; 137:2232–2236.

120. Glyn-Ballinger JR, Bernardini GL, Lipton JM. Alpha-MSH injected into the septal region reduces fever in rabbits. Peptides (Fayetteville) 1983; 4:199.

121. Murphy MT, Richards DB, Lipton JM. Antipyretic potency of centrally administered alpha-melanocyte stimulating hormone. Science 1983; 221: 192–193.

122. Sundar SK, Becker KJ, Cierpial MA, Carpenter MD, Rankin LA, Fleener SL, Ritchie JC, Simson PE, Weiss JM. Intracerebroventricular infusion of interleukin 1 rapidly decreases peripheral cellular immune responses. Proc Natl Acad Sci USA 1989; 86:6398–6402.

123. Robertson B, Dostal K, Daynes RA. Neuropeptide regulation of inflammatory and immunologic responses. The capacity of α-melanocyte-stimulating hormone to inhibit tumor necrosis factor and IL-1-inducible biologic responses. J Immunol 1988; 140:4300–4307.

124. Goelst K, Mitchell D, Laburn H. Effects of α-melanocyte stimulating hormone on fever caused by endotoxin in rabbits. J Physiol 1991; 441:469–476.

125. Goelst K, Laburn H. The effect of α-MSH on fever caused by staphylococcus-aureus cell walls in rabbits. Peptides 1991; 12:1239–1242.

126. Stefano GB. Role of opioid neuropeptides in immunoregulation. Prog Neurobiol 1989; 33:149–159.

127. Weber RJ, Pert A. The periaqueductal gray matter mediates opiate-induced immunosuppression. Science 1989; 245:188–190.

128. Gilmore W, Weiner LP. β-Endorphin enhances interleukin-2 (IL-2) production in murine lymphocytes. J Neuroimmunol 1988; 18:125–138.

129. Apte RN, Durum SK, Oppenheim JJ. Opioids modulate interleukin-1 production and secretion by bone-marrow macrophages. Immunol Lett 1990; 24:141–148.

130. Millar DB, Hough CJ, Mazorow DL, Gootenberg JE. β-Endorphin's modulation of lymphocyte proliferation is dose, donor, and time dependent. Brain Behav Immun 1990; 4:232–242.

131. Chiappelli F, Nguyen L, Bullington R, Fahey JL. β-Endorphin blunts phosphatidylinositol formation during invtro activation of isolated human lymphocytes: Preliminary report. Brain Behav Immun 1992; 6:1–10.

132. Claman HN. Corticosteroids—immunologic and anti-inflammatory effects. In: Berczi I, Kovacs K, eds. Hormones and Immunity. Lancaster, UK: MTP Press; 1987:38–42.

133. Homo-Delarche F, Duval D. Glucocorticoid receptors in lymphoid tissue. In: Berczi I, Kovacs K, eds. Hormones and Immunity. Lancaster, UK: MTP Press; 1987:1–19.

134. McConkey DJ, Hartzell P, Nicotera P, Orrenius S. Calcium-activated DNA fragmentation kills immature thymocytes. FASEB J 1989; 3:1843–1849.

135. Emilie D, Crevon MC, Auffredou MT, Galanaud P. Glucocorticosteroid-dependent synergy between interleukin-1 and interleukin-6 for human lymphocyte-B differentiation. Eur J Immunol 1988; 18:2043–2047.

136. Munck A, Naray-Fejes-Toth A, Guyre PM. Mechanisms of glucocorticoid actions on the immune system. In: Berczi I, Kovacs K, eds. Hormones and Immunity. Lancaster, UK: MTP Press; 1987:20–37.

137. Nieto MA, Lopez-Rivas A. Il-2 protects T lymphocytes from glucocorticoid induced DNA fragmentation and cell death. J Immunol 1989; 143: 4166–4170.

138. Fuggetta MP, Graziani G, Aquino A, D'Atri S, Bonmassar E. Effect of hydrocortisone on human natural killer activity and its modulation by beta interferon. Int J Immunopharmacol 1988; 10:687–694.

139. Masera R, Gatti G, Sartori ML, Carignola R, Salvadori A, Magro E, Angeli A. Involvement of Ca^{2+}-dependent pathways in the inhibition of human natural killer (NK) cell activity by cortisol. Immunopharmacology 1989; 18:11–22.

140. Rouabhia M, Chakir J, Deschaux P. Interaction between the immune and endocrine systems: Immunomodulatory effects of luteinizing hormone. Prog Neuroendocrinimmunol 1991; 4:86–91.

141. Berczi I. Gonadotropins and sex hormones. In: Berczi I, ed. Pituitary Function and Immunity. Boca Raton, FL: CRC Press; 1986:185–211.

142. Grossman CJ. Interactions between the gonadal steroids and the immune system. Science 1985; 227:257–261.

143. Stimson WH. Sex steroids, steroid receptors, and immunity. In: Berczi I, Kovacs K, eds. Hormones and Immunity. Lancaster, UK: MTP Press; 1987:43–53.

144. Stimson WH. Oestrogen and human T lymphocytes: Presence of specific receptors in the T-suppressive/cytotoxic subset. Scand J Immunol 1988; 28:345–350.

145. Nelson JL, Steinberg AD. Sex steroids, autoimmunity, and autoimmune disease. In: Berczi I, Kovacs K, eds. Hormones and Immunity. Lancaster, UK: MTP Press; 1987:93–119.

146. Raveche ES, Steinberg AD. Sex hormones in autoimmunity. In: Berczi I, ed. Pituitary Function and Immunity. Boca Raton, Florida: CRC Press; 1986:283–301.

147. Fried W, Morley C. Effects of androgenic steroids on erythropoiesis. Steroids 1985; 46:799–826.

148. Sullivan DA. Endocrine regulation of the ocular secretory immune system. In: Berczi I, Kovacs K, eds. Hormones and Immunity. Lancaster, UK: MTP Press; 1987:54–92.

149. Seaman WE, Gindhart TD, Greenspan JS, Blackman MA, Talal N. Natural killer cells, bone, and the bone marrow: Studies in estrogen-treated mice and in congenitally osteopetrotic (mi/mi) mice. J Immunol 1979; 122: 2541–2547.

150. Cohen JHM, Danel L, Cordier G, Saez S, Revillard JP. Sex steroid receptors in peripheral T cells: Absence of androgen receptors and restriction of estrogen receptors to OKT8-positive cells. J Immunol 1983; 131:2767–2771.

151. Bick PH, Tucker AN, White KL Jr, Holsapple MP. Effect of subchronic exposure to diethylstilbestrol on humoral immune function in adult female $(C_3B_6)F_1$ mice. Immunopharmacology 1984; 7:27–39.

152. Harbour DV, Leon S, Keating C, Hughes K. Thyrotropin modulates B-cell function through specific bioactive receptors. Prog Neuroendocrinimmunol 1990; 3:266–276.

153. Coutelier JP, Kehrl JH, Bellur SS, Kohn LD, Notkins AL, Prabhakar BS. Binding and functional effects of thyroid stimulating hormone on human immune cells. J Clin Immunol 1990; 10:204–210.

154. Todd I, Pujol-Borrell R, Hammond LJ, McNally JM, Feldman M, Bottazzo GF. Enhancement of thyrocyte HLA class II expression by thyroid stimulating hormone. Clin Exp Immunol 1987; 69:524–531.

155. Barlow JW, DeNayer P. Characterization of thyroid hormone receptors in human IM-9 lymphocytes. Acta Endocrinol 1988; 117:327–332.

156. Kvetny J, Matzen LE, Blochert-Toft M, Watt-Boolsen S, Date J. Nuclear thyroid hormone receptor binding in human mononuclear blood cells after goiter resection. Horm Metab Res 1989; 21:142–144.

157. Fabris N, Mocchegiani E. Endocrine control of thymic serum factor production in young adult and old mice. Cell Immunol 1985; 91:325–335.

158. Fabris N, Mocchegiani E, Mariotti S, Pacini F, Pinchera A. Thyroid function modulates thymic endocrine activity. J Clin Endocrinol Metab 1986; 62:474–478.

159. Mocchegiani E, Amadio L, Fabris N. Neuroendocrine-thymus interactions. I. In vitro modulation of thymic factor secretion by thyroid hormones. J Endocrinol Invest 1990; 13:139–147.

160. Dainiak N, Sutter D, Kreczko, S. L-Triiodothyronine augments erythropoietic growth factor release from peripheral blood and bone marrow leukocytes. Blood 1986; 68:1289–1297.

161. Weetman AP, McGregor AM, Ludgate M, Hall R. Effect of tri-iodothyronine on normal human lymphocyte function. J Endocrinol 1984; 101: 81–86.

162. Bachman SE, Mashaly MM. Relationship between circulating thyroid hormones and humoral immunity in immature male chickens. Dev Comp Immunol 1986; 10:395–403.

163. Bachman SE, Mashaly MM. Relationship between circulating thyroid hormones and cell-mediated immunity in immature male chickens. Dev Comp Immunol 1987; 11:203–213.

164. Mashaly MM, Youtz SL, Wideman RF Jr. Hypothyroidism and antibody production in immature male chickens. Immunol Commun 1983; 12:551–563.

165. Haddad EE, Mashaly MM. In vivo effects of TRH, T3, and cGH on antibody production and lymphocytes-T and lymphocytes-B proliferation in immature male chickens. Immunol Invest 1991; 20:557–568.

166. Stein-Streilein J, Zakarija M, Papic M, McKenzie JM. Hyperthyroxinemic mice have reduced natural killer cell activity. Evidence for a defective trigger mechanism. J Immunol 1987; 139:2502–2507.

167. Turaihi K, Khan FA, Baron DN, Dandona P. Effect of short term triiodothyronine administration on human leukocyte Rb(K) influx and Na efflux. J Clin Endocrinol Metab 1987; 65:1031–1034.

168. Ruben LN, Clothier RH, Murphy GL, Marshall JD, Lee R, Pham T, Nobis C, Shiigi S. Thyroid function and immune reactivity during metamorphosis

in Xenopus laevis, the South African clawed toad. Gen Comp Endocrinol 1989; 76:128–138.

169. Chandel AS, Chatterjee S. Effect of thyroid hormones on delayed type hypersensitivity reaction. Indian J Exp Biol 1989; 27:408–411.

170. Torres BA, Johnson HW. Arginine vasopressin (AVP) replacement of helper cell requirement in IFN-γ production. Evidence for a novel AVP receptor on mouse lymphocytes. J Immunol 1988; 140:2179–2183.

171. Elands J, Van Woudenberg A, Resink A, de Kloet ER. Vasopressin receptor capacity of human blood peripheral mononuclear cells is sex dependent. Brain Behav Immun 1990; 4:30–38.

172. Bell J, Adler MW, Greenstein JI. The effect of arginine vasopressin on the autologous mixed lymphocyte reaction. Int J Immunopharmacol 1992; 14: 93–103.

173. Kavelaars A, Ballieux RE, Heijnen CJ. The role of IL-1 in the corticotropin-releasing factor and arginine-vasopresin-induced secretion of immunoreactive β-endorphin by human peripheral blood mononuclear cells. J Immunol 1989; 142:2338–2342.

174. Kavelaars A, Ballieux RE, Heijnen CJ. β-Endorphin secretion by human peripheral blood mononuclear cells: Regulation by glucocorticoids. Life Sci 1990; 46:1233–1240.

175. Malkinson TJ, Bridges TE, Lederis K, Veale WL. Perfusion of the septum of the rabbit with vasopressin antiserum enhances endotoxin fever. Peptides 1987; 8:385–389.

176. LeBoeuf RD, Burns JN, Bost KL, Blalock JE. Isolation, purification, and partial characterization of suppressin, a novel inhibitor of cell proliferation. J Biol Chem 1990; 265:158–165.

177. LeBoeuf RD, Carr DJJ, Green MM, Blalock JE. Cellular effects of suppressin: A biological response modifier of cells of the immune system. Prog Neuroendocrinimmunol 1990; 3:176–187.

178. Hadden JW, Galy A, Chen H, Hadden EM. A pituitary factor induces thymic epithelial cell proliferation in vitro. Brain Behav Immun 1989; 3: 149–159.

179. Calabresi P, Parks RE Jr. Antiproliferative agents and drugs used for immunosuppression. In: Gilman AG, Goodman LS, Gilman A, eds. The Pharmacological Basis of Therapeutics. New York: Macmillan; 1980:1256–1313.

180. Daughaday WH. The adenohypophysis. In: Williams RH, ed. Textbook of Endocrinology. Philadelphia: Saunders; 1981:73–116.

181. Kelley KW, Brief S, Westly HJ, Novakofski J, Bechtel PJ, Simon J, Walker EB. GH₃ pituitary adenoma cells can reverse thymic aging in rats. Proc Natl Acad Sci USA 1986; 83:5663–5667.

182. Huggins C, Oka H. Regression of stem-cell erythroblastic leukemia after hypophysectomy. Cancer Res 1972; 32:239–242.

183. Huggins CB, Ueda N. Regression of myelocytic leukemia in rats after hypophysectomy. Proc Natl Acad Sci USA 1984; 81:598–601.

184. Fleming WH, Murphy PR, Murphy LJ, Hatton TW, Matusik RJ, Friesen HG. Human growth hormone induces and maintains c-*myc* gene expression in Nb2 lymphoma cells. Endocrinology 1985; 117:2547–2549.

185. Klein G. Specific chromosomal translocations and the genesis of B-cell-derived tumors in mice and men. Cell 1983; 32:311–315.

186. Berczi I, Nagy E, de Toledo SM, Matusik RJ, Friesen HG. Pituitary hormones regulate c-*myc* and DNA synthesis in lymphoid tissue. J Immunol 1991; 146:2201–2206.

187. Langdon WY, Harris AW, Cory S, Adams JM. The c-*myc* oncogene perturbs B-lymphocyte development in Eu-*myc* transgenic mice. Cell 1986; 47:11–18.

188. Morse HC III, Hartley JW, Fredrickson TN, Yetter RA, Majumdar C, Cleveland JL, Rapp UR. Recombinant murine retroviruses containing avian v-*myc* induce a wide spectrum of neoplasms in newborn mice. Proc Natl Acad Sci USA 1986; 83:6868–6872.

189. Stiles CD, Capone GT, Scher CD, Antoniades HN, Van Wyk JJ, Pledger WJ. Dual control of cell growth by somatomedins and platelet-derived growth by somatomedins and platelet-derived growth factor. Proc Natl Acad Sci USA 1979; 76:1279–1283.

190. Armelin HA, Armelin MCS, Kelly K, Stewart T, Leder P, Cochran BH, Stiles CD. Functional role for c-*myc* in mitogenic response to platelet-derived growth factor. Nature 1984; 310:655–660.

191. Pardee AB. Molecules involved in proliferation of normal and cancer cells: Presidental address. Cancer Res 1987; 47:1488–1491.

192. Tanaka T, Shiu RPC, Gout PW, Beer CT, Noble RL, Friesen HG. A new sensitive and specific bioassay for lactogenic hormones: Measurement of prolactin and growth hormone in human serum. J Clin Endocrinol 1980; 51:1058–1063.

193. Berczi I, Cosby H, Hunter T, Baragar F, McNeilly AS, Friesen HG. Decreased bioactivity of circulating prolactin in patients with rheumatoid arthritis. Br J Rheum 1987; 26:433–436.

194. McNeilly AS, Friesen HG. Presence of a nonlactogenic factor in human serum which synergisticaly enhances prolactin-stimulated growth of Nb2 rat lymphoma cells in vitro. J Clin Endocrinol Metab 1985; 61:408–411.

195. Paul WE. The immune system: An introduction. In: Paul WE, ed. Fundamental Immunology, 2nd ed. New York: Raven; 1989:3–19.

196. Audhya T, Kroon D, Heavner G, Viamontes G, Goldstein G. Tripeptide structure of bursin, a selective B-cell-differentiation hormone of the bursa of Fabricius. Science 1986; 231:997–999.

197. Clark SC, Kamen R. The human hematopoietic colony-stimulating factors. Science 1987; 236:1229–1237.

198. Goldstein AL, Low TLK, Zatz MM, Hall NR, Naylor PH. Thymosins. Clin Immunol Allergy 1983; 3:119–132.

199. Metcalf D. The granulocyte-macrophage colony-stimulating factors. Science 1985; 229:16–21.

200. Sachs L. The molecular control of blood cell development. Science 1987; 238:1374–1379.

201. von Boehmer H, Kishi H, Scott B, Borgulya P, Teh HS, Kisielow P. Self–nonself discrimination by the immune system. In: Melchers F, Albert ED, von Boehmer H, Dierich MP, DuPasquier L, Eichman K, Gemsa D, Götze O, Kalden JR, Kaufmann SHE, Kirchner H, Resch K, Riethmüller G, Schimpl A, Sorg C, Steinmetz M, Wagner H, Zachau HG, eds. Progress in Immunology VII. Berlin: Springer-Verlag; 1989:297–301.

202. MacDonald HR, Lees RK. Programmed death of autoreactive thymocytes. Nature 1990; 343:642–644.

203. Quesenberry PJ. Synergistic hematopoietic growth factors. Int J Cell Cloning 1986; 4:3–15.
204. Brook CGD, Hindmarsh PC, Stanhope R. Review: Growth and growth hormone secretion. J Endocrinol 1988; 119:179–184.
205. Dardenne M, Savino W, Gagnerault MC, Itoh T, Bach JF. Neuroendocrine control of thymic hormonal production. I. Prolactin stimulates in vivo and in vitro the production of thymulin by human and murine thymic epithelial cells. Endocrinology 1989; 125:3–12.
206. Goff BL, Roth JA, Arp LH, Incefy GS. Growth hormone treatment stimulates thymulin production in aged dogs. Clin Exp Immunol 1987; 68: 580–587.
207. Mick CCW, Nicoll CS. Prolactin directly stimulates the liver in vivo to secrete a factor (synlactin) which acts synergistically with the hormone. Endocrinology 1985; 116:2049–2053.
208. Spangelo BL, MacLeod RM. Thymic stromal elements contain prolactin and growth hormone releasing activities. Prog Neuroendocrinimmunol 1988; 1:9–10.
209. Goya RG, Quiqley KL, Takahashi S, Reichhart R, Meites J. Differential effect of homeostatic thymus hormone on plasma thyrotropin and growth hormone on plasma thyrotropin and growth hormone in young and old rats. Mech Ageing Dev 1989; 49:119–128.
210. Malarkey WB, Zvara BJ. Interleukin-1-beta and other cytokines stimulate adrenocorticotropin release form cultured pituitary cells of patients with Cushing's disease. J Clin Endocrinol Metab 1989; 196–199.
211. Balkwill FR, Burke F. The cytokine network. Immunol Today 1989; 10: 299–304.
212. Gillis S. Interleukin-2: Biology and biochemistry. J Clin Immunol 1983; 3:1–13.
213. Bretscher P, Cohn M. A theory of self–nonself discrimination. Science 1970; 169:1042–1049.
214. Schwartz RA. A cell culture model for T lymphocyte clonal anergy. Science 1990; 248:1349–1356.
215. Chen W, Reese V, Cheever MA. Adoptively transferred antigen-specific T cells can be grown and maintained in large numbers in vivo for extended periods of time by intermittent restimulation with specific antigen plus IL-2. J Immunol 1990; 144:3659–3666.
216. Bateman A, Singh A, Kral T, Solomon S. The immune-hypothalamic-pituitary-adrenal axis. Endocr Rev 1989; 10:92–112.
217. Berkenbosch F, van Oers J, del Rey A, Tilders F, Besedovsky H. Corticotropin-releasing factor-producing neurons in the rat activated by interleukin-1. Science 1987; 238:524–526.
218. Bernton EW, Beach JE, Holaday JW, Smallridge RC, Fein HG. Release of multiple hormones by a direct action of interleukin-1 on pituitary cells. Science 1987; 238:519–521.
219. del Rey A, Besedovsky HO. Immune-neuroendocrine feedback regulatory signals. In: Berczi I, Kovacs K, eds. Hormones and Immunity. Lancaster, UK: MTP Press; 1987:215–230.
220. Sapolsky R, Rivier C, Yamamoto G, Plotsky P, Vale W. Interleukin-1 stimulates the secretion of hypothalamic corticotropin-releasing factor. Science 1987; 238:522–524.

221. Monroy RL, Davis TA, MacVittie TJ. Granulocyte-macrophage colony-stimulating factor: More than a hemopoietin. Clin Immunol Immunopathol 1990; 54:333–346.

222. Carr DJJ, Blalock JE. 'Classical' neuroendocrine peptide hormones produced by cells of the immune system. Brain Behav Immun 1988; 2:328–334.

223. Goetzl EJ, Sreedharan SP, Harkonen WS. Pathogenetic roles of neuro-immunologic mediators. Immunol Allergy Clin North Am 1988; 8:183–200.

224. Costa O, Mulchahey JJ, Blalock JE. Structure and function of luteinizing hormone-releasing hormone (LHRH) receptors on lymphocytes. Prog Neuroendocrinimmunol 1990; 3:55–60.

225. Emanuele NV, Emanuele MA, Tentler J, Kirsteins L, Azad N, Lawrence AM. Rat spleen lymphocytes contain an immunoactive and bioactive luteinizing hormone-releasing hormone. Endocrinology 1990; 126:2482–2486.

226. Hattori N, Shimatsu A, Sugita M, Kumagai S, Imura H. Immunoreactive growth hormone (GH) secretion by human lymphocytes: Augmented release by exogenous GH. Biochem Biophys Res Commun 1990; 168:396–401.

227. Standaert FE, Chew BP, Wong TS, Michal JJ. Porcine lymphocytes secrete a bioactive and immunoreactive LH-like factor in response to LHRH and concanavalin-A. Am J Reprod Immunol 1991; 25:175–180.

228. Weigent DA, Riley JE, Galin FS, Le Boeuf RD, Blalock JE. Detection of growth hormone and growth hormone-releasing hormone-related messenger RNA in rat leukocytes by the polymerase chain reaction. Proc Soc Exp Biol Med 1991; 198:643–648.

229. Blalock JE, Smith EM. A complete regulatory loop between the immune and neuroendocrine systems. Fed Proc 1985; 44:108–111.

230. Dinarello CA. Biology of interleukin-1. FASEB J 1988; 2:108–115.

231. Scarborough DE, Reichlin S. Cytokines, the brain and aging. Prog Neuroendocrinimmunol 1988; 1:10–15.

232. Ohalloran DJ, Jones PM, Bloom SR. Neuropeptides synthesized in the anterior pituitary—possible paracrine role. Mol Cell Endocrinol 1991; 75: C7–C12.

233. Vankelecom H, Carmeliet P, Van Damme J, Billiau A, Denef C. Production of interleukin-6 by folliculo-stellate cells of the anterior pituitary gland in a histiotypic cell aggregate culture system. Neuroendocrinology 1989; 49:102–106.

234. Spangelo BL, MacLeod RM, Isakson PC. Production of interleukin-6 by anterior pituitary cells in vitro. Endocrinology 1990; 126:582–586.

235. Koenig JI. Presence of cytokines in the hypothalamic-pituitary axis. Prog Neuroendocrinimmunol 1991; 4:143–153.

236. Geenen V, Robert F, Fatemi M, Martens H, Defresne MP, Boniver J, Legros JJ, Franchimont P. Neuroendocrine-immune interactions in T-cell ontogeny. Thymus 1989; 13:131–140.

237. Smith EM, Morrill AC, Meyer WJ III, Blalock JE. Corticotropin releasing factor induction of leukocyte-derived immunoreactive ACTH and endorphins. Nature 1986; 321:881–882.

238. Hokfelt T, Elfvin LG, Elde R, Schultzberg M, Goldstein M, Luft R. Occurrence of somatostatin-like immunoreactivity in some peripheral sympathetic noradrenergic neurons. Proc Natl Acad Sci USA 1977; 74:3587–3591.

239. Germain G, Ferre F. Hormones et parturition chez les primates. Ann Endocrinol (Paris) 1987; 48:311–321.

240. Green DR, Wegmann TG. Beyond the immune system: The immunotrophic role of T cells in organ generation and regeneration. Prog Immunol 1986; 6:1100–1112.

241. Rivier C, Vale W. In the rat, interleukin-1-alpha acts at the level of the brain and the gonads to interfere with gonadotropin and sex steroid secretion. Endocrinology 1989; 124:2105–2109.

242. Yamashita S, Kimura H, Ashizawa K, Nagayama Y, Hirayu H, Izumi M, Nagataki S. Interleukin-1 inhibits thyrotrophin-induced human thyroglobulin gene expression. J Endocrinol 1989; 122:177–183.

243. Brown R, Li Z, Vriend CY, Nirula R, Janz L, Falk J, Nance DM, Dyck DG, Greenberg AH. Suppression of splenic macrophage interleukin-1 secretion following intracerebroventricular injection of interleukin-1β—evidence for pituitary adrenal and sympathetic control. Cell Immunol 1991; 132: 84–93.

244. Beutler B, Milsark IW, Cerami A. Passive immunization against cachectin/tumor necrosis factor protects mice from lethal effects of endotoxin. Science 1985; 229:869–871.

245. Beutler B, Cerami A. Cachectin (tumor necrosis factor): A macrophage hormone governing cellular metabolism and inflammatory response. Endocr Rev 1988; 9:57–66.

246. Gulick T, Chung MK, Pieper SJ, Lange LG, Schreiner GF. Interleukin 1 and tumor necrosis factor inhibit cardiac monocyte beta-adrenergic responsiveness. Proc Natl Acad Sci USA 1989; 86:6753–6757.

247. Sharp BM, Matta SG, Peterson PK, Newton R, Chao C, Mcallen K. Tumor necrosis factor-alpha is a potent ACTH secretagogue: Comparison to interleukin-1. Endocrinology 1989; 124:3131–3133.

248. Woloski BMRNJ, Jamieson JC. Rat corticotropin, insulin, and thyroid hormone levels during the acute phase response to inflammation. Comp Biochem Physiol [A] 1987; 86:15–19.

249. Woloski BMRNJ, Smith EM, Meyer WJ III, Fuller GM, Blalock JE. Corticotropin-releasing activity of monokines. Science 1985; 230:1035–1037.

250. Nagayama Y, Izumi M, Ashizawa K, Kiriyama T, Yokohama N, Morite S, Ohtakara S, Fukuta T, Eguchi K, Morimoto I, Okamoto I, Ihikawa N, Ito K, Nagataki S. Inhibitory effect of interferon-gamma on the response of human thyrocytes to thyrotropin (TSH) stimulation: Relationship between the response to TSH and the expression of DR antigen. J Clin Endocrinol Metab 1987; 64:949–953.

251. Orava M, Cantell K, Kauppia A, Vihko R. Interferon and serum thyroid hormones. Int J Cancer 1983; 31:671–672.

252. Orava M, Voutilainew R, Vihko R. Interferon-gamma inhibits steroidogenesis and accumulation of mRNA of the steroidogenic enzymes P450scc and P450c17 in cultured porcine Leydig cells. Mol Endocrinol 1989; 3: 887–894.

253. Pestka S, Langer JA, Zoon KC, Samuel CE. Interferons and their actions. Annu Rev Biochem 1987; 56:727–777.

254. Roosth J, Pollard RB, Brown SL, Meyer WJ. Cortisol stimulation by recombinant interferon-alpha₂. J Neuroimmunol 1986; 12:311–316.

255. Shimizu F, Shimizu M, Kamiayama K. Inhibitory effect of interferon on the production of insulin. Endocrinology 1985; 117:2081–2084.

256. Stanton GJ, Weigent DA, Fleischmann WR, Dianzani F, Baron S. Interferon review. Invest Radiol 1987; 22:259–273.
257. Berczi I, ed. Pituitary Function and Immunity. Boca Raton, Florida: CRC Press; 1986.
258. Dantzer R, Kelley KW. Minireview. Stress and immunity: An integrated view of relationships between the brain and the immune system. Life Sci 1989; 44:1995–2008.
259. Marcos MAR, Sundblad A, Grendien A, Huetz F, Avrameas S, Coutinho A. The physiology of autoimmune reactivities. In: Melchers F, et al., eds. Progress in Immunology VII. Berlin: Springer-Verlag; 1989:793–804.
260. Hess AD, Fischer AC. Immune mechanisms in cyclosporine-induced syngeneic graft-versus-host disease. Transplantation 1989; 48:895–900.
261. Butenandt O. Rheumatoid arthritis and growth retardation in children: Treatment with human growth hormone. Eur J Pediatr 1979; 130:15–28.
262. Allen RC, Jimenez M, Cowell CT. Insulin-like growth factor and growth hormone secretion in juvenile chronic arthritis. Ann Rheum Dis 1991; 50:602–606.
263. Asa SL, Bilbao JM, Kovacs K, Josse RG, Kreines K. Lymphocytic hypophysitis of pregnancy resulting in hypopituitarism: A distinct clinocopathologic entity. Ann Intern Med 1981; 95:166–171.
264. Ferrari C, Boghen M, Paracchi A, Rampini P, Raiteri F, Benco R, Romussi M, Codecasa F, Mucci M, Bianco M. Thyroid autoimmunity in hyperprolactinaemic disorders. Acta Endocrinol (Copenh) 1983; 104:35–41.
265. Lever EG, McKerron CG. Auto-immune Addison's disease associated with hyperprolactinaemia. Clin Endocrinol 1984; 21:451–457.
266. Hedner LP, Bynke G. Endogenous iridocyclitis relieved during treatment with bromocriptine. Am J Ophthalmol 1985; 100:618–619.
267. Lavalle C, Loyo E, Paniagua R, Bermudez JA, Herrera J, Graef A, Gonzalez-Barcena D, Fraga A. Correlation study between prolactin and androgens in male patients with systemic lupus erythematosus. J Rheumatol 1987; 14:268–272.
268. Schauenstein K, Fassler R, Dietrich H, Schwarz S, Kromer G, Wick G. Disturbed immune–endocrine communication in autoimmune disease. Lack of corticosterone response to immune signals in obese strain chickens with sponaneous autoimmune thyroiditis. J Immunol 1987; 139:1830–1833.
269. MacPhee IAM, Antoni FA, Mason DW. Spontaneous recovery of rats from experimental allergic encephalomyelitis is dependent on regulation of the immune system by endogenous adrenal corticosteroids. J Exp Med 1989; 169:431–445.
270. Sternberg EM, Hill JM, Chrousos GP, Kamilaris T, Listwak SJ, Gold PW, Wilder RL. Inflammatory mediator-induced hypothalamic-pituitary-adrenal axis activation is defective in streptococcal cell wall arthritis-susceptible Lewis rats. Proc Natl Acad Sci USA 1989; 86:2374–2378.
271. Sternberg EM, Young WS III, Bernardini R, Calogero AE, Chrousos GP, Gold PW, Wilder RL. A central nervous system defect in biosynthesis of corticotropin-releasing hormone is associated with susceptibility to streptococcal cell wall-induced arthritis in Lewis rats. Proc Natl Acad Sci USA 1989; 86:4771–4775.
272. Cutolo M, Balleari E, Giusti M, Monachesi M, Accardo S. Sex hormone status of male patients with rheumatoid arthritis—evidence of low serum

concentrations of testosterone at baseline and after human chorionic gonadotropin stimulation. Arthritis Rheum 1988; 31:1314–1317.

273. Feher KG, Feher T, Meretey K. Interrelationship between the immunological and steroid hormone parameters in rheumatoid arthritis. Exp Clin
Endocrinol 1986; 87:38–42.

274. Sambrook PN, Eisman JA, Champion GD, Pocock NA. Sex hormone status
and osteoporosis in postmenopausal women with rheumatoid arthritis.
Arthritis Rheum 1988; 31:973–978.

275. McMurray R, Keisler D, Kanuckel K, Izui S, Walker SE. Prolactin influences autoimmune disease activity in the female B/W mouse.
J Immunol 1991; 147:3780–3787.

276. Jara-Quezada L, Graef A, Lavalle C. Prolactin and gonadal hormones
during pregnancy in systemic lupus erythematosus. J Rheumatol 1991; 18:
349–353.

277. Folomeev M, Prokaeva T, Nassaonova V, Nassonov E, Masenko E, Ovtraht
N. Prolactin levels in men with SLE and RA. J Rheumatol 1990; 17:
1569–1570.

278. Asa SL. The pathology of autoimmune endocrine disorders. In: Berczi I,
Kovacs K, eds. Hormones and Immunity. Lancaster, UK: MTP Press;
1987:247–271.

279. Bottazzo GF, Mirakian R, De Lazzari F, Mauerhoff T, Todd I, Pujol-
Borrell R. Autoimmune endocrine/organ-specific disorders: Clinical diag-
nostic relevance and novel approaches to pathogenesis. In: Berczi I, Kovacs
K, eds. Hormones and Immunity. Lancaster, UK: MTP Press; 1987:296–
311.

280. Jankovic BD. Neuroimmunomodulation: Facts and dilemmas. Immunol Lett
1989; 21:101–118.

281. Welsh JB, Szabo M. Impaired suppression of growth hormone release by
somatostatin in cultured adenohypophyseal cells of spontaneously diabetic
BB/W rats. Endocrinology 1988; 123:2230–2234.

282. Leff AR. Toward the formulation of a theory of asthma. Perspect Biol Med
1990; 33:292–302.

283. Szentivanyi A. The beta-adrenergic theory of the ectopic abnormality in
bronchial asthma. J Allergy 1968; 42:203–232.

284. Walker KB, Serwonska MH, Valone FH, Harkonen WS, Frick OL, Scriven
KH, Ratnoff WD, Browning JG, Payan DG, Goetzi EJ. Distinctive
patterns of release of primary afferent neuropeptides after nasal challenge
of allergic subjects with rye grass antigen. J Clin Immunol 1988; 8:108–
113.

285. Kidd BL, Mapp PI, Gibson SJ, Polak JM, O'Higgins F, Buckland-Wright
JC, Blake DR. A neurogenic mechanism for symmetrical arthritis. Lancet
1989; 2:1128–1130.

286. Frayn KN. Hormonal control of metabolism in trauma and sepsis. Clin
Endocrinol (Oxf) 1986; 24:577–599.

287. Leshin LS, Malven PV. Bacteremia-induced changes in pituitary hormone
release and effect of naloxone. Am J Physiol 1984; 247:E585–E591.

288. Smith BB, Wagner WC. Effect of Escherichia coli endotoxin and thyrotropin-releasing hormone on prolactin in lactating sows. Am J Vet Res 1985;
46:175–180.

289. Yki-Jarvinen H, Sammalkorpi K, Koivisto VA, Nikkila EA. Severity, duration, and mechanisms of insulin resistance during acute infections. J Clin Endocrinol Metab 1989; 69:317–323.
290. Banck G, Forsgren A. Many bacterial species are mitogenic for human blood lymphocytes. Scand J Immunol 1978; 8:347–354.
291. Cavaillon JM. The role of bacterial polyclonal activators in autoimmunity. Nouv Presse Med 1982; 11:3125–3129.
292. Denicoff KD, Rubinow DR, Papa MZ, Simpson C, Seipp CA, Lotze MT, Chang AE, Rosenstein D, Rosenberg SA. The neuropsychiatric effects of treatment with interleukin-2 and lymphokine activated killer cells. Ann Intern Med 1987; 107:293–300.
293. McDonald EM, Mann AH, Thomas HC. Interferons as mediators of psychiatric morbidity. Lancet 1987; 2:1175–1177.
294. Grau GE, Fajardo LF, Piguet PF, Allet B, Lambert PH, Vassalli P. Tumor necrosis factor (cachectin) as an essential mediator in murine cerebral malaria. Science 1987; 237:1210–1212.
295. Havell EA. Evidence that tumor necrosis factor has an important role in antibacterial resistance. J Immunol 1989; 143:2894–2899.
296. Sheppard BC, Fraker DL, Norton JA. Prevention and treatment of endotoxin and sepsis lethality with recombinant human tumor necrosis factor. Surgery 1989; 106:156–161.
297. Ramachandra RN, Sehon AH, Berczi I. Neuro-hormonal host defence in endotoxin shock. Brain Behav Immun 1992; 6:157–169.
298. Bertini R, Bianchi M, Ghezzi P. Adrenalectomy sensitizes mice to the lethal effects of interleukin-1 and tumor necrosis factor. J Exp Med 1988; 167:1708–1712.
299. Zuckerman SH, Shellhaas J, Butler LD. Differential regulation of lipopolysaccharide-induced interleukin-1 and tumor necrosis factor synthesis. Effects of endogenous and exogenous glucocorticoids and the role of the pituitary-adrenal axis. Eur J Immunol 1989; 19:301–305.
300. Bertok L. Bacterial endotoxins and nonspecific resistance. In: Ninnemann JL, ed. Traumatic Injury. Baltimore: University Park Press; 1983:119–123.
301. Nagy E, Chalmers IM, Baragar FD, Friesen HG, Berczi I. Prolactin deficiency in rheumatoid arthritis. J Rheum 1991; 18:1662–1668.
302. Tracey KJ, Lowry SF, Cerami A. Cachectin: A hormone that triggers acute shock and chronic cachexia. J Infect Dis 1988; 157:413–420.
303. Berczi I. Cancer immunology—quo vadis? An overview. J Exp Clin Cancer Res 1983; 2:135–144.
304. Harbour D, Blalock JE. Lymphocytes and lymphocytic hormones in pregnancy. Prog Neuroendocrinimmunol 1989; 2:55–63.
305. Potter EL, Craig JM. Pathology of the Fetus and the Infant, 3rd ed. Chicago: Year Book; 1975.
306. Jerne NK. Towards a network theory of the immune system. Ann Immunol (Paris) 1974; 125C:373–389.
307. Berthelsen S, Pettinger WA. Functional basis for classification of alpha-adrenergic receptors. Life Sci 1977; 21:595–606.
308. Motulsky HJ, Insel PA. Adrenergic receptors in man direct identification, physiologic regulation, and clinical alterations. N Engl J Med 1982; 307:18–29.

309. Crabtree GR. Contingent genetic regulatory events in T lymphocyte activation. Science 1989; 243:355–361.
310. Tordai A, Sarkadi B, Gorog G, Gardos G. Inhibition of the CD3-mediated calcium signal by protein kinase C activators in human T (Jurkat) lymphoblastoid cells. Immunol Lett 1989; 20:47–52.
311. Rebor RW, Miyake A, Low TLK, Goldstein AL. Thymosin stimulates secretion of luteinizing hormone releasing factor. Science 1981; 214:699–673.
312. Malaise MG, Hazee-Hagelstein MT, Reuter AM, Vrinds-Gevaert Y, Goldstein G, Franchimont P. Thymopoietin and thymopentin enhance the levels of ACTH, beta-endorphin, and beta-lipotropin from rat pituitary cells in vitro. Acta Endocrinol 1987; 115:455–460.
313. Milenkovic L, McCann SM. Effects of thymosin alpha-1 on pituitary hormone release. Neuroendocrinology 1992; 55:14–19.
314. Badamchian M, Spangelo BL, Damavandy T, MacLeod RM, Goldstein AL. Complete amino acid sequence analysis of a peptide isolated from the thymus that enhances release of growth hormone and prolactin. Endocrinology 1991; 128:1580–1588.
315. Nakamura H, Motoyoshi S, Kadokawa T. Anti-inflammatory action of interleukin 1 through the pituitary-adrenal axis in rats. Eur J Pharmacol 1988; 141:67–73.
316. Tsagarakis S, Gillies G, Rees LH, Besser M, Grossman A. Interleukin-1 directly stimulates the release of corticotrophin releasing factor from rat hypothalamus. Neuroendocrinology 1989; 49:98–101.
317. Uehara A, Gottschall PE, Dahl RR, Arimura A. Interleukin-1 stimulates ACTH release by an indirect action which requires endogenous corticotropin releasing factor. Endocrinology 1987; 121:1580–1582.
318. Weidenfeld J, Abramsky O, Ovadia H. Effect of interleukin-1 on ACTH and corticosterone secretion in dexamethasone and adrenalectomized pretreated male rats. Neuroendocrinology 1989; 50:650–654.
319. Yamaguchi M, Yoshimoto Y, Komura H, Koike K, Matsuzaki N, Hirota K, Miyake A, Tanizawa O. Interleukin-1-beta and tumour necrosis factor-alpha stimulate the release of gonadotropin-releasing hormone and interleukin-6 by primary cultured rat hypothalamic cells. Acta Endocrinol 1990; 123: 476–480.
320. Kalra PS, Fuentes M, Sahu A, Kalra SP. Endogenous opioid peptides mediate the interleukin-1-induced inhibition of the release of luteinizing hormone (LH)-releasing hormone and LH. Endocrinology 1990; 127:2381–2386.
321. Bernton EW, Beach JE, Holaday JW, Smallridge RC, Fein HG. Release of multiple hormones by a direct action of interleukin-1 on pituitary cells. Science 1987; 238:519–521.
322. Spangelo BL, Jarvis WD, Judd AM, MacLeod RM. Induction of interleukin-6 release by interleukin-1 in rat anterior pituitary cells invitro—evidence for an eicosanoid-dependent mechanism. Endocrinology 1991; 129:2886–2894.
323. Fukata J, Usui T, Naitoh Y, Nakai Y, Imura H. Effects of recombinant human interleukin-1α, -1β, -2, and -6 on ACTH synthesis and release in the mouse pituitary tumour cell line AtT-20. J Endocrinol 1989; 122: 33–39.

324. Fagarasan MO, Aiello F, Muegge K, Durum S, Axelrod J. Interleukin 1 induces β-endorphin secretion via Fos and Jun in AtT-20 pituitary cells. Proc Natl Acad Sci USA 1990; 87:7871–7874.

325. Karanth S, McCann SM. Anterior pituitary hormone controlled by interleukin-2. Proc Natl Acad Sci USA 1991; 88:2961–2965.

326. Smith LR, Brown SL, Blalock JE. Interleukin-2 induction of ACTH secretion: Presence of an interleukin-2 receptor alpha-chain-like molecule on pituitary cells. J Neuroimmunol 1989; 21:249–254.

327. Denicoff KD, Durkin TM, Lotze MT, Quinlan PE, Davis CL, Listwak SJ, Rosenberg SA, Rubinow DR. The neuroendocrine effects of interleukin-2 treatment. J Clin Endocrinol Metab 1989; 69:402–410.

328. Lissoni P, Barni S, Archili C, Cattaneo G, Rovelli F, Conti A, Maestroni GJ, Tancini G. Endocrine effects of a 24-hour intravenous infusion of interleukin-2 in the immunotherapy of cancer. Anticancer Res 1990; 10: 753–758.

329. Lyson K, Milenkovic L, McCann SM. The stimulatory effect of interleukin 6 on corticotropin-releasing hormone and thyrotropin-releasing hormone release in vitro. Prog Neuroendocrinimmunol 1991; 4:161–165.

330. Vankelecom H, Carmeliet P, Heremans H, Van Damme J, Dijkmans R, Billian A, Denef C. Interferon-γ inhibits stimulated adrenocorticotropin, prolactin, and growth hormone secretion in normal rat anterior pituitary cell cultures. Endocrinology 1990; 126:2919–2926.

331. Gonzalez MC, Riedel M, Rettori V, Yu WH, McCann SM. Effect of recombinant human γ-interferon on the release of anterior pituitary hormones. Prog Neuroendocrinimmunol 1990; 3:49–54.

332. Gonzalez MC, Aguila MC, McCann SM. In vitro effects of recombinant human γ-interferon on growth hormone release. Prog Neuroendocrinimmunol 1991; 4:222–227.

333. Pang XP, Hershman JM, Mirell CJ, Pe Kary AE. Impairment of hypothalamic-pituitary-thyroid function in rats treated with human recombinant tumor necrosis factor-α (cachectin). Endocrinology 1989; 125:76–84.

334. Yamaguchi M, Sakata M, Matsuzaki N, Koike K, Miyake A, Tanizawa O. Induction by tumor necrosis factor-alpha of rapid release of immunoreactive and bioactive luteinizing hormone from rat pituitary cell in vitro. Neuroendocrinology 1990; 52:468–472.

335. Gaillard RC, Turnill D, Sappino P, Muller AF. Tumor necrosis factor α inhibits the hormonal response of the pituitary gland to hypothalamic releasing factors. Endocrinology 1990; 127:101–106.

336. D'Urso R, Falaschi P, Canfalone G, Carusi E, Proietti A, Barnaba V, Balsano F. Neuroendocrine effects of recombinant α-interferon administration in humans. Prog Neuroendocrinimmunol 1991; 4:20–25.

337. Muller H, Hammes E, Hiemke C, Hess G. Interferon-alpha-2-induced stimulation of ACTH and cortisol secretion in man. Neuroendocrinology 1991; 54:499–503.

338. Bernardini R, Kamilaris TC, Calogero AE, Johnson EO, Gomez MT, Gold PW, Chrousos GP. Interactions between tumor necrosis factor-α, hypothalamic corticotropin-releasing hormone, and adrenocorticotropin secretion in the rat. Endocrinology 1990; 126:2876–2881.

339. Murata T, Ying SY. Transforming growth factor-β and activin inhibit basal secretion of prolactin in a pituitary monolayer culture system. Proc Soc Exp Biol Med 1991; 198:599–605.

340. Delidow BC, Billis WM, Agarwal P, White BA. Inhibition of prolactin gene transcription by transforming growth factor-β in GH3 cells. Mol Endocrinol 1991; 5:1716–1722.

341. Elsasser TH, Caperna TJ, Fayer R. Tumor necrosis factor-α affects growth hormone secretion by a direct pituitary interaction. Proc Soc Exp Biol Med 1991; 198:547–554.

342. Camoratto AM, Grandison L. Platelet-activating factor stimulates prolactin release from dispersed rat anterior pituitary cells in vitro. Endocrinology 1989; 124:1502–1506.

343. Bernardini R, Calogero AE, Ehrlich YH, Brucke T, Chrousos GP, Gold PW. The alkyl-ether phospholipid platelet-activating factor is a stimulator of the hypothalamic-pituitary-adrenal axis in the rat. Endocrinology 1989; 125: 1067–1073.

344. Rougeot C, Junier MP, Minary P, Weidenfeld J, Braquet P, Dray F. Intracerebroventricular injection of platelet-activating factor induces secretion of adrenocorticotropin, beta-endorphin, and corticosterone in conscious rats: A possible link between the immune and nervous systems. Neuroendocrinology 1990; 51:267–275.

345. Sullivan NJ, Tashjian AH Jr. Platelet-derived growth factor selectively decreases prolactin production in pituitary cells in culture. Endocrinology 1983; 113:639–645.

346. Drouhault R, Abrous N, David JP, Dufy B. Bradykinin parallels thyrotropin-releasing hormone actions on prolactin release from rat anterior pituitary cells. Neuroendocrinology 1987; 46:360–364.

347. Jones TH, Brown BL, Dobson PRM. Bradykinin stimulates phosphoinositide metabolism and prolactin secretion in rat anterior pituitary cells. J Mol Endocrinol 1989; 2:47–53.

348. Knigge U, Bach FW, Matzen S, Bang P, Warberg J. Effect of histamine on the secretion of pro-opiomelancortin derived peptides in rats. Acta Endocrinol 1988; 119:312–319.

349. Kjaer A, Knigge U, Warberg J. The prolactin releasing effect of histamine is unrelated to its vascular action. Acta Endocrinol 1990; 122:49–54.

350. Donoso AE, Zarate MB. Release of prolactin and luteinizing hormone by histamine agonists in ovariectomized, steroid-treated rats under ether anesthesia. Exp Brain Res 1983; 52:277–280.

7
Hormonal Interactions Between the Thymus and the Pituitary

MIREILLE DARDENNE AND WILSON SAVINO

The existence of a physiological immunoneuroendocrine network working in fine harmony, and clearly contributing to homeostasis, has now been demonstrated. In this context, nervous, endocrine, and immune systems communicate with each other, using common mediators and respective receptors.[1]

An interesting aspect of this network involves the interactions between the thymus and the pituitary. In this chapter we shall discuss these interactions, focusing on the effects of pituitary hormones on the thymic microenvironment, and more particularly on its endocrine function. Before presenting the recent contributions to this field, we shall briefly discuss some general aspects of the microenvironmental compartment of the thymus, and its involvement in intrathymic T-cell differentiation.

Intrathymic T-Cell Differentiation

The thymus is a central lymphoid organ in which bone marrow-derived T-cell precursors undergo a complex process of maturation, eventually leading to the migration of positively selected thymocytes to the T-dependent areas of peripheral lymphoid organs.[2] This differentiation process allows T lymphocytes to distinguish self from nonself proteins, representing the vast majority of the so-called T-cell repertoire, which is generated following the occurrence of T-cell receptor gene rearrangements.

Key events of intrathymic T-cell differentiation are driven by the influence of the thymic microenvironment, which is a tridimentional network composed of distinct cell types comprising epithelial cells, macrophages, and dendritic cells, as well as extracellular matrix elements.

The thymic epithelium is the major component of the thymic microenvironment and exerts important and multifaceted influences on early events of T-cell differentiation. This is accomplished, at the least, in two distinct ways: (1) cell-to-cell contacts, including those occurring through classical adhesion molecules,[3] and the paramount interactions with differentiating thymocytes that are mediated by the major histocompatibility complex products, highly expressed on thymic epithelial cell membranes;[4-7] and (2) secretion of interleukins 1, 3, and 6,[8,9] granulocyte/macrophage colony-stimulating factor,[10] and various thymic hormones.[11]

Thymic Hormonal Function

It is now well established that some stages of T-lymphocyte maturation are regulated by a group of thymus-derived polypeptides called thymic hormones, in association with other signals.[11] Several thymic hormones have been described but it is not yet known how many molecules intervene physiologically as mediators of thymic humoral function. Several polypeptides have been extracted from the thymus. Those which have been chemically well defined constitute a series of molecular entities with no apparent relationship. This series presently includes 4 distinct peptides: thymosin-α1, thymopoietin, thymulin, and thymic humoral factor γ2. Their molecular weights range between 800 and 5000 d.

Thymosins

Thymosins constitute a family of polypeptides isolated from the thymus. A partially purified thymosin preparation from calf thymus, termed thymosin fraction 5 (TF5),[12] has been studied extensively for biological activities and in clinical trials.[13] It is composed of a group of 20–40 polypeptides with molecular weights under 15,000 d. This first peptide to be isolated from fraction 5 was thymosin-α1 (T-α1), an acidic peptide (pI = 4.2) containing 28 amino acid residues with a molecular weight of 3108 d and an acetylated HN_2 terminus. T-α1 has been synthesized by recombinant techniques. It has been shown to induce the expression of some T-cell differentiation antigens, Thy-1, and, Lyt-1, -2, and -3, to increase murine lymphocyte mitogenic responses, stimulate antibody and lymphokine production, and modulate terminal deoxynucleotidyl-transferase expression.[14] Some evidence suggests that T-α1 is a fragment of a larger native polypeptide, prothymosin, a precursor of T-α1, which is found in highest concentrations in the thymus but also in the spleen, lung, kidney, and brain.[15] Some other peptides such as thymosin-β4, composed of 43 aminoacid residues with a molecular weight of 4982 d and a pI of 5.1,[16] which increases terminal deoxynucleotidyl transferase (TDT) activity, and thymosin-α7, which in vitro enhances suppressor T cells, were also isolated from TF5. Other peptides, such as thymosin-β8 and -β9 have also been isolated, but no biological activity has been described.

Thymopoietin

Thymopoietin was isolated from calf thymus by G. Goldstein,[17] by means of its neuromuscular effect rather than its action on the immune system, but thymopoietin was shown ultimately to induce various T-cell specific alloantigens in vitro. The entire aminoacid sequences of bovine and human thymopoietin have been established.[17] Thymopoietin is a polypeptide of 49 aminoacids. Its biological activity is comprised in the pentapeptide thymopentin (TP5), including residues 32 to 36 (Arg-Lys-Asp-Val-Tyr).[18] In addition, another peptide related to thymopoietin has also been extracted from spleen. This peptide, named splenin, differs from thymopoietin by two minor changes, one being located in the active site.

Thymopoietin binds cell membrane receptors present on prothymocytes and mature T cells, resulting in stimulation of adenylate or guanydilate cyclase. Recent studies have shown that thymopoietin binds with high affinity to the acetylcholine receptor. Thymopoietin or TP5 has been shown to enhance several T-cell functions in vivo (rejection of 3LL carcinoma, prevention of autoimmunity in mice, and generation of cytotoxic T cells).

Thymic Humoral Factor (THF)[19]

THF was isolated by N. Trainin from the calf thymus using a graft-versus-host biological assay in vitro. THF restores immune competence in neonatally thymectomized mice.[19] Subsequently, the same authors, using various chromatographic systems, isolated THF2 from crude THF extract and reported that it is an octapeptide (Leu-Glu-Asp-Gly-Pro-Lys-Phe-Leu).[20] Both natural and synthetic peptides have the same biological activity in vivo and in vitro, inducing an increase in lymphocyte proliferation and interleukin (IL)-2 production by spleen cells from neonatally thymectomized (Tx) mice as well as from lymphocytes from patients treated for immune impairment.

Thymulin

Thymulin, initially called FTS, was purified from pig serum using the rosette assay. Thymulin was also isolated from human serum and calf thymus, and is now known to be a nonapeptide (<Glu-Ala-Lys-Ser-Gln-Gly-Gly-Ser-Asn) produced exclusively by the thymic epithelium.[21] Both natural and synthetic products bind zinc with a Kd about 10^{-7} M, and the presence of this metal is necessary for the expression of the biological activity of the peptide.[22] Nuclear magnetic resonance (NMR) studies

demonstrated that the Ser 4 and 8, and Asn 9 residues are implicated in the metal binding. Thymulin has no species specificity and is found in the circulation of a wide range of species, and its level is strictly age dependant.

Thymulin appears to act exclusively on T lymphocytes by binding to T-cell membrane receptors with high affinity. It is noteworthy that this peptide has been shown to be involved in the process of T-cell antigen differentiation, and to enhance the functions of various T-cell subsets. Thymulin acting at high doses targets mainly suppressor cells, and in normal recipients appears to be particularly involved in the prolongation of skin graft survival, the suppression of autoantibody production, and the abrogation of delayed-type hypersensitivity. At low doses it also produces a helper effect on the immune system, increasing the release of IL-2 by normal thymocytes or nude mouse spleen cells, enhancing the antibody production in aging mice and stimulating the mitogen-induced responsiveness in thymectomized animals.[11]

It has been shown that thymulin production by thymic epithelial cells (TEC) is under the control of classical regulatory mechanisms involving the levels of thymulin itself and of other hormones such as thyroid steroid, and pituitary hormones.[23]

Modulation of Pituitary Hormones by Thymic Peptides

In addition to their immunopotentiating properties, some thymic peptides (mainly thymosins and thymopoietin) are also able to regulate pituitary gland function. This line of evidence was initially suggested by the observation that in mice, neonatal thymectomy induced a marked degranulation of the acidophilic cells of the anterior pituitary.[24] Moreover, the acidophilic cells found in anterior pituitary glands from athymic nude animals were smaller, and the number of granules was lower than those found in pituitaries of normal littermates.[25] In addition, the levels of prolactin found in these animals were reduced, but were restored to normal after neonatal thymus grafting.[26] The levels of growth hormone (GH) were also affected by thymus ablation, since neonatal thymectomy in mice induced a decrease in GH level in adulthood.[27]

In addition to the influence exerted on GH and prolactin (PRL) release, it was also demonstrated that the thymus may also act to regulate gonadotropin secretion. Thus, neonatal thymectomy performed in mice induced an ovarian dysgenesis that could be reversed by thymic grafting performed by day 7.[28] Moreover, concentrations of serum and pituitary luteinizing hormone (LH) and follicle-stimulating hormone (FSH) were significantly reduced in nude mice,[29,30] and could by restored to normal by thymic implantation at birth.[31] These results strongly suggested that the thymus could regulate pituitary hormone release. Studies using purified thymic peptides confirmed these findings.[32–37]

Stimulation of Pituitary Peptide Release by Thymosins

Recently, a number of in vitro and in vivo studies have demonstrated that thymosins exert a direct effect on anterior pituitary function. Thus, certain peptides extracted from TP5 were able to regulate some hypothalamic neuroendocrine circuits. In perfusion studies of medial basal hypothalamic and anterior pituitary tissues, TF5 and one of its peptide constituants, thymosin-β4 (T-β4), were able to stimulate the release of LH-releasing factor from the hypothalamus, and LH from the pituitary.[32] In addition, intracerebro-ventricular injection of T-β4 increased LH release in the mouse.[33]

More recent studies indicated that components of TF5 were also able to stimulate the production of ACTH, β-endorphin, PRL, and GH by cultured pituitary cells,[34,35] and enhance in vivo the release of ACTH, β-endorphin, and cortisol in prepubertal monkeys.[36] Moreover, TF5 induced the release of PRL from GH3 cells in a time- and dose-dependent manner.[37] However, this effect was not observed with either T-α1 or T-β4, suggesting that another peptide could be involved in this specific effect.

Using simple reverse phase high performance liquid chromatography (HPLC), Badamchian et al. recently isolated and characterized an unidentified peptide component, named MB-35, which is able to stimulate the in vitro release of GH and PRL from the anterior pituitary more effectively than does TF5.[38] Structurally this peptide is a basic molecule of 35 amino acid residues with a molecular weight of 3756 d, and is identical to a fragment of a nuclear protein (histone H2A) isolated from human, rat, chicken, and bovine thymus. The significance of the relationship between peptide MB-35 and histone H2A remains unclear. However, recent reports suggest that certain histones may exhibit some types of hormone-like activity.[39]

Interestingly, another thymic peptide, homeostatic thymus hormone (HTH), consisting of 2 polypeptide chains (HTH-α and HTH-β), has recently been purified, and the primary structures of the polypeptide chains were found to be identical to those of histones H2A and H2B, respectively.[40] This histone dimer was shown to markedly reduce GH secretion, an effect that was much weaker in old animals,[41] activate the adrenal axis in young rats and to a lesser extent in old rats,[42] and to possess thyrotropin (TSH)-inhibiting activity in young but not in aging animals.[41] These effects would seem to suggest the existence of an age-dependent desensitization of the neuroendocrine system to these hormonal signals.

Stimulation of ACTH and
β-Endorphin Release by Thymopentin

The two thymic polypeptides, thymopoietin and thymopentin, have been shown to influence immunoregulation by several mechanisms.[43] Thymopentin has been proposed as a therapy in diseases producing major immune abnormalities, such as rheumatoid arthritis. This treatment induced an improvement, within 2 weeks, of some clinical parameters such as pain and joint swelling,[44] possibly mediated through interactions with antiinflammatory (ACTH) and pain-relieving (β-endorphin) hormone producing cells. This hypothesis was tested in vitro on isolated rat pituitary cells.

Thymopentin was able to enhance the in vitro levels of ACTH, β-endorphin, and β-lipotropin in a time- and dose-dependant fashion, in a range of physiological concentrations.[45] This effect was restricted to molecular fragments of the common precursor preproopiomelanocortin (POMC); the levels of other hormones such as GH, PRL, LH, TSH, and FSH were not altered.

The Thymic Epithelium: A Target for
Neuroendocrine Control

Much data have recently accumulated showing that the thymic microenvironment is under neuroendocrine control.[23] Treatment of mice with triiodothyronine in vivo and in vitro induces an increase in thymulin production,[23,46,47] a finding in keeping with those studies demonstrating that the thyroid hormone status in humans modulates thymulin serum levels.[47] Additionally, we demonstrated that thymic hormone production is modulated by adrenal and sexual steroids.[48] Interestingly, we found that glucocorticoid hormones also modulate cytokeratin expression and extracellular matrix production.[49]

In Vivo and In Vitro Modulation of the
Thymic Epithelium by Growth Hormone

In addition to thyroid and steroid hormones, pituitary hormones such as PRL and GH can affect some aspects of TEC physiology. Initial data concerning the role of GH on the thymic endocrine function came from studies on the dwarf mouse, which exhibits a precocious age-dependent decline of thymulin serum levels.[50] These findings were supported by those of Goff et al.[51] who showed that treatment with bovine GH partially restored the low thymulin serum levels observed in aged dogs. More recently, we found that GH treatment increased thymulin serum levels in both young and aging mice.[52]

In addition to its action on thymulin secretion, GH was shown to have a stimulatory role on the thymus. This demonstration came from experiments in which GH-secreting GH3 pituitary tumor cells, grafted into old rats, restored thymus structure as well as T-cell proliferation and IL-2 synthesis.[53] These findings were in agreement with previous data showing that treatment of dwarf mice with GH and thyroxine reconstituted their thymic function and markedly prolonged the lifespan of these animals.[54]

The role of GH in TEC physiology apparently depends on a direct action of the hormone upon the epithelial cells, since in vitro GH can stimulate thymulin production by pure TEC cultures.[55,56] Additionally, GH receptors have been demonstrated in both human and murine TEC.[57] However, it should be kept in mind that such GH effects are likely mediated by the production of insulin-like growth factor 1 (IGF-1). This hypothesis is supported by the fact that the in vitro GH-induced increase in thymulin production can be prevented by anti-IGF-1 or anti-IGF-1 receptor antibodies.[56] Moreover, IGF-1 alone enhances thymic hormone production and TEC proliferation. Lastly, increased thymulin levels in acromegalic patients are positively correlated to IGF-1 levels, but not necessarily to circulating values of GH.[56,58] Taken together, these data support the hypothesis that TEC constitutively produce IGF-1 and express IGF-1 receptors, both of which are involved in an autocrine IGF-1 dependent circuit (linked to the GH-related endocrine pathway) modulating TEC physiology.

Prolactin: A Pleiotropic Modulator of the Thymic Epithelium

Pioneer work by Russel and coworkers demonstrated that in vivo injection of anti-PRL serum resulted in changes in thymocyte subpopulations, as expressed by an increase in the percentages of CD4+ single-positive cells.[59] Moreover, injection of bromocriptine, which blocks endogenous PRL production, promoted a similar effect. More recently, we carried out studies searching for potential influences of PRL upon the thymic epithelium. We first observed that injections of PRL into young, normal mice increased serum thymulin levels, and conversely, hypoprolactinemia induced by bromocriptine had opposite effects. Moreover, PRL treatment of old individuals or dwarf mice, both having low thymulin serum levels, significantly augmented thymic hormone production.[55] This resulted from a direct effect of PRL upon the epithelial cells since this result could be reproduced in vitro using human and murine TEC cultures.[55]

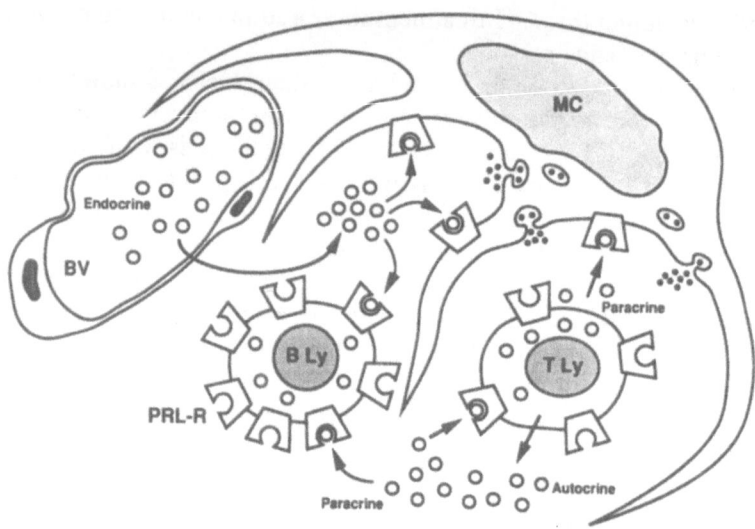

FIGURE 7.1. Proposed endocrine, paracrine, and autocrine pathways for prolactin (PRL) to modulate the thymic lymphoid and microenvironmental compartments. In this hypothetical model, PRL secreted by pituitary cells or thymocytes (T Ly), acts upon the distinct cell types, via specific receptors (PRL-R), which are known to be expressed on the membranes of both thymocytes and TEC. BV: blood vessel.

Our results are of special interest because we clearly demonstrated that PRL effects upon TEC are not restricted to thymic endocrine function, since this hormone is also able to enhance the expression of high molecular weight cytokeratins, and increase TEC proliferation in vitro.[55] Furthermore, PRL augments extracellular matrix production by growing TEC, and increases thymocyte/TEC adhesion (Mello-Coelho et al., in preparation).

The Thymic Epithelium Expresses GH and PRL Receptors

To further validate the various experimental and human data discussed above, it appeared necessary to demonstrate specific receptors for GH and PRL in thymic epithelial cells. Binding experiments using radio-labeled GH allowed us to prove the existence of GH receptors in both human and murine TEC.[57] In addition, using immunochemistry and molecular biology, we found that the thymic epithelium also expresses a PRL receptor (PRL-R), both in situ and in vitro. Interestingly, appropriate amounts of anti-PRL-R monoclonal antibodies, once in contact with cultured TEC, revealed a PRL agonist or antagonist effect, in terms of modulating thymulin production and TEC proliferation.[60]

Conclusions

Taken together, the data summarized above clearly indicate that pituitary hormones, namely prolactin and growth hormone, should be regarded as relevant modulators of the thymic microenvironment, and more particularly of its epithelial component. It is noteworthy that these hormones augment at least one thymocyte differentiation factor, such as thymulin, and in vitro enhance TEC-thymocyte adhesion, thus leading to the more general hypothesis that intrathymic events of T-cell differentiation may be under pituitary hormone control (Figure 7.1).

Conversely, the possibility that thymic hormones can modulate the physiology of pituitary cells is attractive and should be more extensively investigated. We hope such studies will provide additional arguments for the existence of a bidirectional thymus/pituitary physiological circuitry.

Acknowledgments. This work was partially funded by grants from CNP$_q$ (Brazil) and INSERM (France), grant 492 NS 2.

References

1. Blalock JE. Neuroimmunoendocrinology. Chem Immunol 1992; 52:1–190.
2. Van Ewijk W. T-cell differentiation is influenced by thymic microenvironments. Annu Rev Immunol 1991; 9:591–615.
3. Nonoyama S, Nakayama M, Shiohara T, Yata J. Only dull CD3+ thymocytes bind to thymic epithelial cells. The binding is elicited by both CD2/LFA-3 and LFA-1/ICAM-1 interactions. Eur J Immunol 1989; 19:1631–1635.
4. Janossy G, Thomas JA, Bollum FL, Granzer G, Pizzolo G, Bradstock KF, Wong L, Ganeshagun K, Hoffbrand AB. The human thymic microenvironment: An immunohistologic study. J Immunol 1980; 125:202–212.
5. Jenkinson EJ, Van Ewijk W, Owen JJ. Major histocompatibility complex antigen expression on the epithelium of developing thymus in normal and nude mice. J Exp Med 1981; 153:280–292.
6. Savino W, Manganella G, Verley JM, Wolff A, Berrih S, Levasseur P, Binet JP, Dardenne M, Bach JF. Thymoma epithelial cells secrete thymic hormone but do not express class II antigens of the major histocompatibility complex. J Clin Invest 1985; 76:1140–1146.
7. Van Ewijk W, Ron Y, Monaco J, Kapplier J, Marrack P, Le Meur H, Gerlinger P, Durand B, Benoist C, Mattis D. Compartimentalization of MHC class II gene expression in transgenic mice. Cell 1988; 53:357–370.
8. Le PT, Tuck DT, Dinarello CA, Haynes BF, Singer KH. Thymic epithelial cells produce interleukin 1. J Immunol 1988; 138:2520–2525.
9. Le PT, Lazorich S, Whichard LP, Yang YC, Clarck SC, Haynes BF, Singer KH. Human thymic epithelial cells produce IL-6, granulocyte-monocye CSF, and leukemia inhibitory factor. J Immunol 1990; 145:3310–3315.
10. Le PT, Kurtzberg J, Brant SL, Nieldel JE, Haynes BH, Singer KH. Human thymic epithelial cells produce granulocyte and macrophage colony-stimulating factors. J Immunol 1988; 141:1211–1218.

11. Bach JF. Thymic hormones. Clinical Immunology and Allergy 1983; 3:133–156.
12. Low TLK, Goldstein AL. Thymic hormones: An overview. In: Di sabata G, Langone JJ, Van vunakis H, eds. Immunological Techniques. Orlando: Acad. Press; 1985:213–219.
13. Low TLK, Goldstein AL. Thymosins. Isolation, structural studies, and biological activities. In: Goldstein AL, eds. Thymic hormones and lymphokines. Basic Chemistry and clinical applications. New York: Plenum Press; 1984:21–35.
14. Low TLK, Goldstein AL. Thymosin alpha1 and polypeptide beta1. In: Di sabato G, Langone JJ, Vanvunakis H, eds. Immunochemical techniques. Orlando: Acad. Press; 1985; 116:233–255.
15. Haritos AA, Gooddall GJ, Horecker BL. Distribution of prothymosin alpha in rat tissues. Proc Natl Acad Sci USA 1984; 81:1391–1396.
16. Low TLK, Goldstein AL. Chemical characterization of thymosin beta 4. J Biol Chem 1982; 257:1000–1006.
17. Andhya T, Schlesinger DH, Goldstein G. Complete aminoacid sequences of bovine thymopoietin I, II, III: Closely homologous polypeptides. Biochemistry 1981; 20:6195–6202.
18. Goldstein G, Scheid MP, Boyse EA, Schlesinger DH, Van Wauve J. A synthetic pentapeptide with biological activity characteristic of the thymic hormone thymopoietin. Science 1979; 204:1309–1313.
19. Trainin N, Handzell ZV, Pecht M. Biological and clinical properties of THF. Thymus 1985; 7:137–150.
20. Burstein Y, Buchner V, Pecht M, Trainin N. Thymic humoral factor gamma2: Purification and aminoacid sequence of an immunoregulatory peptide from calf thymus. Biochemistry 1988; 27:4066–4071.
21. Bach JF, Dardenne M, Pleau JM, Rosa J. Biochemical characterization of a serum thymic hormone. Nature 1977; 266:55–56.
22. Dardenne M, Pleau JM, Nabarra B, Lefrancier P, Derrien M, Choay J, Bach JF. Contribution of zinc and other metals to the biological activity of the serum thymic factor (FTS). Proc Natl Acad Sci USA 1982; 79:5370–5373.
23. Dardenne M, Savino W. Neuroendocrine control of thymic epithelium: Modulation of thymic endocrine function, cytokeratin expression, and cell proliferation by hormones and neuropeptides. Prog Neuroendocrinimmunol 1990; 3:18–25.
24. Baroni C. Thymus, peripheral lymphoid tissues, and immunological responsiveness of the pituitary dwarf mouse. Experientia 1967; 23:282–284.
25. Ruitenberg EJ, Berkvens JM. The morphology of the endocrine system in congenitally athymic (nude) mice. J Pathol 1977; 121:225–231.
26. Pierpaoli W, Kopp HG, Bianchi E. Interdependence of thymic and neuroendocrine functions in ontogeny. Clin Exp Immunol 1976; 24:501–506.
27. Michael SD, Taguchi O, Nishizuka Y. Effect of neonatal thymectomy on ovarian development and plasma LH, FSH, GH, and PRL in the mouse. Biol Reprod 1980; 22:343–350.
28. Nishizuka Y, Sakakura T. Thymus and reproduction: Sex-linked dysgenesis of the gonad after neonatal thymectomy in mice. Science 1969; 166:753–755.

29. Rebar RW, Morandini IC, Erickson GF, Petze JE. The hormonal basis of reproductive defects in athymic mice: Diminished gonadotropin concentrations in prepubertal females. Endocrinology 1981; 108:120–126.

30. Rebar RW, Morandini IC, Petze JE, Erickson GF. Hormonal basis of reproductive defects in athymic mice: Gonadotropins and testosterone in males. Biol Reprod 1982; 27:1267–1276.

31. Rebar RW, Morandini IC, Bernirschke K, Petze JE. Reduced gonadotropins in athymic mice: Prevention by thymic transplantation. Endocrinology 1980; 107:2130–2132.

32. Rebar RW, Miyake A, Low TL, Goldstein AL. Thymosin stimulates secretion of luteinizing hormone-releasing factor. Science 1981; 214:669–671.

33. Hall JR, Mcgillis JP, Spangelo BL, Palaszynzki E, Moody T, Goldstein AL. Evidence for a neuroendocrine-thymus axis mediated by thymosin polypeptides. In: Serrou B, Rosenfeld C, Daniels JC, Saunders JP, eds. Current Concepts in Human Immunology and Cancer Immunomodulation. Amsterdam: Elsevier; 1982:653–660.

34. Spangelo BL, Judd AM, Ross PC, Login IS, Jarvis WD, Badamchian M, Goldstein AL, Mac Leod RM. Thymosin fraction 5 stimulates prolactin and growth hormone release from anterior pituitary. Endocrinology 1987; 121: 2035–2043.

35. Farah JM, Hall NR, Bishop JF, Goldstein AL, O'Donohue TL. Thymosin fraction 5 stimulates secretion of immunoreactive beta-endorphin in mouse tumor cells. J Neurosci Res 1987; 18:140–146.

36. Healy DL, Hodgen GD, Schulte HM, Chrousos GP, Loriaux DL, Hall NR, Goldstein AL. The thymus-adrenal connection: Thymosin has corticotropin-releasing activity in primates. Science 1983; 222:1353–1355.

37. Spangelo BL, Hall NR, Dunn AJ, Goldstein AL. Thymosin fraction 5 stimulates the release of prolactin from cultured GH_3 cells. Life Sci 1987; 40:283–288.

38. Badamchian M, Spangelo BL, Damavandy T, Mac Leod RM, Goldstein AL. Complete amino acid sequence analysis of a peptide isolated from the thymus that enhances release of growth hormone and prolactin. Endocrinology 1991; 128:1580–1588.

39. Reichhart R, Jornvall H, Carlquist M, Zeppezauer M. The primary structure of two polypeptide chains from preparations of homeostatic thymus hormone (HTH alpha and HTH bet) entire-chain identifies to two histones. FEBS Lett 1985; 188:63–67.

40. Reichhart R, Zeppezauer M, Jornvall H. Preparations of hemeostatic thymus hormone consist predominantly of histones 2A and 2B and suggest additional histone functions. Proc Natl Acad Sci USA 1985; 82:4871–4875.

41. Goya RG, Quigley KL, Takahashi S, Reichhart R, Meites J. Differential effect of homeostatic thymus hormone on plasma thyrotropin and growth hormone in young and old rats. Mech Ageing Dev 1989; 49:119–128.

42. Goya RG, Sosa YE, Quigley KL, Reichhart R, Meites J. Homeostatic thymus hormone stimulates corticosterone secretion in a dose- and age-dependent manner in rats. Neuroendocrinology 1990; 51:59–63.

43. Goldstein G, Audhya T. Thymopoietin to thymopentin experimental studies. In: Sundal E, eds. Thymopentin experimental and clinical medicine. (Survey Immunology Research). Basel: Karger; 1985:1–21.

44. Malaise MG, Hauwaert C, Franchimont P, Danneskiold-Samsoe B, Bach-Andersen R, Gross D, Gerber H, Gerschpacher H, Stocker H, Bolla K. Treatment of active rheumatoid arthritis with slow intravenous injections of thymopentin. A double-blind placebo-controlled randomised study. Lancet 1985; 1:832–836.

45. Malaise MG, Hazee-Hagelstein MT, Reuter AM, Vrinds-Gevaert Y, Goldstein G, Franchimont P. Thymopoietin and thymopentin enhance the levels of ACTH, beta-endorphin and beta-lipotropin from rat pituitary cells in vitro. Acta Endocrinol 1987; 115:455–460.

46. Savino W, Wolff B, Aratan-Spire S, Dardenne M. Thymic hormone containing cells. IV. Fluctuations in the thyroid hormone levels in vivo can modulate the secretion of thymulin by the epithelial cells of young mouse thymus. Clin Exp Immunol 1984; 55:629–635.

47. Fabris N, Mocchegiani E, Mariotti S, Pacini F, Pinchera A. Thyroid function modulates thymic endocrine activity. J Clin Endocrin Metab 1986; 62:474–478.

48. Savino W, Bartoccioni E, Homo-Delarche F, Gagnerault MC, Itoh T, Dardenne M. Thymic hormone containing cells—IX. Steroids in vitro modulate thymulin secretion by human and murine thymic epithelial cells. J Steroid Biochem 1988; 29:135–140.

49. Lannes-Vieira J, Dardenne M, Savino W. Extracellular matrix components of the mouse thymus microenvironment: Ontogenetic studies and modulation by glucocorticoid hormones. J Histochem Cytochem 1991; 39:1539–1546.

50. Pelletier M, Montplaisir S, Dardenne M, Bach JF. Thymic hormone activity and spontaneous autoimmunity in dwarf and their littermates. Immunology 1976; 30:783–788.

51. Goff BL, Roth JA, Arp LH, Incefy GS. Growth hormone treatment stimulates thymulin production in aged dogs. Clin Exp Immunol 1987; 68:580–587.

52. Goya RG, Gagnerault MC, Leite de Moraes MC, Savino W, Dardenne M. In vivo effects of growth hormone on thymus function in aging mice. Brain Behav Immun 1992; 6:341–354.

53. Kelley KW, Brief S, Weatly HJ, Novakofski J, Bechtel PJ, Simon J, Walker EB. GH$_3$ pituitary adenoma cells can reverse thymic aging in rats. Proc Natl Acad Sci USA 1986; 83:5663–5667.

54. Fabris N, Pierpaoli W, Sorkin E. Hormones and the immunological capacity. IV. Restorative effects of developmental hormones lymphocytes on the immunodeficiency syndrome of the dwarf mouse. Clin Exp Immunol 1971; 9:227–240.

55. Dardenne M, Savino W, Gagnerault MC, Itoh T, Bach JF. Neuroendocrine control of thymic hormonal production. I. Prolactin stimulates in vivo and in vitro the production of thymulin by human and murine thymic epithelial cells. Endocrinology 1989; 125:1251–1260.

56. Timsit J, Savino W, Safieh W, Chanson P, Gagnerault MC, Bach JF, Dardenne M. Growth hormone and insulin-like growth factor-1 stimulate hormonal function and proliferation of thymic epithelial cells. J Clin Endocrin Metab 1992; 75:183–188.

57. Ban E, Gagnerault MC, Jammes H, Postel-Vinay MC, Haour F, Dardenne M. Specific binding sites for growth hormone in cultured mouse thymic epithelial cells. Life Sci 1991; 48:2141–2148.

58. Mocchegiani E, Paolucci P, Balsamo A, Cacciari E, Fabris N. Influence of growth hormone on thymic endocrine activity in humans. Horm Res 1990; 33:248–255.
59. Russell DH, Kibler R, Matrisian L, Larson DF, Poulos B, Magun BE. Prolactin receptors on human and B lymphocyte: Antagonisms of prolactin binding by cyclosporine. J Immunol 1985; 134:3027–3031.
60. Dardenne M, Kelly PA, Bach JF, Savino W. Identification and functional activity of prolactin receptors in thymic epithelial cells. Proc Natl Acad Sci USA 1991; 88:9700–9704.

8
Neuroendocrine–Thymus Interactions During Development and Aging

NICOLA FABRIS

A good body of experimental evidences now supports the existence of numerous interactions among the nervous, endocrine, and immune systems. Communication between these networks is regulated by mediator substances, such as hormones, neurotransmitters, and immune-derived cytokines, which are to a large extent shared by the different homeostatic systems. In addition, receptor sites, sensitive to such signals are common to nervous, neuroendocrine, and immune cells (for review see[1-4]).

The existence of signals generated within the immune system, capable of modulating various nervous-neuroendocrine functions, have been suggested by lymphoid ablation studies,[5,6] or through treatment with immunogenic or tolerogenic doses of antigen.[7] The discovery that the majority of such effects could be mimicked by various immune-derived factors, such as thymic peptides and lymphokines, has given a molecular support to those findings.[8,9] Furthermore, the fact that lymphoid and accessory cells may, after antigenic stimulation, synthesize and secrete neurohormonal factors (i.e., adrenocorticotropic hormone (ACTH), growth hormone (GH), thyreotropic stimulating hormone (TSH), prolactine (PRL), gonadotropins, and endogenous oppioid[3]) lends additional support to common signals shared by the immune and the neuroendocrine systems.

Hormones, neurotransmitters, and immune cytokines may exert developmental actions,[8,10] as well as affect the actual performance of mature cells (such as those required to counteract stressful conditions, or antigenic insults).[3,4] The findings related to neuroendocrine–immune interactions responsible for developmental steps should, therefore, be clearly distinguished from those related to emergency events in fully matured systems. The stimuli required to activate a given pathway as well as the end effects, may be quite different, either quantitatively or qualitatively, according to the functional demand, 'morphogenetic' or 'of actual performance' of the organism.

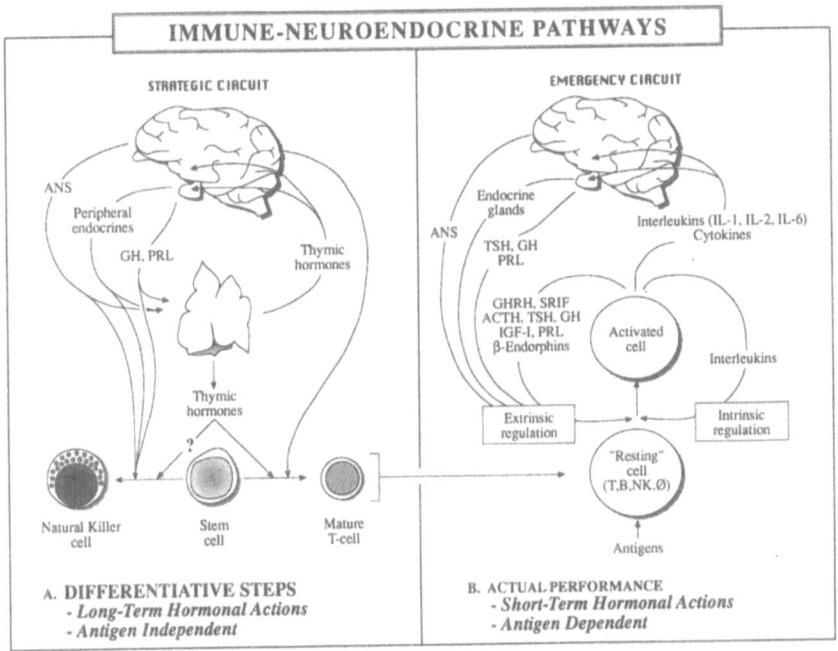

FIGURE 8.1. Schematic representation of the two major pathways of neuroendocrine–immune interactions: A, Strategic circuit; B, Emergency circuit. For explanation see text.

These considerations appear to suggest at least two levels of neuroendocrine–immune interrelationships.[1,10] The first level (strategic circuit) is based on the interactions between the neuroendocrine system and the thymus (Figure 8.1A), an organ reputed to induce proliferation and differentiation of stem cells into mature T lymphocytes. Such interactions should take into account the fact that the thymus is synthesizing and secreting various hormone-like peptides with differentiative properties on the T-cell lineage. The second level (emergency circuit) of interaction is at the periphery (Figure 8.1B), between neuroendocrine signals and the humoral products which are secreted by immune cells during specific reactions to various antigens. The rationale for discriminating these two levels is based on various orders of considerations. The first level of interactions is primarily involved in steps taking place during maturation of both immune and neuroendocrine systems, which in absence of pathological events, are independent with respect to the degree of antigenic stimulation. In fact, neuroendocrine–thymus interactions are observable also in animals maintained under germ-free conditions. On the contrary, the second level of interaction requires the presence of fully differentiated immune cells and the occurrence of a specific antigenic or stress-mediated hormonal stimulus. The main role played by these particular interactions appears to be the normalization of neuroendocrine or immune balance after a sudden alteration by a stressful cognitive or noncognitive event.[10]

The neuroendocrine network is in dynamic change during the life of the individual, since: (1) it develops according to an ordered sequence of events during ontogeny, (2) it shows different profiles during maturity according to sex and biological rhythms, and (3) it suffers from progressive alterations with advancing age.[11]

Also, the immune system and particularly the thymus show sex- and age-dependent modifications from early ontogeny to old age.[12]

This chapter aims to summarize the data available on the possible integration between the neuroendocrine network and thymic function in the development and aging of the strategic circuit.

Neuroendocrine – Thymus Interactions During Ontogeny

During the course of fetal life, humoral factors from both homeostatic systems impact ontogenic steps in an orderly sequence. The interplay of neuroendocrine–immune interactions are believed to be central to this development.

The available data cannot, at present, give a definite and comprehensive picture of these interconnections during ontogeny, but some suggestions can certainly be proposed. Figure 8.2, is a simple overview of two transparencies dealing with neuroendocrine and immune development during ontogeny in the human species. The orderly sequence of events during neuroendocrine and immune development seems to be quite compatible with the existence of bidirectional interactions between the two systems. In fact, the precocious appearance of some pituitary hormones (GH, follicle stimulating hormone, leutinizing hormone, TSH) and insulin in the fetal blood is closely related to the growth of thymus, the appearance of thymic factors, and the increase in lymphoid cells bearing T and B markers. It is interesting to note that the later development of thyroid function is strictly coupled to the acquisition of natural killer (NK) cell cytotoxicity, thereby suggesting an important role of the pituitary-thyroid axis in the development of NK cells.

With regard to thymus–neuroendocrine interactions, initial evidence was based on the discovery that congenital mutation affecting pituitary dwarf mice caused concomitant alterations in the thymus and in the thymus dependent system.[13] In addition, the early involution of the thymus was also responsible for alterations in extraimmunological function resulting in an early aging syndrome.[14] Furthermore, studies carried out in thymectomized athymic nude mice have also confirmed the existence of such thymic influence on extraimmunological functions, and

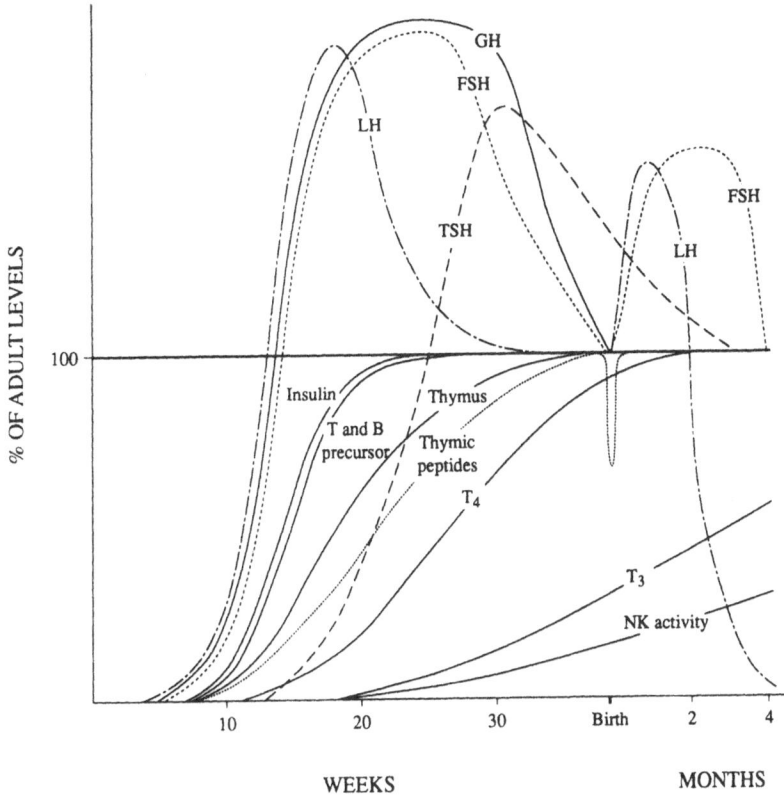

FIGURE 8.2. Comparison between the degree of maturity of neuroendocrine and immune systems during ontogeny.

primarily on the neuroendocrine profile, thus suggesting that thymus–neuroendocrine relationships might be bidirectional.[6,15]

Neuroendocrine Influences on Thymus Development

Pituitary dwarf mice show a normal development of the lymphoid system during the first 2 weeks of life. After this time not only is the usual further development not observed but such mice undergo a progressive involution of the entire immune system, and mainly of the thymus. This thymic involution is characterized by a reduction in size, and histologically by a decrease in the cellularity in the cortex and a loss of the corticomedullary distinction.[13,16]

Such thymic involution causes underdevelopment of the thymus-dependent system, resulting in prolonged allogeneic skin-graft survival and the depressed capability of spleen cells to induce graft-vs-host reactions. In addition, these cells do not appropriately react to T mitogens or give rise in vitro to T-cell colonies, resulting in a reduced humoral antibody response to thymus-dependent antigens. On the other hand the synthesis of immunoglobulins remains within normal range (Figure 8.3).

The only unusual finding in this context was the observation of a 'normal' take of transplantable tumors in dwarf mice at variance with adult hypophysectomized animals, which show a reduced take when compared with healthy controls. This finding has been interpreted in the light of the endocrinological as well as immunological surveillance on tumor growth. In fact, in hormonally reconstituted dwarfs, after the hormonal treatment has been interrupted, the take of tumor is much reduced in respect to both untreated dwarf and normal siblings, as if in these animals there is a prevalence of immune surveillance over the hormonal stimulation of tumor growth which is lacking.

The relevance of the pituitary–thymus interactions for the immunodeficiency state of the dwarf mouse is supported by the findings that this thymic underdevelopment (and the immunologic deficiencies) may be completely corrected by daily treatment of those mice for 30 days with growth hormone and thyroxine. However this intervention will only work provided the thymus has not been previously removed.[17]

These findings have been confirmed in a strain of dwarf dogs (Wiemaraner dogs) that show retarded growth, small thymi, absence of thymic cortex, and deficiency in lymphocyte mitogen response.[18] All these immunological defects can be corrected by growth hormone treatment.[19]

Further support for the view that thymic development is not autonomous with respect to other homestatic systems can be found in the lethargic mutant mouse (Lh/Lh) model. This naturally occurring mutant mouse has a hypotrophic thymus at birth, and neurological abnormalities develop in these animals at preweaning time and last for 1 to 2 months.[20] However, as soon as neural alterations disappears, the thymus reverts to normal status.[20]

A number of experimental designs have further supported these findings obtained in experiments of nature. The majority of them have been based on the removal of endocrine glands and on the observation of the consequent functional modification of the thymus, and of the peripheral efficiency of the thymus-dependent lymphoid system.[21–23]

The discovery that some thymic factors are secreted into the blood stream has offered a new technical approach to evaluate neuroendocrine–thymus interactions both in animals and humans. Certainly the circulating level of at least one of them, the facteur thymique serique (FTS),[24] (more recently called thymulin in its zinc-bound form[25]) strictly reflects the functional activity of the thymus.

It has been demonstrated that congenital hypopituitarism, experimental diabetes, and thyroidectomy, all cause a rapid reduction of plasma level of thymulin, whereas removal of the gonads or of the adrenals does not induce any significant modification. Reconstitution experiments by means

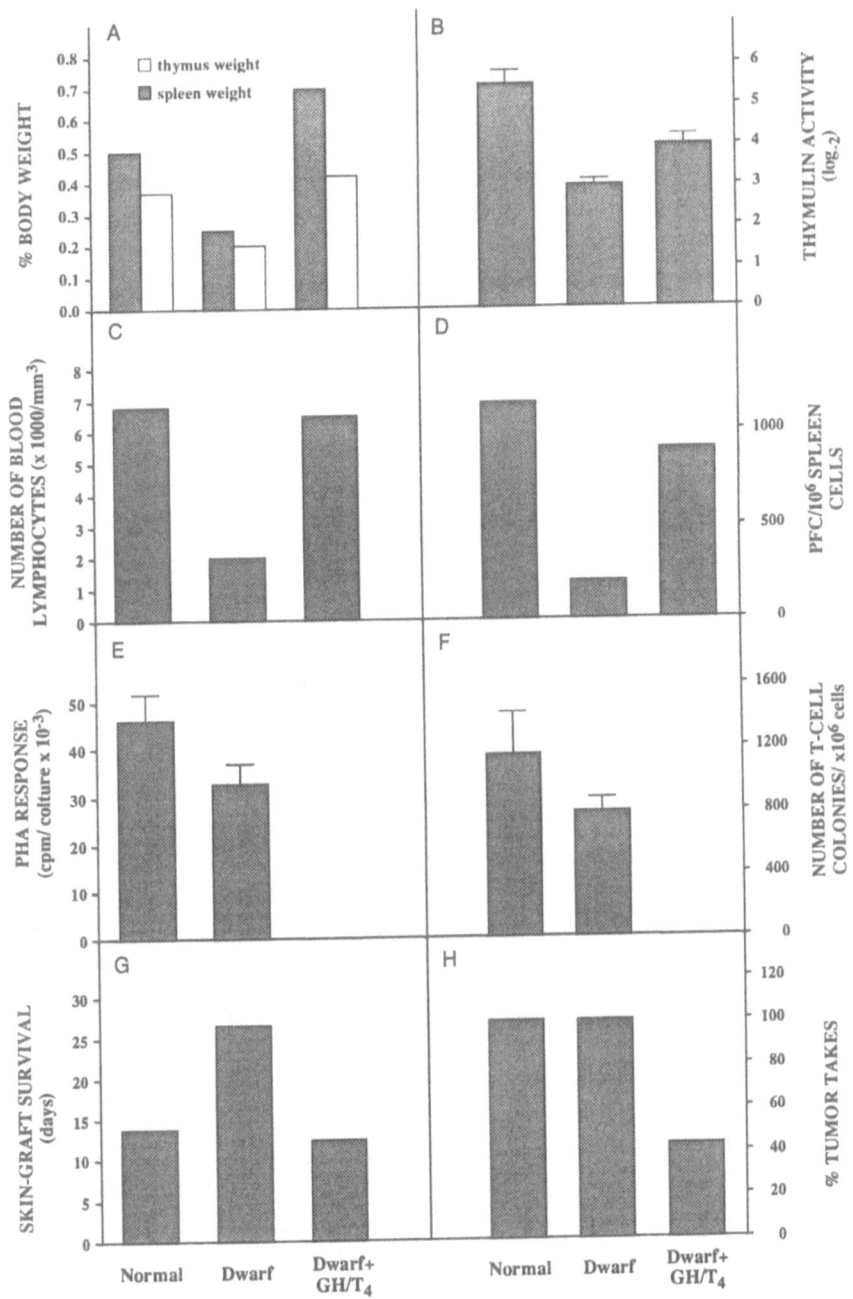

FIGURE 8.3. Alteration of various immunological parameters in 60-day-old dwarf mice when compared with normal littermates, and with dwarf mice treated with growth hormone and thyroxine for 20 days. A, relative thymus and spleen weight;[10] B, blood concentration of thymulin;[27] C, number of peripheral blood lymphocytes;[10] D, Spleen plaque-forming-cells (PFCs) against sheep red blood cells;[10] E, PHA response of spleen cells;[100] F, number of T-cell colonies after PHA stimulation;[100] G, survival of allogeneic skin graft;[10] H, % of tumor takes after 10^4 fibrosarcoma cell implantation (unpublished data).

of specific substituting hormonal therapy have demonstrated that the circulating level of thymulin returns to normal levels only a few days after the beginning of the hormonal treatment.[26]

Also in humans, many disendocrinopathies occurring during development are associated with alterations of circulating thymulin. Thus, GH-deficiency, due to congenital defect,[27,28] and hypothyroidism[29] are associated with consistent reduction of thymulin level; by contrast, hyperthyroidism is associated with high levels of thymulin.[29]

Also, functional alterations of thyroid hormone turnover, such as the 'low T_3' syndrome associated with premature birth, show reduced thymulin levels. In these studies a positive correlation has been found between thymulin concentrations and T_3, but not T_4 levels. This appears to suggest that T_3 rather than T_4 is the hormone exerting its action on the thymus.[30]

With regard to GH-deficiency, it has been recently demonstrated that the low thymulin levels present in these conditions significantly rebound following growth hormone injection. In these last studies no correlation has been found between GH and thymulin levels, but a significant positive correlation was found between insulin-like-growth factor (IGF-1) and thymulin blood concentrations, suggesting that GH probably acts on the thymus through somatomedins.[28,31]

Another hormonal disturbance that appears to be relevant for thymic function, is insulin alteration. Here low thymulin blood levels have been observed in type 1 juvenile diabetes, but this defect does not depend on thymic failure, but instead on reduced zinc ion availability, with consequent incomplete saturation (and biological activation) of thymulin molecules.[32]

Although these observations may substantially support the existence of neuroendocrine–immune interactions during ontogenetic development, they do not define the orderly sequence of events that may condition the development of a given function. At present, little information is available, but it may certainly be indicative of the validity of such an approach. In fact, the timing of an experimental ectomy may have quite different end-effects. Thus, neonatal adrenalectomy causes a retarded development of thymus-dependent humoral antibody responses when performed during the first days of life. However the same adrenalectomy performed at 20 days of age has no effects and, if performed later, may actually induce an increase in the immune responses.[10]

On the other hand, neonatal thyroidectomy causes a profound underdevelopment of the thymus and of thymus-dependent functions, whereas adult thyroidectomy has minor effects and more time is required after surgery in order to detect them.[33]

In supplementation studies it was demonstrated that the neonatal administration of GH to normal mice accelerates the development of thymus-dependent immune reactions when compared to untreated animals.[5] Similar accelerated development is caused by treatment with thyroxine, whereas administration of insulin does not modify the physiological pattern of immunological maturation.[34]

On the contrary, the administration of testosterone to chicken embryos causes underdevelopment of the bursa of Fabricius with consequent defect in B-cell responses which can not be corrected by the appearance of sexual hormones during physiological development.[35] Perinatal treatment of female mice with the nonsteroidal estrogen diethylstilbestrol (DES) gives rise to persistent alterations in immunological functions, mainly through its interference with T-cell differentiation.[36]

Another example of the influence of sex steroids on immune development is offered by New Zealand mice. The female New Zealand mouse frequently develops a lethal glomerulonephritis between 8 and 14 months of age. Castration or testosterone treatment of females prolongs survival, whereas castration or estradiol treatment of males has opposite effects.[37,38] It is important to note that castration of males results in accelerated mortality for autoimmune disease only if performed at 2–3 weeks of age, with minor effects at 5 weeks of age. The effects disappear when castration is performed at 14–15 weeks of age.[38]

More recently, evidence has been gathered showing that sequential activation mechanisms also cooperate in the ontogenetic development of NK function. It has been reported that interleukin-2 (IL-2) acts mainly on the growth and differentiation of NK cells from nonlytic precursors, while interferon (IFN) exerts its action on later steps of NK cell differentiation.[39,40] In mice, early in life, NK lytic activity is very low and progressively increases afterwards.

A different kinetics of appearance of responsiveness to IL-2 and IFN is present during ontogenetic development, the sensitivity to IL-2 preceding that for IFN. Both lymphokines are unable to stimulate spleen cells from 15-day-old mice, but only IL-2 can boost NK cell activity in 25-day-old animals. On the other hand, both of them act on the cytotoxicity of spleen cells in mice over 50 days of age.[41] The in vitro administration of physiological concentrations of thyroxine (T_4) induces an earlier development of IFN-responsiveness of NK cells from 25-day-old mice. Neither the basal nor the IL-2 induced NK activities are affected by T_4 treatment. Furthermore, the IFN sensitivity increases after T_4 administration in 50-day-old mice, while spleen cells from 15-day-old mice remain unresponsive.[42] The specific effect of thyroid hormones on IFN sensitivity of NK cells is further demonstrated by studying the effect of experimentally induced hypothyroidism on IFN-boosted NK activity.

The treatment of mice from birth to 60 days of age with propylthyouracil (PTU) abrogates the IFN responsiveness without modifying the IL-2 induced NK cytotoxicity. The interruption of PTU treatment completely reverses the sensitivity of NK cells to IFN.[43] On the other hand, the preincubation of spleen cells with TSH determines an earlier development of IL-2 responsiveness of NK cells, so that the spleen cells from 15-day-old mice become responsive to IL-2 after 2-day incubation with physiologic TSH concentrations. Interestingly, however, IFN sensitivity is not affected by TSH treatment.

Influence of the Thymus on Neuroendocrine Development

The immune system, and particularly the thymus, may act, particularly during early stages of life, on the physiologic development of non-immunologic functions. Such a hypothesis has originated from the observation that post-thymectomy wasting disease, in addition to the obvious immunological disturbances, is characterized by pathological signs that can hardly be linked to the direct effect of immune deficiency itself. In fact, mice thymectomized at birth, show a progressive impairment of body growth with reduced length of ears and tail, microsplancnia, microsomia, thinness of the skin and lack of subcutaneous fat, osseal alterations (particularly evident in the vertebrae, with consequent hunched posture), and hypotrophy of various tissues including submaxillary gland, hair follicles, and bone marrow.

At the pituitary level it was demonstrated that thymectomized mice show a progressive degranulation of pituitary acidophilic GH-producing cells, whereas other cell lineages in the hypophysis are unmodified.[5] Degranulation of GH- and PRL-producing cells has also been observed in thymusless nude mice.[44] Determination of blood levels of pituitary hormones has demonstrated a reduction of ACTH (transient), GH, PRL plasma level, and an increased level of luteotropic hormone (LH) (Figure 8.4).[22]

In nude mice, features of hypotrophy of thyroid gland, with reduced T_4 plasma levels, have been reported.[15] Unpublished data from our laboratory have confirmed these data and show that a syngenic neonatal thymus transplant completely reverses such a defect (Figure 8.4).

Both neonatally thymectomized and nude mice have been reported to show an abnormal histological picture of the adrenals, accompanied by a transient increase of plasma levels of corticosterone. On the contrary, according to other authors, neonatal thymectomy in rats induces reduction of corticosterone plasma levels, which, in the presence of the concomitant low levels of ACTH, would suggest an action of the thymus on the adrenals via the hypophysis.[22]

Gonadal function in thymus-deprived animals has been extensively investigated since it was demonstrated that neonatal thymectomy in hamster can be expressed quite differently with respect to sex (males undergo wasting diseases, females do not). In mice, thymectomy causes sterility in females but not in males.[45] Further investigations in both thymectomized and athymic nude mice have shown that both thymus-deprived conditions are characterized by a delayed vaginal opening time, with deeper sexual underdevelopment in nude mice than in thymectomized animals,[6] and with alteration in the profiles of sex hormones (Figure 8.4).

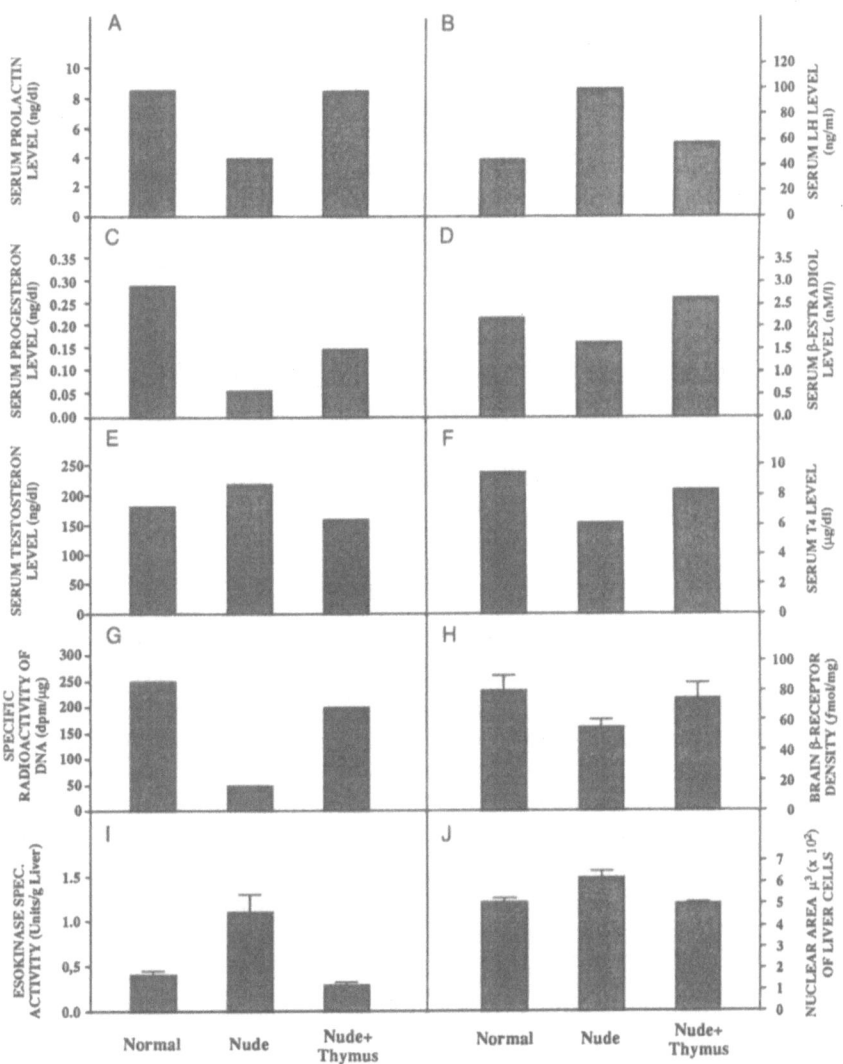

FIGURE 8.4. Alteration in various hormonal profiles and extraimmunological functions in 60-day-old athymic nude mice when compared with normal littermates and with nude mice grafted with neonatal syngenic thymus graft 20 days before sacrifice. A–F, serum levels of different hormones;[44] G, submandibular gland cells response to isoproterenol injection;[46] H, beta-adrenergic receptor density in brain cells;[47] I, esokinase activity in liver cells (unpublished data); J, nuclear area of liver cells.[101]

With regard to the endocrine pancreas, very little is presently known. Preliminary experiments in nude mice have shown that, while there are no differences in the basal levels of plasma insulin between nude and normal litter mates, the insulin-dependent esokinase pattern in the liver is strongly altered in nude animals (Figure 8.4).

Finally, some physiological reactions induced by the stimulation of β-adrenergic receptors (such as the increased rate of DNA synthesis in submandibular glands, or the increment of total water intake shortly after the injection of isoproterenol) are significantly reduced both in thymectomized and nude mice, and are restored to normal values by a syngenic neonatal thymus transplant.[46] Moreover, further data from our laboratory have demonstrated that the β-adrenoceptor density in different tissues (submandibular glands, brain) is reduced in thymusless mice, and it can be recovered by syngenic thymus transplant (Figure 8.4).[47]

Neuroendocrine–Immune Interactions in Aging

A sizeable body of experimental and clinical evidence has demonstrated that with advancing age, both the neuroendocrine and the immune system undergo a progressive deterioration in their efficiency.

Neuroendocrine and Thymus Aging

With regard to the neuroendocrine system, aging may affect all steps of the endocrine cascade.[48] Thus, the alterations observed, regardless of the endocrine gland specificity, in general follow these characteristics: (1) The basal hormonal blood levels are generally found to be unmodified by aging, whereas the secretory response to an appropriate stimulus is frequently decreased: (2) Many protein hormones (particularly those secreted by the pituitary gland), even at a young age, show a biochemical and antigenic polymorphism, which is generally accentuated with advancing age. The functional activity of the different forms and the significance of the increased polymorphism with age remain to be established: (3) Secretory and clearance rates appear diminished: (4) Since a given hormone may act on various cell types, it is not unusual to find that aging may affect the response of one or more cell types, leaving others unaffected. This phenomenon being due to the different rate at which aging may affect receptor availability and hormone-receptor binding.[49]

With regard to the 'master' glands (i.e., the pineal and the pituitary), no significant intrinsic alterations seem to be present in old age, in many species examined. In addition, in these species, the pituitary hormonal content and the basal blood levels of most pituitary hormones do not show significant alterations in old age. Hormones that are altered with age include prolactin, which is usually found increased in the elderly, and gonadotropins, whose pituitary release is much augmented, particularly in females, due to alterations in ovarian function. With regard to protein hormones, no substantial variations have been observed in old age in the pituitary content or in the blood basal levels, whereas the circadian rhythmicity and the secretory response to specific stimuli are significantly modified.[50]

The pineal gland produces various hormones, in particular melatonin, derived from the neurotransmitter serotonin. A major function of melatonin relates to the control of the cyclicity of daily as well as seasonal rhythms. With advancing age, the gland undergoes calcification with loss of pinealocytes, which is not associated with major alterations of the secretory capacities. The night and time amplitude of peak secretion is, however, generally altered with aging,[51] and such an alteration may be responsible for the modified night-time profile of other hormones such as ACTH, GH, PRL, and TSH. A major consequence of this phenomenon is that the 24-hour total secretion rate of these hormones, with the exception of PRL, is generally decreased.

With regard to the immune system, the stem-cell compartment, the efficiency of B-cells, and the function of macrophages and of antigen-presenting cells are not significantly affected by age. Other components, such as the thymus and the T-cell compartment, as well as the efficiency of NK cells are more or less altered during aging.

The thymus attains its maximum size at puberty, after which it undergoes a progressive involution characterized by a decrease in weight, due essentially to the depletion of cortical lymphocytes and an infiltration of fat.[52] Fat cells are most abundant in the cortex and differentiate in situ during involution. There is a decrease in the number of thymocytes, and of those present, many are picnotic in old age.[53] Also, the epithelial cells (which are believed to synthesize and secrete thymic factors[54]) are decreased in number during aging and show cystic changes and reduction of intracellular granules.[55,56] This has led to the conclusion that the thymus 'is the only gland whose progressive involution with age is a common feature of animals and man'.[57] There are some exceptions in nature of this age-dependent thymic involution. Thus, hens do not show consistent thymic involution,[58] nor do germ-free animals.[59]

Measurement of the circulation level of thymic factors has demonstrated, both in other animals and humans, that the plasma level of one of the best known thymic peptides (thymulin) declines progressively from birth to old age. Certainly, in mice past the 18th months of age, and in humans past 60 years of age thymulin levels become virtually undetectable. According to a recent more precise determination of thymulin,

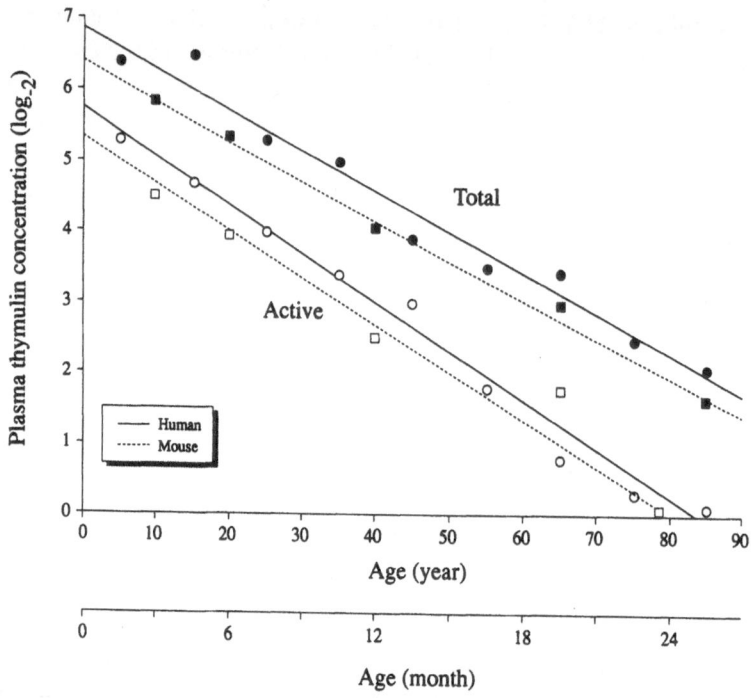

FIGURE 8.5. Age-dependency of plasma level of active zinc-bound (ZnFTS) and total (ZnFTS + FTS) in human and mice.

which takes into account the interference due to a marginal zinc deficiency[60] present with advancing age, the decline of thymulin levels is less pronounced than previously reported (Figure 8.5). Even in very old age, a residual production of thymulin is detectable.[29,60]

The age-associated decline of thymic endocrine activity seems to be one of the major causes for the deterioration of the peripheral T-cell compartment. Additional deterioration is seen in the efficiency of T cells with cytotoxic properties, as well as of T cells with helper and suppressor activity. In fact, treatments of old mice with thymic hormone preparations have demonstrated the reversibility of age-associated defects in peripheral T-cell functions.[61] From this brief review, it appears that alterations do occur with advancing age both in the neuroendocrine and in the immune system, but the data available do not give information on whether such alterations are intrinsic and irreversible.

Neuroendocrine–Thymus Plasticity During Aging

It has been demonstrated that modifications induced by experimental manipulation of the thymus (and of the immune system) can alter the neuroendocrine system and vice-versa. Therefore, it may also be

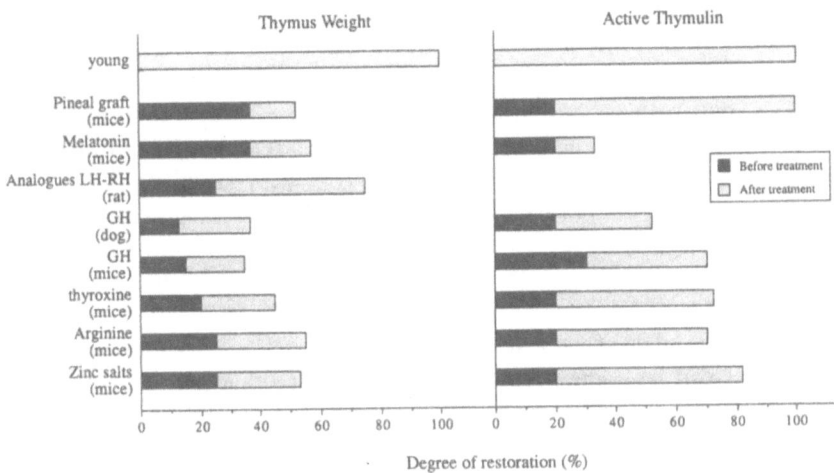

FIGURE 8.6. Restoration of thymus weight and plasma level of active thymulin by different neuroendocrinological or nutritional interventions. The degree of restoration is calculated as the mean value of young individuals (= 100).

expected that the physiological decline with advancing age of either the immune or the neuroendocrine system may, in part, be responsible for the alterations observed in the other partner.

As a matter of fact, regrowth of an old thymus with recovery of its endocrine activity was observed when the thymus was implanted into young syngenic recipients. This appears to confirm the suggestion that the 'old' microenvironment cannot support thymic function.[62] Following this observation, experiments have been addressed to obtain similar results by various endocrine manipulations. Thus, it has been demonstrated that regrowth of the thymus may be achieved in old animals by treatment with thyroid hormones,[63] with growth hormone,[64,65] with analogues of LH-RH,[66,67] and with melatonin or intrathymic graft of young syngenic pineal gland (Figure 8.6).[68]

Interestingly, similar thymic 'rejuvenation' was obtained in mice by treatment with arginine[69] which has a secretagogue activity on pituitary GH. A similar effect can be obtained with zinc salts[70] which certainly may have a direct action on the thymus, but are also capable of acting on the pituitary-thyroid axis[70,71] hormone production.

In humans, very few trials have been done, but, at least with regard to thymic endocrine activity, both arginine[60,72] and zinc[73] are still effective in old age. On the other hand, the capacity of thyroid hormones and of growth hormone to restore thymic function in old age is further supported by the clinical observation that hyperthyroidism in old humans is associated with thymic enlargement.[74] Additionally, both hyperthyroidism and acromegaly in old subjects are associated with high circulating plasma levels of thymic hormones.[29,75]

Restoration of thymic function by endocrine or nutritional interventions is associated with recovery of peripheral immune T-dependent functions. Such functions may include mitogen-induced lymphocyte proliferation which is enhanced by treatments with GH,[74] with arginine,[69,72] or with zinc salts.[70] With regard to NK activity, relationships of activity to thymic function is still controversial. It is of interest to note, however, that both GH[64] and β-endorphins[76] are able to increase basal NK activity. On the other hand, treatments with TSH only increased IL-2 induced NK cytotoxicity, while T_3 boosted IFN NK activity.[77,78] The major deductions that can be gained from these findings are that age-related thymic involution is not an irreversible process, and that functional recovery can be achieved even in old age. Further, reconstitution of thymic efficiency in old mice greatly influences neuroendocrine functions.

In mice, with advancing age, there are modifications of the plasma levels of some hormones (such as an increased insulin and a decreased T_3 level) and reduction of the adaptive reaction to β-adrenergic stimuli.[46] This latter change is probably due to a decreased density of β-adrenoceptors on cell membranes of various tissues, including the submandibular gland and some parts of the brain.[47] All of these deficits are fully restored in old animals by neonatal thymus grafts. Furthermore, a neonatal thymus graft can also correct the increased polyploidy present in aged liver cells.[79]

The majority of the neuroendocrine changes demonstrated in these studies are strictly age-dependent (i.e., they display a linear progression starting early in life). Therefore, their interconnection with the thymus, which shows quite a similar age-dependent progressive deterioration, does not seem to be merely coincidental. Focusing on the 'strategic' circuit described in Figure 8.1A with advancing age, there does not seem to be any single intrinsic and critical event that can account for the progressive deterioration of the neuroendocrine-thymus functions in old age.

Mechanisms of Neuroendocrine–Thymus Interactions

The effect of hormones on thymic cell maturation may be mediated by a direct action on thymocytes or through the action exerted on thymic epithelial cells (TEC). Evidence does exist for the presence of receptors on thymocytes for prolactin,[80] for LH-RH,[67] and for β-agonists.[81] On a functional basis, much evidence supports the idea that other pituitary/CNS products (such as GH, thyroid hormones, and endogenous oppioid[82–84]) may regulate thymocytes or mature T cells.

With regard to thymic epithelial cells, many hormones and neuropeptides are capable of modulating thymulin secretion. Among the neuropeptides, leu-enkephalin and β-endorphin are able to increase thymulin production by TEC, whereas met-enkephalin, α-endorphin, and γ-endorphin are inactive.[85] Among hormones, GH, PRL, adrenal and sex steroids, and thyroid hormones can act as specific stimulators of thymulin production in vitro.[85,86] Such an in vitro effect clearly supports the idea that TEC possess specific receptors for these hormones and neuropeptides. At present, experimental demonstration of receptors on TEC has been obtained for glucocorticoids, progesterone, GH, PRL, and T_3.[85]

Recent findings have shown that human thymic cells are capable of secreting neuropeptides (oxytocin, vasopressin, neurophysins).[87] These substances have been found particularly in thymic nurse cells.[88] The significance of such neuropeptides is still unclear, but it has been proposed that their role is that of offering a criptocrine signal for the induction of immune tolerance to the neurohypophyseal-related peptide system.[89]

However, it is most important to realize that such secretions may significantly contribute to thymic function. Certainly both vasopressin and oxytocin were shown to replace IL-2 for IFN-γ production by mouse splenocytes and by cultured human peripheral lymphocytes.[90] Thus, thymic vasopressin and oxytocin may exert IL-2 like properties on targets, and this could be of relevance with regard to the recent observation of IL-2 receptor expression as a differentiation marker on intrathymic stem cells.[91] Certainly this is supported by the demonstration that IL-2, synergizing with IL-1, can alter the proliferation rate of thymic 'double-negative' cells (Thy 1.2^+, $Ly2^-$, $L3T4^-$) cells.[91,92] Interleukins are also produced at intrathymic level, while IL-1 is secreted by thymic epithelial cells,[92] but the intrathymic source of IL-2 requires further confirmation. The intrathymic production of these interleukins does not, however, exclude the possibilities that peripherally produced interleukins may modulate thymic cell maturation. In vivo experimental models have clearly shown that intravenously injected IL-1 and IL-2 synergistically act to enhance the maturation of T cells by marker and functional criteria. This fact has been interpreted to mean that the expression of a feedback control on thymic function acts via 'signals from the periphery leading to replenishment of the peripheral pool whenever required'.[92]

With regard to the mechanism of thymus action on the neuroendocrine network, both thymic humoral factors as well as the cellular product of the thymus (i.e., the mature T lymphocytes) might be involved. Such a hypothesis is predicated firstly on the hormone-like nature of the inter-actions and, secondly on the fact that these neuroendocrine interactions may produce lymphokines capable of influencing some pituitary functions, or even pituitary hormone-like substances, such as ACTH, TSH, PRL, GH, and gonadotropins.[3]

The relevance of these products of mature T cells in the context of the above reported experimental designs can be questioned. Firstly, because such products are secreted upon stimulation with specific antigens and therefore might exert only a temporarily limited action. Secondly, because thymus–neuroendocrine interactions also work under germ-free conditions, where even the background antigenic stimulation is supposed to be nearly absent.

Furthermore, at least with respect to some altered neuroendocrine patterns in thymus-deprived animals (such as isoproterenol (IPR) response and reduced T_3 and T_4 plasma levels), no recovery has been achieved when mature lymphocytes have been used instead of neonatal thymus grafts.[46]

On the contrary, a possible role played by thymic factors may be supported by the following considerations: (1) In order to act, they do not require any specific antigenic stimulation: (2) Some neuroendocrine abnormalities, such as the degranulation of GH-producing cells in the pituitary of thymus deprived mice, can be prevented by injection of thymic extracts[93]: (3) Evidence has been recently gathered of a direct effect of some thymosins at the hypothalamic level on corticotropin-releasing factor (CRF) and luteotropin-releasing factor (LRF) release, thus modulating both the pituitary-adrenal and pituitary-gonadal axes.[94] By using single peptides it has also been shown that thymosin-α1 acts preferentially on the pituitary-adrenal axis, whereas thymosin-β4 acts on the pituitary-gonadal axis. This would appear to suggest a specific effect of these compounds.[94] Furthermore, in vitro effects of thymosins on the release of PRL and GH from pituitary cells have also been reported.[9]

Neuroendocrine–Immune Interactions: Theoretical and Practical Implications

The findings discussed above clearly demonstrate that some functional activities of the neuroendocrine and the immune networks are not intrinsic to the specific domain, but instead depend on the interaction with the other domains of the homeostasis of the organism. The generally accepted assumption of a genetically determined hierarchy among the three homeostatic systems is no longer tenable. This is of peculiar relevance to the systemic theories of aging (i.e., the immune[95,96] or the neuroendocrine theory[97]), since they are based on the occurrence of primary, intrinsic, and irreversible events at the level of each single system.

The mechanism involved in age-associated dysfunction seems to result, not from a breakdown in a single homeostatic system, but rather, from disruption of the complex neuroendocrine–immune interactions. Certainly, available experimental findings would support this hypothesis.

According to such an approach, we may assume that neuroendocrine–immune interactions are continuously modified during life by external

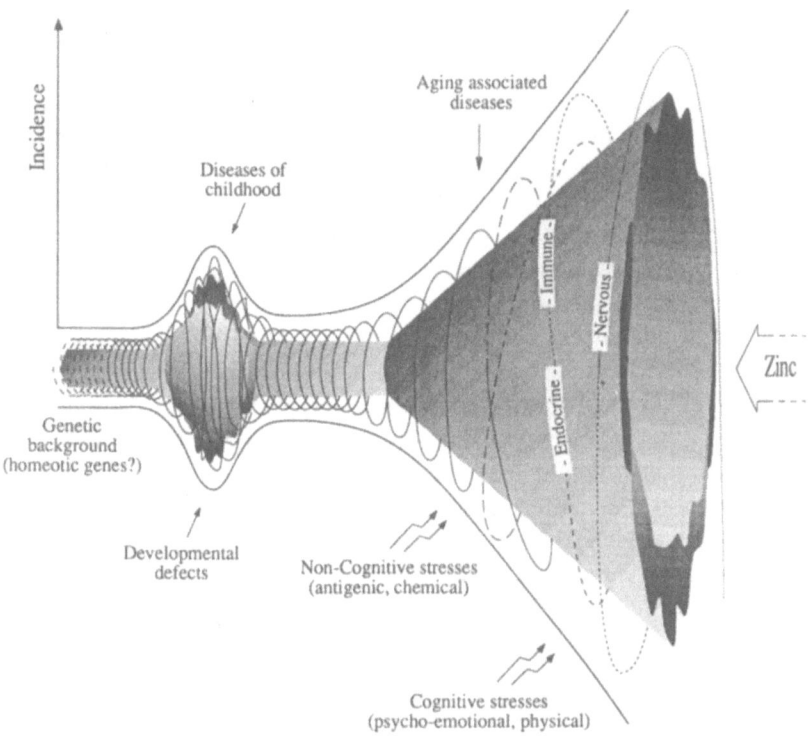

Figure 8.7. The neuroendocrine–immune theory of aging.

stressors which may be either cognitive (psycho-emotional, social, etc.) or noncognitive (chemical, antigenic, etc.). The original balance may undergo a progressive exhaustion, which may vary in its time course, depending on the quality and quantity of stressor events that each individual experienced (Figure 8.7). The individual diversity of life experience may account for variations of a single homeostatic mechanism, both in early ontogeny and in aging in different individuals. The interaction, however, with the other networks, may explain the global alterations usually observed in these situations. In other words, priority in the appearance of age-related phenomena among nervous, neuroendocrine, and immune systems is not a strictly genetically determined phenomenon, but develops in an individual according to personal life experience. This assumption can explain the increased incidence of diseases in ontogeny as due to defective development of the interactions among those homeostatic systems and/or to abnormal stressor events. In aging, such increases in disease may be due to the accumulation of individually different 'collages' of various noncognitive or cognitive stressor consequences.

Alternatively, we cannot exclude the possibility that the deterioration of neuroendocrine–immune interactions both during development and aging, in addition to depending on alterations at the level of one of the homeostatic systems involved, might also depend on modifications of some basic mechanisms capable of influencing all of the homeostatic systems. A putative factor in this context is zinc metabolism,[46] since it has been demonstrated that zinc is required for the functional efficiency of the nervous, the neuroendocrine, and the immune systems.[98]

In fact, alterations in zinc turnover during development cause profound disturbances on all the homeostatic network. In addition to more recent experimental evidences,[70] the original observations of stunted growth, mental retardation, defective sexual maturation, and increased infectious diseases in children with low zinc intake,[98] clearly pin-point the relevance that such a trace element has for the development of the major homeostatic networks. The recent demonstration that children with Down's syndrome suffer from zinc abnormalities and that zinc supplementation can correct both immunological and neuroendocrine alterations[71] may support our hypothesis.

Also, aging is characterized by altered zinc turnover: plasma zinc levels decline progressively with age, this being due most likely to a defect in absorption.[99] Also, in this situation zinc supplementation is able to restore thymic function, restore various immune deficiencies, and correct some age-related hormonal defects.[70] These findings clearly support the idea that zinc can play a crucial role in neuroendocrine–immune interactions both during development and aging, though the exact nature and extent of this role remains to be established.

References

1. Fabris N, Mocchegiani E, Muzzioli M, Provinciali M. Neuroendocrine–thymus interactions: Perspectives for intervention in aging. Ann NY Acad Sci USA 1988; 521:72–87.
2. Bulloch K, Lucito R. The effect of cortisone on acetylcholenesterase (AChE) in the neonatal and aged thymus. Ann NY Acad Sci USA 1988; 521:59–71.
3. Blalock JE. Production of neuroendocrine peptide hormones by the immune system. In: Blalock JE, Bost KL, eds. Neuroimmunendocrinology. Progress in Allergy, vol. 43, Basel: Karger; 1988:1–13.
4. Besedovsky HO, Del Rey A. Immune-neuroendocrine circuits: Integrative role of cytokines. Front Neuroendocrinology 1992; 13(1):61–94.
5. Pierpaoli W, Fabris N, Sorkin E. Developmental hormones and immunological maturation. In: Wolstenholme GEW, Knight J, eds. Hormones and the Immune Response. (Ciba study group No. 36) London: Churchill; 1970: 126–143.
6. Besedovsky HO, Sorkin E. Thymus involvement in female sexual maturation. Nature 1974; 249:356–358.

7. Besedovsky HO, Sorkin E, Keller M. Changes in blood hormone levels during the immune response. Proc Soc Exp Med 1975; 50:466–502.

8. Bernton EW, Beach JE, Holaday JW, Smallridge R, Fein HG. Release of multiple hormones by a direct action of interleukin 1 on pituitary cells. Science 1987; 238:519–525.

9. Spangelo BL, Judd AM, Ross PC, Login IS, Jarvis WD, Badamchian M, Goldstein AL, MacLeod RM. Thymosin fraction 5 stimulates prolactin and growth hormone release from anterior pituitary cells in vitro. Endocrinology 1987; 121:2035–2040.

10. Fabris N. Biomarkers of aging in the neuroendocrine–immune domain: Time for a new theory of aging. Ann NY Acad Sci 1992; 663:335–348.

11. Meites J, Goya R, Takahashi S. Why the neuroendocrine system is important in aging processes. A review. Exp Gerontol 1986; 22:1–15.

12. Grossman CJ. The role of sex steriods in immune system regulation. In: Grossman CJ, ed. Bilateral Communication Between the Endocrine and Immune Systems. New York: Springer-Verlag; 1993.

13. Fabris N, Pierpaoli W, Sorkin E. Hormones and the immunological capacity. III. The immunodeficiency diseases of the hypopituitary Snell-Bagg dwarf mouse. Clin Exp Immunol 1971; 9:209–225.

14. Fabris N, Pierpaoli W, Sorkin E. Lymphocytes, hormones, and aging. Nature 1972; 240:557–559.

15. Pierpaoli W, Sorkin E. Alteration of adrenal cortex and thyroid in mice with congenital absence of the thymus. Nature N Biol 1972; 238:282–286.

16. Baroni CD, Fabris N, Bertoli G. Synergistic action of thyroxin and somatotropic hormone in pituitary dwarf mice. Immunology 1969; 17:303–306.

17. Fabris N, Pierpaoli W, Sorkin E. Hormones and the immunological capacity. IV. Restorative effects of developmental hormones or of lymphocytes on the immunodeficiency syndrome of the dwarf mouse. Clin Exp Immunol 1971; 9:227–240.

18. Roth JA, Lamax LG, Alszuler N, Hampshire J, Laeberle ML, Shelton M, Draper DD, Ledet AE. Thymic abnormatilities and growth hormone deficiency in dogs. Am J Vet Res 1980; 41:1256–1262.

19. Roth JA, Laeberle ML, Grier DL, Hopper JG, Spiegel HE, Macallister HA. Improvement in clinical condition and thymus morphological features associated with growth treatment of immuno-deficient dwarf-dogs. Am J Vet Res 1984; 45:1151–1155.

20. Dung HC. Deficiency in the thymus-dependent immunity in 'lethargic' mutant mice. Transplantation 1977; 23:39–44.

21. Fabris N. Ontogenetic and phylogenetic aspects of neuroendocrine–immune network. Dev Comp Immunol 1981; 5:49–60.

22. Fabris N, Piantanelli L. Thymus–neuroendocrine interactions during development and aging. In: Adelman RC, Roth GS, eds. Endocrine and Neuroend Mechanics of Aging. (CRC Press Series) Boca Raton, Florida; 1982:186–195.

23. Provinciali M, Fabris N. Models and mechanism of neuroendocrine–immune interactions during ontogeny. Adv Neuroimmunol 1991; 1:124–138.

24. Bach JF, Dardenne M, Pleau JM, Bach AM. Isolation, biochemical characteristics, and biological activity of a circulating thymic hormone in the mouse and in the human. Ann NY Acad Sci 1975; 249:186–191.

25. Dardenne M, Pleau JM, Nabama B, Lefancier P, Denien M, Choay J, Bach JF. Contribution of zinc and other metals to the biological activity of the serum thymic factor. Proc Natl Acad Sci USA 1982; 79:5370–5373.
26. Fabris N, Mocchegiani E. Endocrine control of thymic serum factor production in young-adult and old mice. Cell Immunol 1985; 91:325–335.
27. Fabris N, Mocchegiani E, Muzzioli M, Imberti R. Thymus–neuroendocrine network. In: Fabris N, Garaci E, Hadden J, Mitchison NA, eds. Immunoregulation. New York: Plenum Press; 1983:341–362.
28. Mocchegiani E, Paolucci P, Balsamo A, Cacciari E, Fabris N. Influence of growth hormone on thymic endocrine activity in humans. Horm Res 1990; 33:248–255.
29. Fabris N, Mocchegiani E, Mariotti S, Pacini F, Pinchera A. Thyroid function modulates thymus endocrine activity. J Clin Endocrinol Metab 1986; 62:474–478.
30. Fabris N, Mocchegiani E, Mariotti S, Caramia G, Bracilli T, Pacini F, Pinchera A. Thymulin deficiency and low 3,5,3'-triiodothyronine syndrome in infants with low birth weight syndromes. J Clin Endocrinol Metab 1987; 65:247–253.
31. Mocchegiani E, Fabris N. Growth hormone influence on thymic endocrine activity in humans. Int J Neurosci 1990; 51:253–254.
32. Mocchegiani E, Boemi M, Fumelli P, Fabris N. Zinc-dependent low thymic hormone level in type I diabetes. Diabetes 1989; 38(7):932–937.
33. Fabris N. Immunodepression in thyroid-deprived animals. Clin Exp Immunol 1973; 15:601–609.
34. Pierpaoli W, Fabris N, Sorkin E. The effects of hormones in the development of the immune capacity. In: Cellular Interactions in the Immune Response. Basel: Karger; 1971:25–29.
35. Glick B. The bursa of Fabricius and the development of immunologic competence. In: Good RA, Gabrielson AE, eds. The thymus in Immunobiology. New York: Hoeber Medical Division, Harper and Row; 1964: 343–360.
36. Kalland T, Strand O, Forsberg JG. Long-term effects of neonatal estrogen treatment on mitogen responsiveness of mouse spleen lymphocytes. J Natl Cancer Inst 1979; 63:413–421.
37. Roubinian JR, Tala N, Greenspan JS, Goodman JR, Siteri PK. Effect of castration and sex hormone treatment on survival, antinucleic acid antibodies, and glomerulonephritis in NZB/NZW F_1 mice. J Exp Med 1978; 147:1568–1583.
38. Steinberg AD, Melez KA, Raveche ES, Reeves JP, Boegel WA, Smathers PA, Taurog JD, Weinlein L, Duvic M. Approach to the study of the role of sex hormones in autoimmunity. Arthritis Rheum 1979; 22:1170–1176.
39. Koo GB, Manyak CL. Generation of cytotoxic cells from murine bone marrow by human recombinant IL-2. J Immunol 1986; 137:1751–1756.
40. Kalland T. Generation of Natural killer cells from bone marrow precursors in vitro. Immunology 1986; 57:493–497.
41. Provinciali M, Muzzioli M, Fabris N. Timing of appearance and disappearance of IFN and IL-2 induced natural immunity during ontogenetic development and aging. Exp Gerontology 1989; 24:227–236.
42. Provinciali M, Fabris N. Modulation of lymphoid cell sensitivity to interferon by thyroid hormones. J Endocrinol Invest 1990; 13:187–191.

43. Provinciali M, Muzzioli M, Di Stefano G, Fabris N. Recovery of spleen cell natural killer activity by thyroid hormone treatment in old mice. Nat Immun Cell Growth Regul, 1991; 10:226–236.

44. Pierpaoli W, Kopp HG, Bianchi E. Interdependence of thymic and neuro-endocrine functions in ontogeny. Clin Exp Immunol 1976; 24:501–506.

45. Nishizuka Y, Sakakura T. Thymus and reproduction sex-linked dysgenesis of the gonad after neonatal thymectomy in mice. Science 1969; 166:753–756.

46. Piantanelli L, Basso A, Muzzioli M, Fabris N. Thymus-dependent reversibility of physiological and Isoproterenol-evoked age-related parameters in athymic nude and old normal mice. Mech Ageing Dev 1978; 7:171–179.

47. Piantanelli L, Gentile S, Fattoretti P, Viticchi C. Thymic regulation of brain cortex beta-adrenoceptors during development and aging. Arch Gerontol Ger 1985; 4:179–185.

48. Meites J, ed. Neuroendocrinology of Aging. New York: Plenum Press; 1983.

49. Sowers JR, Felicetta JV, eds. Endocrinology of Aging. New York: Raven Press; 1988:1–348.

50. Van Coevorden A, Mockel J, Laurent E, Kerkhofs M, L'Hermite-Baleriaux M, Decoster C, Nève P, Van Cauter E. Neuroendocrine rhythms and sleep in aging men. Am Physiol Soc 1991; 51–63.

51. Reiter RJ. The pineal gland: An important link to the environment. N Physiol Sci 1986; 1:202–205.

52. Muller-Hermelink HK, Steinman G, Stein H. Structural and functional alteration of the aging human thymus. Adv Exp Med Biol 1984; 17:142.

53. Simpson JF, Gray ES, Beck JS. Age involution in the normal human adult thymus. Clin Exp Immunol 1975; 19:261–268.

54. Savino W, Dardenne M. Thymic hormone-containing cells. VI. Immunohistologic evidence for the simultaneous presence of thymulin, thymopoietin, and thymosin alpha 1 in normal and pathological human thymuses. Eur J Immunol 1984; 14:987–991.

55. Meleg-Smith SN, Ossa-Gomez LJ. A quantitative histologic comparison of the thymus in 100 healthy and diseased adults. Am J Clin Pathol 1981; 76:657–662.

56. Steinmann GG, Klaus B, Muller-Hermelink HK. The involution of aging human thymic epithelium is independent of puberty. Scand J Immunol 1985; 22:536–575.

57. Korenchevski V. Physiological and pathological aging. In: Bourne GH, ed. New York: Hafner; 1961:65.

58. Hammar JA. Die normal morphologische Thymusforschung im letzten Vierteljahrhundert. Leipzig: Barth; 1936.

59. Moore RW. Unpublished observations, cited by Good RA in discussion. In: Wolstenholme GEW, Porter R, eds. The Thymus: Experimental and Clinical Studies. Boston: Little Brown and Co.; 1966:179–181.

60. Fabris N, Mocchegiani E, Amadio L, Zannotti M, Licastro F, Franceschi C. Thymic hormone deficiency in normal ageing and Down's syndrome. Is there a primary failure of the thymus? Lancet 1984; 1:983–986.

61. Zatz MM, Goldstein AL. Thymosin, lymphokines, and the immunology of ageing. Gerontology 1985; 31:263–272.

62. Bach MA, Beaurain G. Respective influence of extrinsic and intrinsic factors on the age-related decrease of thymic secretion. J Immunol 1979; 122:2505–2507.

63. Fabris N, Muzzioli M, Mocchegiani E. Recovery of age-dependent immunological deterioration in Balb/c mice by short term treatment with L-thyroxine. Mech Ageing Dev 1982; 18:327–343.

64. Davila DR, Brief S, Simon J, Hammer RE, Brinster RL, Kelly KW. Role of growth hormone in regulating T-dependent immune events in aged, nude, and transgenic rodents. J Neurosci Res 1987; 18:108–116.

65. Goff BL, Roth JA, Arp LH, Incefy GS. Growth hormone treatment stimulates thymulin production in aged dogs. Clin Exp Immunol 1987; 68:580–587.

66. Greenstein BD, Fitzpatrick FT, Kendall MD, Wheeler MJ. Regeneration of the thymus in old male rats treated with a stable analogue of LHRH. J Endocrinol 1987; 11:345–350.

67. Marchetti B, Morale MC, Batticane N, Gallo F, Farinelli Z, Cioni M. Aging of the reproductive-neuroimmune axis. Ann NY Acad Sci 1991; 621:159–173.

68. Pierpaoli W, Dall'ara A, Pedrinis E, Regelson W. The pineal control of aging. The pineal control of aging. The effects of melatonin and pineal grafting on the survival of older mice. Ann NY Acad Sci 1991; 621:291–313.

69. Fabris N, Mocchegiani E, Muzzioli M. Recovery of age related decline of thymic endocrine activity and PHA response by lysine-arginine combination. Int J Immunopharmacol 1986; 8:677–685.

70. Fabris N, Mocchegiani E, Muzzioli M, Provinciali M. The role of zinc in neuroendocrine–immune interactions during aging. Ann NY Acad Sci 1991; 621:314–326.

71. Licastro F, Mocchegiani E, Zannotti M, Fabris N. Normalisation of thyroid stimulating hormone and reversal triiodothyronine plasmic levels by dietary zinc supplementation in children with Down's syndrome: Evaluation of clinical impact. Int J Neurosci 1992; 65:259–268.

72. Mocchegiani E, Cacciatore L, Talarico M, Lingetti M, Fabris N. Recovery of low thymic hormone levels in cancer patients by lisine-arginine combination. Int J Immunopharmacol 1990; 12(4):365–371.

73. Travaglini P, Moriondo P, Togni E, Venegoni P, Bochicchio D, Conti A, Faglia G, Ambroso G, Ponticelli C, Mocchegiani E, Fabris N. Effect of an oral zinc administration on prolactin and thymulin circulating levels in uremic patients. J Clin Endocrinol Metab 1989; 68(1):186–190.

74. Simpson JC, Gray ES, Michie W, Beck JS. The influence of preoperative drug treatment on the extent of hyperplasia of the thymus in primary thyrotoxicosis. Clin Exp Immunol 1975; 22:249–253.

75. Travaglini P, Mocchegiani E, Togni E, Muratori M, Re T, Bazzoni, Fabris N. Thymulin and zinc circulating level in patient with GH- and PRL-secreting pituitary adenomas. Int J Neurosci 1990; 51:269–271.

76. Solomon GF, Fiatarone MA, Benton D, Morley JE, Bloom E, Makinodan T. Psychoimmunologic and endorphin function in the aged. Ann NY Acad Sci 1988; 521:43–58.

77. Provinciali M, Fabris N. Role of pituitary-thyroid axis on basal and lymphokine-induced NK cell activity in aging. Int J Neurosci 1990; 51:273–274.

78. Provinciali M, Di Stefano G, Bressani N, Fabris N. Sequential activation of hormone/cytokines in the differentiation of NK cells. J Chemother 1991; 3:81–83.

79. Pieri C, Giuli C, Del Moro M, Piantanelli L. Electron microscopic morphometric analysis of mouse liver. II. Effect of aging and thymus transplantation in old animals. Mech Aging Dev 1980; 13:275–280.

80. Hienstand PC, Mekler P, Nordmann R, Grieder A, Permmongkol C. Prolactin as a modulator of lymphocyte responsiveness provides a possible mechanism of action for cyclosporine. Proc Natl Acad Sci USA 1986; 83:335–340.

81. Marchetti B, Morale MC, Pelletier G. Autoradiographic localization of the beta-2 adrenergic receptor in the thymus and presence of a sexual dimorphism during ontogeny, Progress in NeuroEndocrinImmunology (PNEI), 1990; 3(2):103–115.

82. Arrenbrecht S, Sorkin E. Growth hormone-induced T cell differentiation. Eur J Immunol 1973; 3:601–604.

83. Lemarchand-Béraud T. Triiodothyronine and thyroxine nuclear receptors in lymphocytes from normal, hyper-, and hypothyroid patients. Acta Endocrinol 1977; 85:44–51.

84. Wybran J. Enkephalins and endorphins as modifiers of the immune system: Present and future. Neuropeptides 1985; 44:92–94.

85. Dardenne M, Savino W. Hormonal interactions between the thymus and the pituitary. In: Grossman CJ, ed. Bilateral Communication Between the Endocrine and Immune Systems. New York: Springer-Verlag; 1993.

86. Mocchegiani E, Amadio L, Fabris N. Neuroendocrine–thymus interactions. I. In vitro modulation of thymic factor secretion by thyroid hormones. J Endocrinol Invest 1990; 13:139–147.

87. Geenen V, Legros JJ, Franchimont P, Baudrihaye M, Defresnse MP, Boniver J. The neuroendocrine thymus: Coexistence of oxytocin and neurophysin in the human thymus. Science, 1986; 232:508–510.

88. Geenen V, Defrense MP, Robert F, Legros JJ, Franchimont P, Boniver J. Immunocytochemical evidence that thymic nurse cells are neuroendocrine cells. Neuroendocrinology 1988; 47:365–368.

89. Geenen V, Robert F, Martens H, Benhida A, De Giovanni G, Defrense MP, Boniver J, Legros JJ, Martial J, Franchimont P. Biosynthesis and paracrine/cryptocrine actions of 'self' neurohypophysial-related peptides in the thymus. Mol Cell Endocrinol 1991; 76:C27–C31.

90. Johnson HM, Ferrar WL, Torres BA. Vasopressin replacement of interleukin-2 requirement in gamma-interferon production: Lymphokine activity of a neuroendocrine hormone. J Immunol 1982; 129:983–986.

91. Ceredig R, Lowenthal JW, Nahholz M, MacDonald HR. Expression of interleukin-2 receptors as a differentiation marker. Nature 1985; 314:98–100.

92. Hadden JW, Galy A, Chen H, Wang Y, Hadden E. The hormonal regulation of thymus and T lymphocyte development and function. In: Hadden JW, Masek K, Nisticò G, eds. Interactions Among CNS, Neuroendocrine, and Immune Systems. Rome-Milan: Pytagora Press; 1989:147–174.

93. Deschaux P, Massengo B, Fontanges R. Endocrine interaction of the thymus with the hypophysis, adrenals, and testes: Effect of two thymic extracts. Thymus 1979; 1:95–100.

94. Hall NRS, O'Grady MP, Farah JM Jr. Activation of the hypothalamic-pituitary-adrenal axis by thymic peptides. In: Hadden JW, Masek K, Nisticò

G, eds. Interactions Among CNS, Neuroendocrine, and Immune Systems. Rome-Milan: Pythagora Press; 198:114–125.

95. Walford RL. The Immunological Theory of Aging. Copenhagen: Munksgaard; 1969.
96. Burnet FM. An immunological approach to aging. Lancet 1970; ii:358–360.
97. Frolkis VV. Aging and life prolonging process. Vienna, New York: Springer-Verlag; 1982.
98. Prasad AS. Clinical, endocrinological and biochemical effects of zinc deficiency. Clin Endocrinol Metab 1985; 14(3):567–589.
99. Turnlund JR, Durvin N, Costa F, Margen S. Stable isotope studies of zinc absorption and retention in young and elderly men. J Nutr 1986; 116(7): 1239–1247.
100. Fabris N, Muzzioli M, Mocchegiani E. Recovery of age-dependent immunological deterioration in Balb/c mice by short-term treatment with L-thyroxine. Mech Aging Dev 1982; 18:327–338.
101. Giuli C, Pieri C, Piantanelli L, Fabris N. Electron-microscopic morphometric analysis of mouse liver. I. Experimental studies on the morphogenetic significance of the thymus in nude and normal mice. Mech Ageing Dev 1980; 13:265–272.

9
Effects of Cytokines on the Hypothalamic–Pituitary–Adrenal Axis of the Rat

CATHERINE RIVIER

While the concept of bilateral communication between the immune and the neuroendocrine axes has received empirical support from many clinical observations, the biochemical basis for such functional interplay has only recently been determined. It is now well documented that activated immune cells (in particular macrophages) produce proteins, called cytokines or lymphokines, which not only exert stimulatory effects on other immune cells, but can be released into the general circulation and reach neuroendocrine organs. Among the various cytokines, interleukins (IL) are presently considered as playing a major role in communicating to the brain the occurrence of immune activation. This chapter will present an overview of the neuroendocrine effects of IL on the hypothalamic–pituitary–adrenal (HPA) axis of the rat. The reader seeking additional information, or interested in the effects of cytokines on other neuroendocrine functions, should consult recent reviews.[1-5]

Effects of Exogenously Administered Cytokines, and Mechanisms Mediating These Effects

Support for a functional link between immune activation and stimulation of the HPA axis was provided by the observation that rats injected with sheep red blood cells mounted an immune response (as evidenced by increases in antigen-specific gammaglobulins) which reportedly occurred in parallel with increases in circulating corticosterone levels.[6] While the obligatory occurrence of stimulated adrenal function during immune activation has been questioned by work recently carried out in our laboratory,[7] the hypothesis that cytokines (whether released endogenously by activated macrophages or administered exogenously) can stimulate the HPA axis has been convincingly verified.

Indeed, in the rat the exogenous administration of IL-1 (both the α and the β form), IL-6, and tumor necrosis factor-α (TNF-α) causes a rapid

183

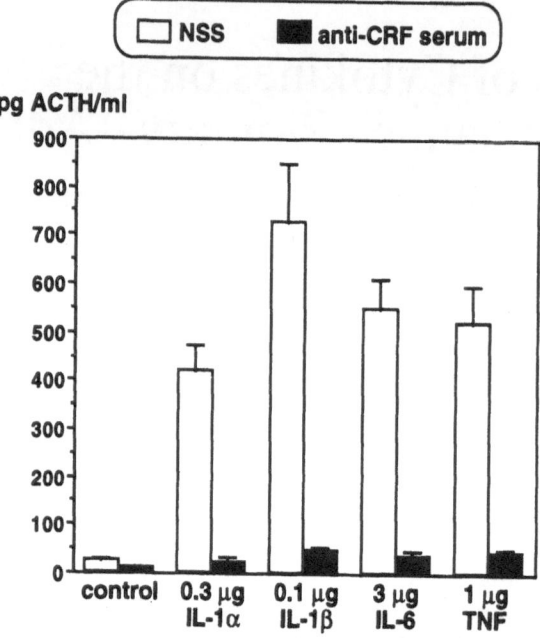

FIGURE 9.1. Effect of immunoneutralization of endogenous CRF on ACTH secretion induced in intact rats by Il-1α, IL-β, IL-6, and TNF-α. Each bar represents the means ± SEM of 6 animals. Blood samples were obtained 15 min after treatment.

and significant increase in plasma adrenocorticotropic hormone (ACTH) and corticosterone levels.[8-11] The inability of cytokines to induce the acute release of ACTH by pituitary cells cultured in the absence of endotoxin[10,12] had suggested that this effect took place primarily at the level of corticotropin-releasing factor (CRF) perikarya and/or CRF nerve terminals. Indeed, the observation that immunoneutralization of endogenous CRF significantly interfered with IL-induced ACTH secretion[10,13,14] demonstrated the major role played by this peptide in modulating the ability of cytokines to activate the HPA axis. The primary role of endogenous CRF was subsequently demonstrated for other cytokines as well[8,9] (Figure 9.1). However, controversy regarding the ability of large proteins to penetrate the brain led to studies designed to investigate the mechanisms through which this stimulatory effect might take place. Several questions therefore needed to be addressed. First, can cytokines cross the blood–brain barrier (BBB), and if not, how do they reach CRF-secreting cells? Second, do cytokines act directly on CRF cells, or do they rely on neurotransmitters known to be released by interleukins, such as prostaglandins (PGs) and catecholamines? And third, do pituitary cells in situ respond to cytokines?

Sites of Action of Cytokines

CNS

The paraventricular nucleus (PVN) of the hypothalamus contains a large proportion of CRF perikarya.[15] Increases in brain cytokine levels, or penetration of cytokines beyond the BBB activate CRF-secreting cells in the PVN.[14,16,17] These perikarya indeed represent a major source of the CRF released by cytokines, as evidenced by our observation that PVN lesions (placed 10 days earlier, and which removed the main source of hypothalamic CRF) significantly blunted the stimulatory action of IL-1β on ACTH release.[18] How, on the other hand, do blood-born cytokines activate the HPA axis? Some investigators have proposed that IL crosses the BBB at sites where this barrier is fenestrated or leaky, such as the organum vasculosum of the lamina terminalis (OVLT).[19–21] Others have provided evidence that these proteins can be actively transported to the hypothalamus.[22,23] Finally the possibility that peripheral cytokines might, through undetermined mechanisms, increase the production of brain cytokines and/or alter their receptors is receiving increasing attention.[24–28]

The immediate early gene c-*fos*, a proto-oncogene expressed in numerous neuron systems after stimulation, is widely used as an anatomical marker of functional neuronal activity.[29] We therefore hypothesized that changes in c-*fos* immunoreactivity would help us to identify brain areas activated by IL-1, and in particular that if IL-1 acted primarily on cells of the PVN, these cells would show increased immunostaining for c-*fos*. We observed that the peripheral injection of IL-1β (which markedly increased plasma ACTH levels) did not measurably increase c-*fos* immunostaining in any brain areas. In contrast, intracerebro-ventricular (icv) administration of a comparable amount of IL-1 (which also significantly released ACTH) significantly increased c-*fos* staining in the PVN. Double staining indicated that these changes took place primarily in CRF perikarya.[30] These results led us to propose that the acute effect of peripherally injected IL-1 takes place primarily at the level of CRF nerve terminals in the median eminence, a hypothesis supported by other investigators.[31,32] It should be noted, however, that some increase in c-*fos* immunoreactivity can be observed 2 h after i.v. injection of IL-1.[33] This suggests that blood-born cytokines can exert a delayed reaction at the level of the PVN which, while being different from that of centrally administered IL-1, probably also participates in the overall activation of the HPA axis. Also, peripheral administration of cytokines does increase CRF expression within the PVN,[34] a phenomenon that may at least partially reflect increased demand on synthesis caused by increased release from the nerve terminals. Thus, we propose that while both iv and icv injected IL-1β activate the HPA axis, the sites at which this effect takes place are different.

Pituitary

As mentioned above, cultured pituitary cells do not release ACTH in response to an acute exposure to IL-1.[10,35] Perifused cells, on the other hand, appear responsive.[36] One possible explanation for this discrepancy lies in the recent findings that cytokines are synthesized within the pituitary itself[37–40] and influence the activity of the corticotrophs. As folliculo-stellate cells represent one source of ILs,[41] it is possible that pituitary preparations that maintain, at least in some degree, the integrity of the intercellular structure, remain responsive to cytokines. Another, not mutually exclusive, hypothesis is that the identity and/or responsiveness of pituitary cytokine receptors[42,43] is altered in cultured cells. Finally, it is important to mention that long-term exposure to cytokines increases proopiomelanocortin (POMC) message,[44] may augment the corticotroph's responsiveness to secretagogues,[45] and measurably stimulates ACTH release. Thus a direct pituitary effect of cytokines is certainly important during prolonged immune activation.[12,44]

Mechanisms of Action

Catecholamines

Do cytokines act directly on CRF cells and/or terminals, or is their effect dependent on the release of neurotransmitters? Studies done in many laboratories have provided evidence that cytokines increase the release of prostaglandins[46,47] and catecholamines,[48,49] which can influence the activity of the HPA axis. In the case of catecholamines, the levels of circulating epinephrine reached by rats injected with IL-1 are comparable to those measured following exposure to various stimuli (Figure 9.2). We have reported that the peripheral administration of the adrenergic receptor blockers prazosin and propanolol, at doses which totally blocked the stimulatory action of catecholamines on ACTH secretion, did not measurably alter IL-1-induced stimulation of the HPA axis.[11] This suggested that peripheral catecholamines are not the primary modulators of the stimulatory action of IL-1 on the HPA axis. The possible role of catecholamine-dependent pathways in the brain was examined by injection of 6-dehydroxydopamine; this treatment, which caused a significant (though not complete) depletion of norepinephrine content in the PVN, significantly reduced the HPA axis' response to IL-1 injected into brain ventricles[50] or into the median eminence.[51] In contrast, these lesions did not alter the stimulatory effect of IL-1 infused directly into the PVN.[52] Thus it is possible that depending on the site to which it is delivered, IL-1 can activate the HPA axis either by a direct effect on CRF neurons in the PVN (in which case stimulation of adrenergic pathways is not required), or through mechanisms which depend on catecholaminergic pathways.

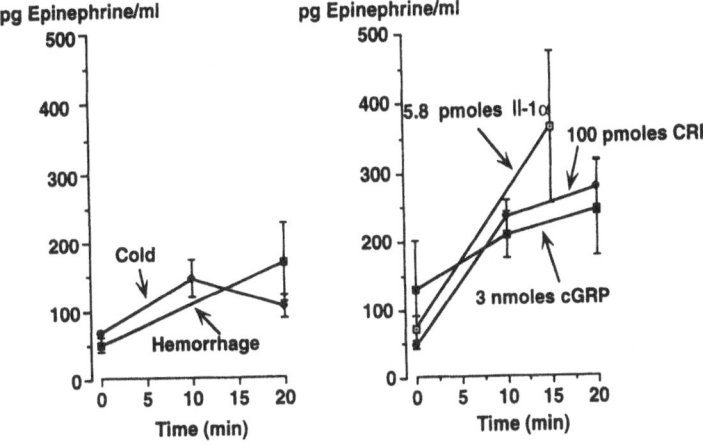

FIGURE 9.2. Comparisons between plasma epinephrine levels measured following exposure to various stimuli or IL-1α. Each point represents the means ± SEM of 6 rats. (Results obtained in collaboration with Dr. Marvin Brown, University of California, San Diego.)

Prostaglandins

Prostaglandins are released by IL-1, and indeed represent important mediators of the thermogenic actions of cytokines.[53-55] In intact rats, acute blockade of PG synthesis by indomethacin completely obliterated the stimulatory effect of IL-1 on ACTH secretion.[56-59] Adrenalectomized rats bearing corticosterone pellets, on the other hand, only exhibited a partial blockade, as did intact animals pretreated with indomethacin for at least 24 hours prior to cytokine injection.[60] These results led us to suggest that while PGs most probably do play a role in modulating the activation of the HPA axis following acute exposure to cytokines, interpretation of findings obtained with indomethacin must take into account a possible effect of negative steroid feedback. Interestingly, there appears to be a species difference with regard to the involvement of PGs. In intact mice, indomethacin markedly suppressed the effect of IL-1 injected i.v., but only attenuated that early phase of the corticosterone response when the cytokine was administered i.p.[61] In contrast in rats indomethacin consistently blocks the early phase, but usually not later phases, of the release of ACTH following i.v. or i.p. injection of at least moderate doses of IL-1β (C. Rivier, unpublished). This discrepancy could be caused, at least in part, by differences in the ability of corticosteroid feedback to modulate the HPA axis of mice and rats, the significant higher dose of IL-1β (on a per kilogram basis) used in the mice study, and/or in differences in involvement of PGs in both species.

Stimulation of Endogenous Cytokines Production: Effects of Endotoxins

The i.v. injection of IL-1 has allowed the investigation of the mechanisms which mediate the ability of this protein to activate the HPA axis, and to study the brain sites at which this effect might take place. However, true immune activation results in the release of a vast array of cytokines, and the i.v. route represents only one of the routes of entry of pathogens into mammalian organisms. We therefore used endotoxins to mimic some of the events occurring during true immune activation. Endotoxins, which are lipopolysaccharides (LPS) present in the walls of Gram-negative bacteria, have been extensively used as experimental tools to stimulate the activity of immune cells. In particular, the injection of endotoxins mimics the events characteristic of the early part of immune activation (called the acute-phase response), and causes the release of endogenous cytokines.[62] The peripheral administration of LPS induces dose-related increases in plasma ACTH and corticosterone levels in the rat[63-67] and the mouse,[3,68] and this response occurs at sub-pyrogenic doses of the endotoxin.[69] The hypothesis that at least part of this effect depended on endogenous cytokines was demonstrated by the ability of antibodies against IL-1 receptors to significantly blunt the stimulatory action of LPS on the HPA axis of mice.[68] As endotoxins exert many effects on metabolism and endocrine functions, it is possible that the stimulatory action of these proteins on the HPA axis may represent multiple sites of action. We have observed that immunoneutralization of endogenous CRF significantly attenuated LPS-induced of ACTH secretion, and that blockade of V_1 vasopressin receptors also interfered with this response.[67] Earlier reports have also suggested an important role for the hypothalamus in modulating the effect of LPS on the HPA axis.[65,66] Nevertheless, there is evidence that other mechanisms, such as histamine release[64,70] and/or activation of structures other than the PVN,[63] may also be important. Indeed, a recent report has indicated that following removal of CRF and vasopressin (VP) by PVN lesions, rats still secreted measurable amounts of ACTH in response to LPS.[71]

As mentioned above, we observed that indomethacin completely prevented the early phase of ACTH secretion regardless of the route of IL-1β administration. Infection is reportedly associated with elevated circulating levels of IL-1, IL-6, and TNF-α,[72,73] and these cytokines gain access to neuroendocrine organs through various routes. We therefore reasoned that if LPS stimulated the HPA axis through mechanisms that did not entirely rely on increased levels of IL-1β, and if eicosanoids were not involved in these other mechanisms, pretreatment with indomethacin might help us better understand the pathways which were activated following either i.v. or i.p. injection of LPS. Our results indicated that

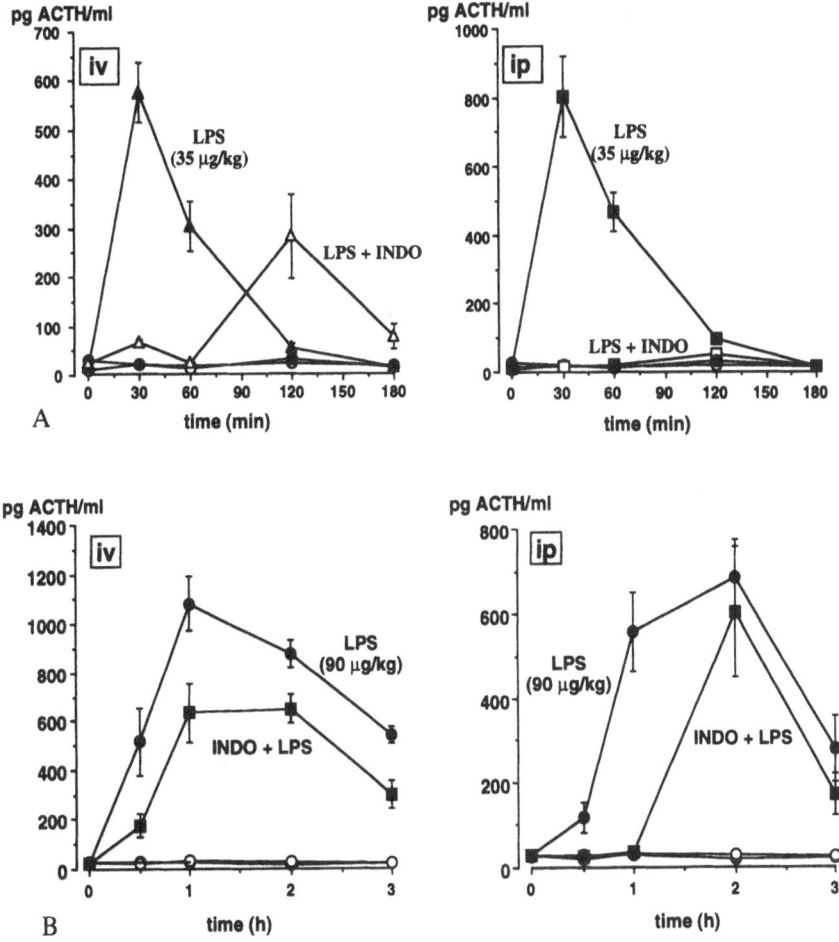

FIGURE 9.3. Effect of indomethacin (INDO, 2.5 mg injected i.v. 15 min before and 60 min after treatment) on ACTH released by the vehicle or endotoxin (LPS) injected (A) intravenously (iv) or (B) intraperitoneally (ip). Each point represents the means ± SEM of 6 rats.

indomethacin totally blocked ACTH secretion induced by the i.p. injection of 35 µg/kg LPS/kg (Figure 9.3A), but only slightly interfered with the stimulatory action of 90 µg/kg (Figure 9.3B). Upon i.v. injection of 35 µg/kg LPS/kg, only the first phase (60 min) of activation of the HPA axis was attenuated by indomethacin, while ACTH levels remained significantly elevated at all times in rats injected with 90 µg/kg LPS/kg. As at least in our hands, indomethacin blocked the activation of the HPA axis caused by either IL-6 or TNF (unpublished results), it appears improbable that these cytokines play a major role in modulating those neuroendocrine effects of LPS which are independent of prostaglandins. At present, the mechanisms responsible for the increased ACTH release caused by the higher dose of LPS in the presence of indomethacin remain unknown.

Sepsis, or increased levels of endotoxins, are accompanied by elevated release of IL-1β, IL-6, and TNF-α into the circulation.[74–76] IL-6, in particular, is emerging as a major factor in mediating the host responses to pathogenic injury.[38,77–80] Though IL-6 stimulates the HPA axis (albeit at much higher doses than IL-1β[81]), it has been suggested that the primary role of this cytokine resides in altering the level of responsiveness of both immune and neuroendocrine cells.[38,82] In addition to increasing circulating levels of various cytokines, endotoxins can induce the production of ILs within the pituitary,[83–85] in particular in folliculo-stellated cells.[40,41] Cytokines produced by the pituitary or secreted by macrophages into the general circulation may also alter the corticotrop's responses to CRF,[86] synergize each other's activity on ACTH secretion,[38,82] but also induce the production of IL inhibitors.[87] Thus the activity of the HPA axis during immune activation represents the net effect of synergistic as well as antagonistic actions of various cytokines acting both at the level of the central nervous system (CNS) and the pituitary.

Conclusions

This chapter has summarized our present knowledge of the ability of cytokines to stimulated the HPA axis, an effect considered essential for the coordination of the appropriate neuroendocrine responses to an antigen challenge. During the initial phase of immune activation, cytokines are believed to act primarily at the level of the CNS to release CRF, VP, and neurotransmitters. In later phases, a direct pituitary site of action of cytokines also becomes important. Thus the overall neuroendocrine responses to immune challenges represent complex interplays between central and peripheral mechanisms aimed at restoring, then maintaining homeostasis during exposure to antigens.

Acknowledgments. This work was supported by NIH grant DK-26741 and the Foundation for Medical Research, Inc. The IL-1β used in these studies was generously supplied by Dr. S. Gillis, Immunex, Seattle, WA.

References

1. Bateman A, Singh A, Kral T, Solomon S. The immune-hypothalamic-pituitary-adrenal axis. Endocr Rev 1989; 10:92–112.
2. Weigent DA, Carr DJJ, Blalock JE. Bidirectional communication between the neuroendocrine and immune systems: Common hormones and hormone

receptors. In: Koob GF, Sandman CA, Strand FL, eds. Proceedings of the Tenth Annual Winter Neuropeptide Conference. New York: The New York Academy of Sciences; 1990:17–27.

3. Dunn AJ. Interleukin-1 as a stimulator of hormone secretion. Prog Neuroendocrinimmunol 1990; 3:26–34.

4. Busbridge NJ, Grossman AB. Stress and the single cytokine: Interleukin modulation of the pituitary-adrenal axis. Mol Cell Endocrinol 1991; 82: C209–C214.

5. Rivier C, Rivest S. Effect of stress on the activity of hypothalamic-pituitary-gonadal axis in the rat. Biol Repord 1991; 45:523–532.

6. Besedovsky H, Sorkin E. Changes in blood hormone levels during the immune response. Proc Soc Exp Biol Med 1975; 150:466–470.

7. Stenzel-Poore M, Vale W, Rivier C. Relationship between antigen-induced immune stimulation and activation of the HPA axis in the rat. Endocrinology 1993; 132:1313–1318.

8. Naitoh Y, Fukata J, Tominaga T, Nakai Y, Tamai S, Mori K, Imura H. Interleukin-6 stimulates the secretion of adrenocorticotropic hormone in conscious, freely-moving rats. Biochem Biophys Res Commun 1988; 155:1459–1463.

9. Sharp BM, Matta SG, Peterson PK, Newton R, Chao C, McAllen K. Tumor necrosis factor-α is a potent ACTH secretagogue: Comparison to interleukin-1β. Endocrinology 1989; 124:3131–3133.

10. Sapolsky R, Rivier C, Yamamoto G, Plotsky P, Vale W. Interleukin-1 stimulates the secretion of hypothalamic corticotropin-releasing factor. Science 1987; 238:522–524.

11. Rivier C, Vale W, Brown M. In the rat, interleukin-1α and -β stimulate adenocorticotropin and catecholamine release. Endocrinology 1989; 125: 3096–3102.

12. Kehrer P, Turnill D, Dayer J-M, Muller AF, Gaillard RC. Human recombinant interleukin-1beta and -alpha, but not recombinant tumor necrosis factor alpha stimulate ACTH release from rat anterior pituitary cells in vitro in a prostaglandin E_2 and cAMP independent manner. Neuroendocrinology 1988; 48:160–166.

13. Uehara A, Gottschall PE, Dahl RR, Arimura A. Interleukin-1 stimulates ACTH release by an indirect action which requires endogenous corticotropin releasing factor. Endocrinology 1987; 121:1580–1582.

14. Berkenbosch F, VanOers J, DelRay A, Tilders F, Besedovsky H. Corticotropin-releasing factor-producing neurons in the rat activated by interleukin-1. Science 1987; 238:524–526.

15. Swanson LW, Sawchenko PE, Rivier J, Vale WW. Organization of ovine corticotropin releasing factor (CRF)-immunoactive cells and fibers in the rat brain: An immunohistochemical study. Neuroendocrinology 1983; 36: 165–186.

16. Ju G, Zhang X, Jin B-Q, Huang C-S. Activation of corticotropin-releasing factor-containing neurons in the paraventricular nucleus of the hypothalamus by interleukin-1 in the rat. Neurosci Lett 1991; 132:151–154.

17. Saphier D, Ovadia H. Selective facilitation of putative corticotropin-releasing factor-secreting neurons by interleukin-1. Neurosci Lett 1990; 114:283–288.

18. Rivest S, Rivier C. Influence of the paraventricular nucleus of the hypothalamus in the alteration of neuroendocrine functions induced by physical stress or interleukin. Endocrinology 1991; 129:2049–2057.

19. Katsuura G, Arimura A, Koves K, Gottschall PE. Involvement of organum vasculosum of lamina terminalis and preoptic area in interleukin 1β-induced ACTH release. Am J Physiol 1990; 258:E163–E171.

20. Stitt JT. Passage of immunomodulators accross the blood–brain barrier. Yale J Biol Med 1990; 63:121–131.

21. Shibata M, Blatteis CM. Human recombinant tumor necrosis factor and interferon affect the activity of neurons in the organum vasculosum laminae terminalis. Brain Res 1991; 562:323–326.

22. Banks WA, Kastin AJ, Durham DA. Bidirectional transport of interleukin-1 alpha across the blood–brain barrier. Brain Res Bull 1989; 23:433–437.

23. Banks WA, Ortiz L, Plotkin SR, Kastin AJ. Human interleukin (IL) 1α, murine IL-1α and murine IL-1β are transported from blood to brain in the mouse by a shared saturable mechanism. J Pharmacol Exp Ther 1991; 259:257–259.

24. Fontana A, Weber E, Dayer JM. Synthesis of interleukin 1/endogenous pyrogen in the brain of endotoxin-treated mice: A step in fever induction? J Immunol 1984; 133:1696–1698.

25. Haour F, Ban E, Milon G, Baran D, Fillion G. Brain interleukin 1 receptors: Characterization and modulation after lipopolysaccharide injection. Prog Neuroendocrinimmunol 1990; 3:196–204.

26. Higgins GA, Olschowka JA. Induction of interleukin-1-beta messenger RNA in adult rat brain. Mol Brain Res 1991; 9:143–148.

27. Schettini G. Interleukin 1 in the neuroendocrine system: From gene to function. Prog Neuroendocrinimmunol 1990; 3:157–166.

28. Koenig JI. Presence of cytokines in the hypothalamic-pituitary axis. Prog Neuroendocrinimmunol 1991; 4:143–153.

29. Morgan JI, Curran T. Stimulus-transcription coupling in the nervous system: Involvement of the inductible proto-oncogenes *fos* and *jun*. Annu Rev Neurosci 1991; 14:421–451.

30. Rivest S, Torres G, Rivier C. Differential effects of central and periopheral injection of interleukin-1β on brain c-*fos* expression and neuroendocrine functions. Brain Res 1992; 587:13–23.

31. Watanobe H, Sasaki S, Takebe K. Evidence that intravenous administration of interleukin-1 stimulates corticotropin-releasing hormone secretion in the median eminence of freely moving rats: Estimation by push-pull perfusion. Neurosci Lett 1991; 133:7–10.

32. Spinedi E, Hadid R, Daneva T, Gaillard RC. Cytokines stimulate the CRH but not the vasopressin neuronal system: Evidence for a median eminence site of interleukin-6 action. Neuroendocrinology 1992; 45:46–53.

33. Ericsson A, Sawchenko PE. c-*fos*-Based functional mapping of central pathways subserving the effects of interleukin-1 on the hypothalamo-pituitary-adrenal axis. In: DeSouza EB, eds. Methods in Neuroscience. New York: Academic Press; 1992: in press.

34. Suda T, Tozawa F, Ushiyama T, Sumitomo T, Yamada M, Demura H. Interleukin-1 stimulates corticotropin-releasing factor gene expression in rat hypothalamus. Endocrinology 1990; 126:1223–1228.

35. Uehara A, Gillis S, Arimura A. Effects of interleukin-1 on hormone release from normal rat pituitary cells in primary culture. Neuroendocrinology 1987; 45:343–347.
36. Cambronero JC, Rivas FJ, Borrell J, Guaza C. Interleukin-1-beta induces pituitary adrenocorticotropin secretion: Evidence for glucocorticoid modulation. Neuroendocrinology 1992; 55:648–654.
37. Spangelo BL, MacLeod RM, Isakson PC. Production and function of interleukin-6 in the rat anterior pituitary. Mol Cell Biol Cytokines 1990; 10:433–438.
38. Spangelo BL, MacLeod RM. Regulation of the acute phase response and neuroendocrine function by interleukin 6. Prog Neuroendocrinimmunol 1990; 3:167–175.
39. Carmeliet P, Vankelecom H, Van Damme J, Billiau A, Denef C. Release of interleukin-6 from anterior pituitary cell aggregates: Developmental pattern and modulation by glucocorticoids and forskolin. Neuroendocrinology 1991; 53:29–34.
40. Tatsuno I, Somogyvari-Vigh A, Mizuno K, Gottschall PE, Hidaka H, Arimura A. Neuropeptide regulation of interleukin-6 production from the pituitary: Stimulation by pituitary adenylate cyclase activating polypeptide and calcitonin gene-related peptide. Endocrinology 1991; 129:1797–1804.
41. Vankelecom H, Carmeliet P, VanDamme J, Billiau A, Denef C. Production of interleukin-6 by folliculo-stellate cells of the anterior pituitary gland in a histiotypic cell aggregate culture system. Neuroendocrinology 1989; 49: 102–106.
42. Ohmichi M, Hirota K, Koike K, Kurachi H, Ohtsuka S, Matsuzaki N, Yamaguchi M, Miyaka A, Tanizwa O. Binding sites for interleukin-6 in the anterior pituitary gland. Neuroendocrinology 1992; 55:199–203.
43. Cunningham ET, Wada E, Carter DB, Tracey DE, Battey JF, DeSouza EB. In situ histochemical localisation of type I interleukin-1 receptor messenger RNA in the central nervous system, pituitary, and adrenal gland of the mouse. J Neurosci 1992; 12:1101–1114.
44. Suda T, Tozawa F, Ushiyama T, Tomori N, Sumitomo T, Nakagami Y, Yamada M, Demura H, Shizume K. Effects of protein kinase-C-related adrenocorticotropin secretagogues and interleukin-1 on proopiomelanocortin gene expression in rat anterior pituitary cells. Endocrinology 1989; 124: 1444–1449.
45. Fagarasan MO, Alelrod J, Catt KJ. Interleukin-1 potentiates agonist-induced secretion of beta-endorphin in anterior pituitary cells. Biochem Biophys Res Commun 1990; 173:988–993.
46. Komaki G, Arimura A, Koves K. Effect of intravenous injection of IL-1β on PGE_2 levels in several brain areas as determined by microdialysis. Am J Physiol 1992; 262:E246–E251.
47. Katsuura G, Gottschall PE, Dahl RR, Arimura A. Interleukin-1 beta increases prostaglandin E_2 in rat astrocyte cultures: Modulatory effect of neuropeptides. Endocrinology 1989; 124:3125–3127.
48. Dunn AJ. Systemic interleukin-1 administration stimulates hypothalamic norepinephrine metabolism paralleling the increased plasma corticosterone. Life Sci 1988; 43:429–435.
49. Palazzolo DL, Quadri SK. Interleukin-1 stimulates catecholamine release from the hypothalamus. Life Sci 1990; 47:2105–2109.

194   C. Rivier

50. Weidenfeld J, Abramsky O, Ovadia H. Evidence for the involvement of the central adrenergic system in interleukin 1-induced adrenocortical response. Neuropharmacology 1989; 28:1411–1414.
51. Matta SG, Singh J, Newton R, Sharp BM. The adrenocorticotropin response to interleukin-1β instilled into the rat median eminence depends on the local release of catecholamines. Endocrinology 1990; 127:2175–2182.
52. Barbanel G, Ixart G, Szafarczyk A, Malaval F. Intraphypothalamic infusion of interleukin-1β increases the release of corticotropin-releasing hormone (CRH 41) and adrenocorticotropic hormone (ACTH) in free-moving rats bearing a push-pull cannula in the median eminence. Brain Res 1990; 516: 31–36.
53. LeMay LG, Vander AJ, Kluger MJ. Role of interleukin 6 in fever in rats. Am J Physiol 1990; 258:R798–R803.
54. Stitt JT. Prostaglandin E_2 as the neural mediator of the febrile response. Yale J Biol Med 1986; 59:137–149.
55. Blatteis CM. Neural mechanisms in the pyrogenic and acute phase responses to interleukin-1. Int J Neurosci 1987; 38:223–232.
56. Morimoto A, Murakami N, Nakamori T, Sakata Y, Watanabe T. Possible involvement of prostaglandin E in development of ACTH response in rats induced by human recombinant interleukin-1. J Physiol 1989; 411:245–256.
57. Murakami N, Watanabe T. Activation of ACTH release is mediated by the same molecule as the final mediator, PGE_2, of the febrile response in rats. Brain Res 1989; 478:171–174.
58. Watanabe T, Morimoto A, Sakata Y, Murakami N. ACTH response induced by interleukin-1 is mediated by CRF secretion stimulated by hypothalamic PGE. Experiential 1990; 46:481–484.
59. Katsuura G, Gottschall PE, Dahl RR, Arimura A. Adrenocorticotropin release induced by intracerebroventricular injection of recombinant human interleukin-1 in rats: Possible involvement of prostaglandin. Endocrinology 1988; 122:1773–1779.
60. Rivier C, Vale W. Stimulatory effect of interleukin-1 on ACTH secretion in the rat: It is modulated by prostaglandins? Endocrinology 1991; 129:384–388.
61. Dunn AJ, Chuluyan HE. The role of cyclo-oxygenase and lipoxygenase in the interleukin-1-induced activation of the HPA axis: Dependence on the route of injection. Life Sci 1992; 51:219–225.
62. Dinarello CA. Interleukin-1 and the pathogenesis of the acute-phase response. N Eng J Med 1984; 311:1413–1418.
63. Makara GB, Stark E, Meszaros T. Corticotrophin release induced by E. coli endotoxin after removal of the medial hypothalamus. Endocrinology 1971; 88:412–414.
64. Suzuki S, Oh C, Nakano K. Pituitary-dependent and -independent secretion of CS caused by bacterial endotoxin in rats. Am J Physiol 1986; 250: E470–E474.
65. Moberg GP. Site of action of endotoxins on hypothalamic-pituitary-adrenal axis. Am J Physiol 1974; 220:397–400.
66. Yasuda N, Greer MA. Evidence that the hypothalamus mediates endotoxin stimulatin of adrenocorticotropic hormone secretion. Endocriology 1978; 102:947–953.

67. Rivier C. Role of endotoxin and interleukin-1 in modulating ACTH, LH, and sex steroid secretion. In: *Proceedings of the Symposium on Circulating Regulatory Factors and Neuroendocrine Function*. Porter JC, Jezova D, eds. New York: Plenum Press; 1989:295–301.

68. Rivier C, Chizzonite R, Vale W. In the mouse, the activation of the hypothalamic-pituitary-adrenal axis by a lipopolysaccharide (endotoxin) is mediated through interleukin-1. Endocrinology 1989; 125:2800–2805.

69. Derijk RH, vanRooijen N, Berkenbosch F. The role of macrophages in the hypothalamic-pituitary-adrenal activation in response to endotoxin (LPS). Res Immunol 1992; 143:224–229.

70. Suzuki S, Nakano K. Suppression of endotoxin-induced corticosterone secretion in rats by H_1-antihistamine. Am J Physiol 1985; 248:E26–E30.

71. Elenkov IJ, Kovacs K, Kiss J, Betok L, Vizi ES. Lipopolysaccharide is able to bypass corticotrophin-releasing factor in affecting plasma ACTH and corticosterone levels: Evidence from rats with lesions of the paraventricular nucleus. J Endocrinol 1991; 133:231–236.

72. Frei K, Malipiero UV, Leist TP, Zinkernagel RM, Schwab ME, Fontana A. On the cellular source and function of interleukin 6 produced in the central nervous system in viral diseases. Eur J Immunol 1989; 19:689–694.

73. Ertel W, Morrison MH, Wang P, Ba ZF, Ayala A, Chaudry IH. The complex pattern of cytokines in sepsis—association between prostaglandins, cachectin, and interleukins. Ann Surg 1991; 214:141–148.

74. Shalaby MR, Waage A, Aarden L, Espevik T. Endotoxin, tumor necrosis factor-α and interleukin 1 induce interleukin 6 production in vivo. Clin Immunol Immunopathol 1989; 53:488–498.

75. Bristow AF, Mosley K, Poole S. Interleukin-1β production in vivo and in vitro in rats and mice measured using specific immunoradiometric assays. J Mol Endocrinol 1991; 7:1–7.

76. Butler LD, Layman NK, Riedl PE, Cain RL, Shellhaas J, Evans GF, Zuckerman SH. Neuroendocrine regulation of in vivo cytokine production and effects. I. In vivo regulatory networks involving the neuroendocrine system, interleukin-1, and tumor necrosis factor-α. J Neuroimmunol 1991; 24:143–153.

77. Ramadori G, VanDamme J, Rieder H, Zum Buschenfelde K-HM. Interleukin 6, the third mediator of acute-phase reaction, modulates hepatic protein synthesis in human and mouse. Comparison with interleukin 1β and tumor necrosis factor-α. Eur J Immunol 1988; 18:1259–1264.

78. Geiger T, Andus T, Klapproth J, Hirano T, Kishimoto T, Heinrich PC. Induction of rat acute-phase proteins by interleukin 6 in vivo. Eur J Immunol 1988; 18:717–721.

79. Castell JV, Gomez-Lechon MJ, David M, Andus T, Geiger T, Trullenque R, Fabra R, Heinrich PC. Interleukin-6 is the major regulator of acute phase protein synthesis in adult human hepatocytes. Fed Eur Biochem Soc 1989; 242:237–239.

80. VanSnick J. Interleukin-6: An overview. Annu Rev Immunol 1990; 8:253–278.

81. Besedovsky HO, DelRey A, Klusman I, Furukawa H, Arditi GM, Kabiersch A. Cytokines as modulators of the hypothalamus-pituitary-adrenal axis. J Ster Biochem Mol Biol 1991; 40:613–618.

82. Perlstein RS, Mougey EH, Jackson WE, Neta R. Interleukin-1 and inter-leukin-6 act synergistically to stimulate the release of adrenocorticotropic hormone in vivo. Lymph Cyt Res 1991; 10:141–146.
83. Koenig JI, Snow K, Clark BD, Toni R, Cannon JG, Shaw AR, Dinarello CA, Reichlin S, Lee SL, Lechan RM. Intrinsic pituitary interleukin-1β is induced by bacterial lipopolysaccharide. Endocrinology 1990; 126:3053–3058.
84. Spangelo BL, Judd AM, Isakson PC, MacLeod RM. Interleukin-1 stimulates interleukin-6 release from rat anterior pituitary cells in vitro. Endocrinology 1991; 128:2685–2692.
85. Spangelo BL, Jarvis WD, Judd AM, MacLeod RM. Induction of interleukin-6 release by interleukin-1 in rat anterior pituitary cells in vitro: Evidence for an eicosanoid-dependent mechanism. Endocrinology 1991; 129:2886–2894.
86. Gaillard RC, Turnill D, Sappino P, Muller AF. Tumor necrosis factor α in-hibits the hormonal response of the pituitary gland to hypothalamic releasing factors. Endocrinology 1990; 127:101–106.
87. Dinarello CA. Interleukin-1 and interleukin-1 antagonism. Blood 1991; 77:1627–1652.

10
Role of Growth Factors and Cytokines in the Therapy of Immune Deficiencies

SUDHIR GUPTA

During the 1980s, rapid progress was made in better understanding of the pathogenesis of immunodeficiencies at both cellular and molecular levels. Furthermore, the development of recombinant techniques has led to molecular cloning, expression, and formulation of a number of hematopoietic growth factors and cytokines that have become more affordable and whose potential therapeutic uses have been explored. The purpose of this chapter is to briefly review the scope of certain growth factors and cytokines that have already been used or have future potential in the therapy of immunodeficiency disorders. An attempt is made to summarize the biological and molecular characteristics of these cytokines and growth factors, cellular and molecular defects of pertinent immunodeficiency diseases, and the results of the therapy in these disorders. Among the growth factors, granulocyte-colony stimulating factor (G-CSF) and granulocyte monocyte colony stimulating factor (GM-CSF) will be discussed. Among the cytokines, interleukin 2 (IL-2) and interferon gamma (IFN-γ) will be reviewed.

Growth Factors

Neutrophilic granulocytes and monocytes are of importance in resistance to infections; abnormally low numbers or abnormal functions of granulocytes are associated with susceptibility to recurrent or persistent life-threatening bacterial infections. There are four regulators or growth factors, known as colony stimulating factors (CSFs), that control the production, maturation, and function of granulocytes and monocytes macrophages.[1] The CSFs are produced by multiple cell types, including endothelial cells, fibroblasts, stromal cells, macrophages, lymphocytes, and consist of glycoprotein with molecular masses of 18–19 kd. The serum levels of CSF are low in the healthy state, but the levels are seen to increase in infection. G-CSF, GM-CSF, and multi-CSF or interleukin 3

(IL-3) consist of a single polypeptide chain, whereas macrophage-CSF (M-CSF) is a dimer of two identical subunits. The carbohydrate portion of the CSFs is not required for biological activities; thus recombinant CSFs are active molecules. The CSFs are polyfunctioning; that is, they control differentiation in granulocyte macrophage progenitor cells, and initiate the maturation, proliferation, and functioning of the mature cells.[2] Each CSF initiates proliferation of the responding cell by moving the noncycling cells into mitotic cycle. Once the cell has been moved into mitotic cycle, the concentration of CSF determines the length of the cycle and the total number of progeny produced. Although each CSF can stimulate cell proliferation at a low level, they differ in the cellular pattern of proliferation. Whereas both GM-CSF and IL-3 stimulate the proliferation of granulocyte and macrophage colonies, G-CSF and M-CSF selectively stimulate granulocytic and macrophage colonies respectively. CSFs exert their biological activities through binding to specific membrane receptors. Most granulocyte macrophage progenitors and their maturing progeny express specific membrane receptors for all four CSFs.[2] The receptors of CSFs have an extracellular domain, a transmembrane domain, and an intracellular domain. M-CSF has an intracytoplasmic tyrosine kinase domain,[3] whereas other CSFs lack the tyrosine kinase intracytoplasmic domain and therefore must elicit signal transduction by other mechanisms. It is presumed that these nontyrosine kinase receptors may have additional subunits or associated polypeptides. The human GM-CSF receptor has been shown to contain such an additional subunit.[4] The occupancy of CSF receptors by CSFs can initiate a multiple signaling cascade in the responding cell. However, it appears that the responding cells must themselves be able to determine which signaling cascades are generated and which types of cellular responses are elicited.

G-CSF and GM-CSF in Neutropenias

Neutrophils are the most important phagocytic cells that play a crucial role in defense against bacterial infections. Therefore, individuals suffering from disorders associated with chronic and severe neutropenia are highly susceptible to severe bacterial infections leading to pneumonia, otitis media, subcutaneous abscesses, septicemia, etc. The most common organisms include *Staphylococcus aureus* and Gram-negative bacteria. Although IL-3, GM-CSF, and G-CSF have been shown to increase neutrophil granulocytes[5,6] in vivo in preclinical and in phase I–III clinical studies, the most promising results have been obtained with G-CSF. G-CSF is a glycoprotein of 19,600 kd with 174 amino acids.[7] G-CSF is produced by fibroblasts, endothelial cells, and monoctes and macrophages. It stimulates proliferation and differentiation of myeloid progenitors to the mature neutrophils.[8] G-CSF exerts its biological activity through binding to a high affinity G-CSF receptor[9,10] composed of a single poly-peptide chain consisting of an extracellular immunoglobulin-like domain, a transmembrane domain, and an intracytoplasmic domain.[11] Initial clinical trials with G-CSF were mainly in patients with maligancy in whom neutropenia was a consequence of chemotherapy;[12] however, in this review the main discussion will focus on neutropenias associated with immunodeficiency.

Congenital Neutropenia (Kostmann's Syndrome)

Severe congenital neutropenia is characterized by severe persistent neutropenia (neutrophil count of <500/μl) presenting clinically in early infancy with abscess formation, otitits media, gingivitis, urinary tract infection, pneumonia, and bacterial sepsis. There is a maturational arrest at the promyelocyte/myelocyte stage.[12-14] Bone marrow transplantation (BMT) has been shown to correct this disorder,[15] however, the lack of availability of HLA-matched donors limits the applicability of the BMT approach. In 1989, Bonilla et al.[18] achieved complete response in 5 patients with congenital neutropenia with rG-CSF with a decrease in the number of infectious episodes in all five. Welte et al.[17-18] treated 32 patients with severe congenital neutropenia (absolute neutrophil count <200/μl). These patients exhibited compensatory eosinophilia, mono-cytosis, and hyperimmunoglobulinemia, and no evidence of antineutrophil antibodies. In 30 of 32 patients, rhG-CSF induced an increase of blood neutrophils to above 1000/μl). The neutrophil functions, including phago-cytosis, intracellular killing of staphylycocci, and reactive oxygen pro-duction, were normal; however, chemotaxis towards FMLP and other chemoattractants IL-8, C5a, LTB4, PAF) was reduced[18].* In all patients, the number and severity of bacterial infections were significantly reduced, while in some patients there was a complete resolution of pneumonitis, liver abscess, and anal abscess that had been resistant to intensive anti-biotic therapy. Initially, 5 of these patients with severe congenital neutro-penia were treated with GM-CSF prior to receiving G-CSF. rhGM-CSF was administered at a dose of 3-30 μg/kg per day intravenously, and in all patients, a dose-dependent increase in absolute granulocyte counts was observed. However, in 4 patients this increase was due to an increase in eosinophils, and only in a single patient was an increase in absolute neutrophils observed.

The reported adverse side effects of rhG-CSF included: necrotizing cutaneous vasculitis, generalized severe vasculitis, mesangioproliferative glomerulonephritis (all three side effects were associated with rapid in-

---

*PAF = Platelet-activating factor; C5a = (is a split-product of LTB4 = Leukotriene B4; and 5th component of complement); FMLP = N-formyl-L-methionyl-L-leucyl-L-phenylalanine.

crease in absolute neutrophil counts and not related to dose of rhG-CSF), osteopenia and osteoporosis, splenomegaly, myelodysplastic syndrome, and acute monocytic leukemia in two patients. Patients with congenital neutropenia are predisposed to acute myeloid leukemia; whether they are also predisposed to acute monocytic leukemia or the occurrence of acute monocytic leukemia in two of these patients was related to rhG-CSF therapy, remains to be determined. The side effect of rhGM-CSF treatment was local phlebitis at a 30 μg/kg per day dose.

Despite significant beneficial effect of rhG-CSF on the clinical course of patients, the pathogenesis of severe congenitial neutropenia remains unclear. A number of possibilities have been entertained, including defective production of G-CSF and/or decreased binding to G-CSF receptors or decreased numbers of G-CSF receptors. Neither of these possibilities appears to be present in severe congenital neutropenia. Pietsch et al. have shown normal[19] and Mempel et al.[20] increased levels of G-CSF in patients with severe congenital neutropenia. Kyas et al.[21] have demonstrated that the binding of G-CSF to its receptors on neutrophils from patients with severe congenital neutropenia is normal. Furthermore, they have observed increased numbers of G-CSF receptors on neutrophils from these patients. Therefore, a possibility of defective post intracellular binding signaling events has to be entertained.

In summary, rhG-CSF is most promising and the treatment of choice for patients with severe congenital neutropenia, resulting in a significant improvement in clinical status and, therefore, prolongation of life span, and improvement in the quality of life.

G-CSF and GM-CSF in Cyclic Neutropenia

Cyclic neutropenia is a rare disorder characterized by regular cyclic fluctuations in the numbers of neutrophils, platelets, and reticulocytes,[22,23] presenting clinically with regular recurring fevers, lymphadenopathy, pharyngitis, mucosal ulcers, and numerous infections (especially with *Staphylococcus aureus*) during the period of neutropenia. The precise defect in cyclic neutropenia is unknown, however, the defect appears to be at the level of stem cells, since the onset in some patients is later in life, suggesting that it is an acquired disorder. Hammond et al.[24] treated 6 patients suffering from cyclic neutropenia with rhG-CSF. He reported that while the absolute neurtrophil counts increased the cycling continued. However, the length of neutropenia was reduced from 21 days to 14 days, and the number of days with severe neutropenia was significantly reduced. In addition, there was a fourfold increase in neutrophil turnover. Clinically, a significant reduction in the frequency of fever, oropharyngeal inflammation, and infections was observed; the side effects included splenic enlargement and bone pains. Welte et al.[18] also observed an increase in absolute neutrophil counts and decreased frequency of infections in 4 patients with cyclic neutropenia treated with rhG-CSF. These studies would appear to suggest that rhG-CSF is a relatively safe and effective treatment for reducing the morbidity of patients with cyclic neutropenia. Freund et al.[25] demonstrated a differential effect of GM-CSF and G-CSF in a patient with cyclic neutropenia. The treatment with rhGM-CSF had no effect on absolute neutrophil count, and the patient developed myalgia, arthralgia, and pericarditis. Following discontinuation of rhGM-CSF, rhG-CSF was administered and an increase in absolute neutrophil counts was observed. This differential effect of GM-CSF and G-CSF is similar to that observed in patients with severe congenital neutropenia.

G-CSF and GM-CSF in Acquired Chronic Neutropenia

rhG-CSF has been used in a single patient each with post-infectious mononucleosis chronic neutropenia and severe neutropenia associated with hyper-IgM syndrome.[18] In both subjects, treatment with rhG-CSF resulted in increased neutrophil counts and a decrease in the frequency of infections. Schroten et al.[26] treated 2 patients with chronic neutropenia associated with glycogen storage disease type Ib with rhG-CSF. One of the 2 patients was initially treated with rhGM-CSF at 8 μg/kg per day for 2 weeks. After 3 weeks of such treatment, absolute neutrophil counts were normalized; however, because of severe local painful hyperemia and severe edema of both legs, the treatment with rhGM-CSF was discontinued. Three months after the termination of the rhGM-CSF treatment the patients were placed on rhG-CSF. In both patients, treatment with rhG-CSF resulted in increased neutrophil numbers and normal production of H_2O_2. These effects on neutrophils were associated with decreased frequency and severity of infections, and additionally, no significant side effects were noted.

G-CSF in Chronic Idiopathic Neutropenia

Chronic idiopathic neutropenia can present clinically from infancy to adulthood. The pathophysiology of chronic idiopathic neutropenia is unclear. However, the bone marrow contains normal numbers of myeloid progenitor cells with an arrest of granulopoiesis at a late stage of granulocyte maturation. Welte et al.[18] have treated 12 patients with chronic idopathic neutropenia with rhG-CSF. Ten of those so treated responded with an increase in neutrophil counts, while the number and severity of infections significantly decreased. The remaining 2 patients developed aplastic anemia 1 year following the treatment. In there studies it is unclear whether the aplastic anemia was secondary to treatment with rhG-CSF or a consequence of general bone marrow aplasia as a part of the natural history of the disease in those patients.

GM-CSF and G-CSF in the Acquired Immunodeficiency Syndrome (AIDS)

In a phase I trial, Groopman et al.[27] treated 16 patients suffering from AIDS-associated leukopenia, with a single intravenous dose of rhGM-CSF, followed after 48 hours with a 14-day course of continuous infusion at doses of 0.5 to 8.0 µg/kg per day. A dose-related increase in circulating leukocytes, shared by mature neutrophils, neutrophilic bands, eosinophils, and monocytes, was observed and neutrophil functions were normal. This effect lasted for 3–9 days and, additionally, this treatment did not affect lymphocytes or $CD4^+$ T or $CD8^+$ T cells. In a follow-up study, subcutaneously self-administered rhGM-CSF was well-tolerated and demonstrated beneficial effect in overcoming leucopenia in 15 patients.[28] A threefold increase in absolute neutrophils and eosinophils was observered in all patients, and a twofold increase in absolute monocyte and lymphocyte counts was observed in a majority of patients. However, no significant changes in the CD4/CD8 ratio or delayed type cutaneous hypersensitivity to recall antigens were present. Adverse side effects included local erythema at the injection site, fatigue, fever, myalgia, headache, nausea, and hepatitis, and no consistent effect was reported with respect to HIV activity. Among 13 evaluable patients, serum p24 antigen increased in 4, decreased in 2, and remained unchanged in seven.

While in vitro effects of rGM-CSF on HIV replication remains controversial, Hammer et al.[29] reported marked suppressive effect on HIV replication (lymphocytic strain) in the U937 cell line, but in contrast, Folks et al.[30] showed that GM-CSF stimulates HIV activity (as demonstrated by increased reverse transcriptase [RT]) in U1 cells, a subclone of U937 cell line with minimal constitutive expression of HIV. Additionally Koyanagi et al.[31] reported increased HIV activity in mononuclear phagocytic cultures with GM-CSG, M-CSF, and IL-3. In clinical trials, however, there has not been any acceleration of HIV-associated disease or consistent increase in HIV p24 antigen,[27,28] although Paluda et al.[32] did note an increase in p24 antigen in some patients who received alternate week treatment with GM-CSF and azidothymidine (AZT) on those weeks when GM-CSF was administered alone. Therefore, it is suggested that that two agents be given concurrently. Perno et al.[33] and Hammer et al.[34] have also demostrated in vitro synergism between GM-CSF and AZT on the inhibition of HIV replication.

The effect of combined GM-CSF and AZT treatment was recently evaluated in patients with AIDS or AIDS-related complex (ARC) who developed absolute neutropenia due to AZT treatment.[35] A significant increase in absolute leucocyte counts shared by neutrophils, monocytes, and eosinophils was observed but no stimulation of HIV, as assessed by circulating p24 antigen and in vitro RT activity, was reported. Adverse effects were similar to previous trials with an exception of the additional side effect of thrombocytopenia. These results demonstrate that concurrent treatment of rhGM-CSF and antiretroviral therapy is indicated in patients with HIV infection associated with absolute leukopenia.

G-CSF has also been used in combination with rh-erythropoeitin (rhEPO) and AZT in AIDS patients with neutropenia and anemia to improve tolerance to AZT and antibiotics used for infections in AIDS. Preliminary data are encouraging and show that G-CSF produces a multilineage effect.[36] Here a ninefold increase in neutrophil count was observed and during the therapy neutrophil functions were preserved and the titers of HIV and p24 did not change.

Interferons

Interferons (IFN) have been classified into three major subtypes as follows: IFN-α, IFN-β, and IFN-γ.[37] IFN-α is produced by peripheral blood mononuclear cells and is also known as leucocyte interferon and type I interferon, while IFN-β (fibroblast interferon) was also classified as type I interferon. Both IFN-α and IFN-β are classically produced during viral infection. More than 20 genes for IFN-α and only a single gene for IFN-β have been described. Although both IFNs display 15–30% amino acid sequence homology, they are antigenically distinct, however, both IFN-α and -β bind to the same receptors on the surface of target cells. In contrast, IFN-γ (immune interferon, type II interferon) is molecularly and functionally distinct from IFN-α and -β.[37,38] IFN-γ is exclusively produced by T cells and NK cells,[39] and viral infections do not induce IFN-γ production. Furthermore, IFN-γ displays a twofold lower specific antiviral activity as compared to IFN-α and -β. Furthermore, IFN-γ is 100- to 100,000-fold more active as an immune modulator than IFN-α or IFN-β. Therefore, IFN-γ is believed to act primarily as an immunomodulator with some concomitant antiviral activity. IFN-γ is classified as a nonglycosylated peptide containing 143 amino acid residues, and in its active form it exists as a 34 kd dimer. The molecular and biological description of IFN-γ is beyond the scope of this chapter, and interested readers who require further information are referred to a recent review article by Gallin.[40] In reference to its clinical application in chronic granulomatous disease, IFN-γ induces both macrophages and neutrophils to synthesize products of oxidation, products of tryptophan metabolism, and granule proteins. In addition, IFN-γ stimulates macrophages to produce human leucocyte antigen D-related proteins, especially the Fc-receptor-1 protein.

IFN-γ in the Treatment of Chronic Granulomatous Disease (CGD)

CGD was initially described in children by Bridges and associates in 1959.[41] The polymorphonuclear (PMN) leucocytes from patients with

CGD display normal phagocytosis but express a functional defect in their ability to increase respiration, are altered in their direct oxidation of glucose via the hexose monophosphate shunt, or their production of hydrogen peroxide that occurs during phagocytosis; therefore, PMNs in CGD are unable to adequately kill bacteria.[42] Recently it has been demonstrated that CGD is caused by the absence or deficiency of various proteins required for NADPH oxidase activity.[43] In phagocytic cells, NADPH oxidase consists of at least 4 proteins, one of which is cytochrome b-558. Cytochrome b-558 is a hetrodimer consisting of a 91 kd heavy chain and a 22 kd light chain.[44-46] The most common form (X-linked) is caused by the absence of the 91 kd chain.[44,45] Two cytosolic proteins that are associated with cytochrome b-558 include a 47 kd protein containing phosphorylation sites, and a 67 kd protein that forms a complex with cytochrome b-558.[44-49] The second most common form of CGD, which occurs in 30% of patients, is caused by a deficiency of the 47 kd cytosolic protein.[50] Less common forms of CGD are caused by deficiencies of membrane 22 kd subunit and 67 kd cytosolic protein of the NADPH complex.[46,49]

In two independent preliminary studies, IFN-γ was shown to enhance nitroblue tetrazolum dye reduction, production of superoxide anion, and to stimulate Staphylococcus aureus killing by macrophages from patients with CGD.[51,52] Ezekowitz et al.[52] reported that, in vivo, the respiratory burst was stimulated only in those patients who had X-linked CGD and had mild clinical manifestation of the disease, and additionally that IFN-γ stimulates production of 91 kd protein mRNA. This would suggest that the patients with X-linked CGD, whose phagocytes retain the ability to produce some superoxide, have a defect in the regulation of synthesis of the 91 kd subunit of cytochrome b-558, and IFN-γ stimulates the expression of this gene.

As a result of the preliminary studies, a multicenter trial of IFN-γ for patients with CGD was initiated. Here, 128 patients were randomized to receive placebo or IFN-γ. Both groups were comparable with regards to age and inheritance of CGD, and the daily dose of IFN-γ was 50 μg/m². A dramatic response to IFN-γ was observed with 72% reduction in relative risk for serious infections at all anatomical locations as compared to the placebo group. A significant improvement in in vitro killing of Aspergillus conidia by the neutrophils from patients treated with IFN-γ was observed, with the frequency of fungal infection also decreased in the treatment group. However, in the multicenter study, in contrast to preliminary studies, no significant effect was observed on the killing of Staphylococcus aureus. The reported side effects of this treatment included fever, chills, myalgias, rashes, and mild local erythema. It should also be noted that IFN-γ is now approved by the Food and Drug Administration for clinical use in patients with CGD.

IFN-γ in Hyper IgE Syndrome

The syndrome of hyperimmunoglobulinemia E was first described by Buckley et al.[53] These patients have unusual frequency of recurrent staphylococcal infections and non-atopic dermatitis. A number of variable defects have been reported, including impaired T-cell-mediated response, defect in PMN chemotaxis, and decreased production of IFN-γ.[53,54] Because IFN-γ is an important negative regulator of IgE production, it was reasoned that the hyper IgE state could be a secondary response to the decreased IFN-γ. In two separate, small, uncontrolled studies, treatment with IFN-γ resulted in a 50–60% decrease in IgE levels.[55,56] However, a large, multicenter, randomized, controlled study is needed to establish the efficacy of IFN-γ in hyper IgE syndrome. Side effects treatment included fever and fatigue, which could limit the clinical use of IFN-γ in hyper IgE syndrome. Recently, we have administered intravenous gamma globulin (IVIG) in two patients with high IgE (>2,000 IU) and observed a decrease in serum IgE levels and improvement in skin lesions. Serum IgE levels rose following discontinuation of IVIG, and again decreased upon readministration of IVIG. To establish the possible a role of IVIG in the treatment of hyper IgE syndrome will however require a placebo-controlled, multicenter study.

Interferons in HIV Infection and AIDS

The first clinical trial of IFN-α in AIDS employed human lymphoblastoid IFN-α. Although early trials with IFN-γ in AIDS were disappointing, subsequent trials have now been performed with recombinant IFN-α and IFN-β. Volberding et al.[57] demonstrated that IFN-α has an effect both on HIV and on Kaposi's sarcoma (KS). In this study, patients who responded tended to have higher $CD4^+$ T-cell counts. In subsequent studies, Adams et al.[58] and Kovacs et al.[59] reported that clinical responses were observed with both low and high doses of IFN-α. According to reports, patients with few consitutional symptoms and no opportunistic infections, and those with greater than 200 $CD4^+$ T-cell counts are more likely to respond to treatment. Lane et al.[60] showed efficacy of IFN-α in asymptomatic patients with HIV infection, and although no improvement in $CD4^+$ T-cell counts was observed, in the treatment group no opportunistic infections were present as compared to the placebo group (30% developed opportunistic infections). Because Harshorn et al.[61] demonstrated synergism in vitro between AZT and IFN-α, Berglund et al.[62] enrolled 18 patients with advanced HIV infection (mean CD4 = 139) and long term prior AZT treatment in a 3-month trial of AZT plus IFN-α. Reduced viral titers and p24 antigen levels were reported in 38% of patients who completed the study. Additionally, $CD4^+$ T-cell counts decreased in most patients, and dose-limiting toxicity included fatigue and neutropenia. Preliminary data from another ongoing multicenter study of patients with early ARC also demonstrate that the combination of AZT and IFN-α reduces p24 antigenemia. Although a number of claims have been made regarding efficacy of oral interferon in HIV infection, these observations await confirmation in well-controlled future studies.

In vitro IFN-β has been shown to inhibit HIV replication, prevent syncytium formation of HIV-infected cells, and function synergistically with AZT in inhibiting viral replication.[63] Based on in vitro data of IFN-β, several clinical trials have been initiated to determine if IFN-β may be used in patients with ARC or AIDS. Doses of IFN-β in these trials range from 15 to 150 million units/day subcutaneously, while the side effects include flu-like syndrome, hematologic suppression, elevated liver function tests, and mild proteinuria.

Interleukin-2 (IL-2)

IL-2 is a 15–17 kd sialic acid-rich glycoprotein whose gene has been cloned,[64–66] and a recombinant form of IL-2 has been available for clinical trials for several years. IL-2 plays a central role in immune response, and its biological activity is medicated by binding to a high affinity receptor that has been biochemically and molecularly characterized.[67] The binding of IL-2 to high affinity IL-2 receptor (IL-2R) stimulates cellular proliferation resulting in an expansion of the antigen-reactive clonal T-cell population. This activation process ultimately results in the generation of specific effector cells that mediate helper, suppressor, and cytotoxic functions. The early increase of IL-2R is followed by down-regulation of IL-2R, and therefore, the specificity, magnitude, and duration of the immune response is controlled in part by the variable display of IL-2R. It has also been demonstrated that activated B cells also express high affinity IL-2R, and that IL-2 promotes proliferation and differentiation of B cells in vitro and IL-2 also enhances activity of NK cells.

IL-2 in Primary Immunodeficiency Disorders

A number of immunodeficiencies have been associated with reduced IL-2 production with or without reduced IL-2R expression. Included here are patients suffering from severe combined immnodeficiency, Nezelof's syndrome, hyper IgM syndrome, ataxia telangiectasia, DiGeorge syndrome, and common variable immunodeficiency. IL-2 treatment has been utilized in some of these disorders with variable success as follows:

1. Servere combined immunodeficiency (SCID) is a disorder with X-linked or autosomal recessive inheritance. Clinically it is characterized by failure to thrive, chronic diarrhea, recurrent life-threatening viral,

bacterial, and fungal infections accompanied by both T- and B-cell defects. In a few cases of SCID, deficient IL-2 mRNA, deficient IL-2 secretion, or defective IL-2 responsiveness have been documented.[68,69] Because rIL-2 could restore T cell-mediated immunity in vitro,[70] 6 cases of SCID have been treated with rIL-2.[71,72] In all cases response to mitrogens improved, the frequency of infection decreased, and infants gained weight. However the effect of rIL-2 on B-cell function was not studied.

2. Nezelof's syndrome is similar to SCID and is characterized by severe T-cell defects with abnormal B-cell functions. The most effective treatment of Nezelof's syndrome appears to be bone marrow transplant. The treatment of a 17-month-old child with 1600 U/ml of rIL-2 every 3–4 days for 50 days resulted in an improvement in both the number of T cells and in lymphocyte response to mitogens. On the other hand no effect was observed on specific antibody response.[70]

3. DiGeorge syndrome is characterized by severe T-cell deficiency as a result of thymic aplasia or hypoplasia. In one case of complete DiGeorge syndrome it was reported that 2 months of treatment with rIL-2 (40,000 U/kg of i.v. daily) resulted in the development of phenotypically normal T lymphocytes.[72]

4. The hyper IgM syndrome is a X-linked recessive disorder in which hypogammaglobulinemia is associated with elevated levels of polyclonal IgM. B cells bearing surface IgG and IgA are lacking, and a deficiency of IL-2 production has been documented in several cases of hyper IgM syndrome. However at present no attempt has been made to treat patients with hyper IgM syndrome with rIL-2, although the results might prove to be of great interest.

5. rIL-2 has been reported to be effective in the treatment of ataxia telangiectasia. Here a patient with deficient IL-2 production and recurrent serious infection was treated with 1000–2000 U/kg i.v. per day rIL-2 for 6 weeks. Although substantial improvement was observed in lymphocyte response to mitogens and secretion of IgM, no clinical response was apparent.[73]

6. Common variable immunodeficiency (CVI) represents a disorder characterized by reduced levels of at least two Ig isotypes. A number of patients with CVI have been shown to have decreased production of various cytokines, including IL-2.[74,75] Recently, Cummingham-Rundles[76] treated 5 patients with CVI with polyethyleneglycol-conjugated rIL-2 (PEG-IL-2) given intravenously at a weekly interval at a dose of 250,000 units/m^2 body surface area for 0–4 weeks, 500,000 units/m^2 for weeks 4–8, and 1,000,000 units/m^2 for weeks 8–12. Following treatment no significant changes were observed in the numbers of T, B, or NK cells; mitogen response was slightly reduced, but the proliferative response to recall antigens was increased in 3 patients. However, the most dramatic effect was observed on Ig secretion in response to pokeweed mitogen.

Improvement in Ig secretion continued well beyond cessation of therapy and was observed to remain within the normal range 36–40 weeks after treatment.

IL-2 in HIV Infection

Clinical trials of IL-2 in HIV infected patients were first attempted in 1983.[77] Phase I studies in a small number of patients demonstrated transient immunological improvement and the results of a larger study were published in 1987.[78] Patients with or without KS were treated with rIL-2 intravenously, but only 3 of 55 patients with KS were considered to have responded to IL-2 and no effect was observed on immune functions, including CD4 counts and helper functions. McMahon et al.[79] treated 16 symptomatic HIV$^+$ subjects in a phase I study, using a combination of AZT (600 mg/day) and rIL-2 (200,000 [6 patients], 700,000 [6 patients] or 2,000,000 [4 patients] units/m^2 per day). Lymphopenia occurred by day 2 in patients receiving 700,000 units/m^2 per day. While in 12 subjects a rebound lymphocytosis shared by CD4, CD8, and CD16 cells was noted; no change in T-cell function was observed.

In another study, Schwartz et al.[80] treated 10 HIV-1$^+$ patients with CD4$^+$ T cells >400/mm^3. Patients received AZT 1200 mg/day for 8 weeks, followed by 1,500,000 units/m^2 IL-2 per day by continuous infusion for 4 weeks. Although a transient increase in CD4$^+$ T-cell count was noted during the first 2 weeks of IL-2 alone there was no change in antigenemia or viremia during the period of treatment. The side effects of rIL-2 treatment in HIV infection included mild neutropenia and anemia, chills, fevers, muscle pains, fatigue, headache, nausea, and elevated liver function tests. Thus, according to currently available information, IL-2 appears to have only limited usefulness in patients with HIV infection and AIDS.

References

1. Metcalf D. Control of granulocytes and macrophages: Molecular, cellular, and clinical aspects. Science 1991; 254:529–533.
2. Gasson J. Molecular physiology of granulocyte-macrophage colony stimulating factor. Blood 1991; 77:1131–1145.
3. Sherr CJ. Colony stimulating factor-1 receptor. Blood 1990; 75:1–12.
4. Hayashida K, Kitamura T, Groman DM, Arai K-I, Yokota T, Miyajama A. Molecular cloning of a second subunit of the human GM-CSF receptor. Reconstitution of a high affinity GM-CSF receptor. Proc Natl Acad Sci USA 1990; 87:9655–9659.
5. Andreeff M, Welte K. Hematopoietic colony stiumulating factors. Semin Oncol 1989; 16:221–229.
6. Groopman JE. Status of colony stimulating factors in cancer and AIDS. Semin Oncol 1990; 17:31–37.

7. Welte K, Platzer E, Lu L, Gabrilove J, Levi E, Mertelsmann R, Moore MAS. Purification and biochemical characterization of human pleuripotent hematopoietic colony stimulating factor. Proc Natl Acad Sci USA 1985; 82:1526–1530.
8. Demetri GD, Griffin JD. Granulocyte colony stimulating factor and its receptor. Blood 1991; 78:2791–2808.
9. Fukunaga R, Ishizaka-Ikeda E, Seta Y, Nagata S. Expression cloning of a receptor for murine granulocyte colony stiumulating factor receptor. Cell 1990; 61:341–350.
10. Fukunaga R, Seto Y, Mizushima S, Nagata S. Three different mRNAs encoding human granulocyte colony-stimulating factor receptor. Proc Natl Acad Sci USA 1990; 87:8702–8706.
11. Larson A, Davis T, Curtis BM, Gimpel S, Costman D, Park L, Sorensen E, March C, Smith CA. Expression cloning of a human G-CSF receptor: A structural mosaic of hematopoietin receptor, immunoglobulin, and fibronectin domains. J Exp Med 1990; 172:1559–1570.
12. Kostmann R. Infantile genetic agranulocytosis. A review with presentation of ten new cases. Acta Paediatr Scand 1975; 64:362.
13. Wriedt K, Kauder E, Mauer AM. Defective myelopoiesis in congenital neutropenia. N Engl J Med 1970; 283:1072–1077.
14. Amato D, Freedman MH, Saunders EF. Granulopoiesis in severe congenital neutropenia. Blood 1976; 47:531–538.
15. Rappeport JM, Parkman R, Newburger P, Camitta BM, Chusid M. Correction of infantile agranulocytosis by allogeneic bone marrow transplantation. Am J Med 1980; 68:605–609.
16. Bonilla MA, Gallo AP, Ruggeiro M, Kernan NA, Brochstein JA, Abdoud M, Fumagalli L, Vincent M, Gabrilove JL, Welte K, Souza LM, O'Reilly RJ. Effects of recombinant human granulocyte colony stimulating factor on neutropenia in patients with congenital agranulocytosis. N Engl J Med 1989; 320:1574–1580.
17. Welte K, Zeidler C, Reiter A, Muller W, Odenwald E, Souza L, Riehm H. Differential effects of granulocyte-macrophage colony stimulating factor and granulocyte colony stimulating factor in children with severe congenital neutropenia. Blood 1990; 75:1056–1063.
18. Welte K, Zeidler C, Reiter A, Riehm H. Effect of granulocyte colony stimulating factor in patients with severe chronic neutropenia. In: Gupta S, Griscelli C, eds. New Concepts in Immunodeficiency. London: Wiley Press; 1993:355–369.
19. Pietsch T, Buhrer C, Mempel K, Menzel T, Steffens U, Schrader C, Santos F, Zeidler C, Welte K. Blood mononuclear cells from patients with severe congenital neutropenia are capable of producing granulocyte colony stimulating factor. Blood 1991; 77:1234–1237.
20. Mempel K, Pietsch T, Menzel T, Zeidler C, Welte K. Increased serum levels of granulocyte colony stimulating factor (G-CSF) in patients with severe congenital neutropenia. Blood 1991; 77:1234–1237.
21. Kyas U, Pietsch T, Welte K. Expression of receptors for granulocyte colony stimulating factor on neutrophils from patients with severe congenital neutropenia. Blood 1992; 79:1144–1147.

22. Wright DG, Dale DC, Fauci AS, Wolff SM. Human cyclic neutropenia: Clinical review and follow-up of patients. Medicine 1981; 60:1–13.

23. Dale DC, Hammond WP. Cyclic neutropenia: A clinical review. Blood 1988; 2:178–185.

24. Hammond WP, Price TH, Souza LM, Dale DC. Treatment of cyclic neutropenia with granulocyte colony stimulating factor. N Engl J Med 1989; 320:1306–1311.

25. Freund MRF, Luft S, Schober C, Heussner P, Schrezenmaier H, Porzsolt F, Welte K. Differential effect of GM-CSF and G-CSF in cyclic neutropenia. Lancet 1991; 336:313.

26. Schroten H, Roesler J, Breidenbach T, Wendel U, Elsner J, Schweitzer S, Zeidler C, Burdach S, Lohmann-Matthes ML, Wahn V, Welte K. Granulocyte and granulocyte-macrophage colony stimulating factors for treatment of neutropenia in glycogen storage disease type Ib. J Pediatr 1991; 119:748–754.

27. Groopman JE, Mitsuyasu RT, DeLeo MJ, Oette DH, Golde DW. Effect of recombinant human granulocyte-macrophage colony stimulating factor on myelopoiesis in the acquired immunodeficiency syndome. N Engl J Med 1987; 317:593–598.

28. Mitsuyasu R, Levine J, Miles SA, De Leo M, Oette D, Golde D, Groopman J. Effects of long term subcutaneous (SC) administration of recombinant granulocyte-macrophage colony stimulating factor (GM-CSF) in patients with HIV-related leukopenia (abstract). Blood 1988; 72:356a.

29. Hammer SM, Gillis JM, Groopman JE, Rose RM. In vitro modification of human immunodeficiency virus infection by granulocyte-macrophage colony stimulating factor and gamma interferon. Proc Natl Acad Sci USA 1986; 83:8734–8738.

30. Folks TM, Justment J, Kinter A, Dinarello CA, Fauci AS. Cytokine-induced expression of HIV-1 in a chronically infected promonocytic cell line. Science 1987; 238:800–802.

31. Koyanagi Y, O'Brien WA, Zhao JQ, Golde DW, Gasson JC, Chen ISY. Cytokines alter production of HIV-1 from primary mononuclear phagocytes. Science 1988; 241:1673–1675.

32. Pluda JM, Yarchoan Y, Smith PD, McAtee N, Shay LE, Oette D, Maha M, Wahl SM, Myers CE, Broder S. Subcutaneous recombinant granulocyte-macrophage colony-stimulating factor used as a single agent and in an alternating regimen with azidothymidine in leukopenic patients with severe human immunodeficiency virus infection. Blood 1990; 76:463–472.

33. Perno C-F, Yarchoan R, Cooney DA, Hartman NR, Webb DSA, Hao E, Mitsuya H, Johns DG, Broder S. Replication of human immunodeficiency virus in monocytes. Granulocyte/macrophage colony-stimulating factor (GM-CSF) potentiates viral production yet enhances the antiviral effect mediated by 3'-azido-2'2'-dideoxythymidine (AZT) and other dideoxynucleoside congeners of thymidine. J Exp Med 1989; 169:933–951.

34. Hammer SM, Gillis JM, Synergistic activity of granulocyte- macrophage colony-stimulating factor and 3'-azido-3'-deoxythymidine against human immunodeficiency virus in vitro. Antimicrob Agent Chemother 1987; 31: 1046–1050.

35. Groopman JE. Granulocyte–macrophage colony–stimulating factor in human immunodeficiency virus disease. Semin Hematol 1990; 27:8–14.

36. Miles SA, Mitsuyasu RT, Moreno J, Baldwin N, Alton NK, Souza L, Glaspy JA. Combined therapy with recombinant granulocyte colony-stimulating factor and erythropoietin decreases hematologic toxicity from zidovudine. Blood 1991; 77:2109–2117.

37. Petska S, Langer JA, Zoon KC, Samuel CE. Interferons and their actions. Annu Rev Biochem 1987; 56:727–777.

38. Gray PW, Goeddel DV. Structure of the human immune interferon gene. Nature 1982; 298:859–863.

39. Kasahara T, Hooks JJ, dougherty SF, Oppenheim JJ. Interleukin 2-mediated immune interferon (IFN-gamma) production by human T cell subsets. J Immunol 1983; 130:1784–1789.

40. Gallin JI. Interferon gamma in chronic granulomatous disease. In: Gupta S, Griscelli C, eds. New Concepts in Immunodeficiency Diseases. London: John Willey Press; 1993:371–379.

41. Bridges RA, Berendes H, Good RA. A fatal granulomatosis of childhood: The clinical, pathological, and laboratory features of a new syndrome. Am J Dis Child 1959; 97:387–392.

42. Holmes B, Page AR, Good RA. Studies of the metabolic activity of leukocytes from patients with a genetic abnormality of phagocytic function. J Clin Invest 1967; 46:1422–1432.

43. Gallin JI, Malech HL. Update on chronic granulomatous disease of childhood. Immunotherapy and potential for gene therapy. JAMA 1990; 263:1533–1537.

44. Royer-Pokora B, Kunkel LM, Monaco AP, Goff SC, Newberger PE, Baehner RL, Cole FS, Curnutte JT, Orkin SH. Cloning the gene for an inherited human disorder—chronic granulomatous disease—on the basis of its chromosomal location. Nature 1986; 322:32–38.

45. Dinauer MC, Orkin SH, Brown R, Jesaitis AJ, Parkos CA. The glycoprotein encoded by X-linked chronic granulomatous disease locus is a component of the neutrophil cytochrome b complex. Nature 1987; 327:717–720.

46. Dinauer MC, Pierce EA, Bruns GAP, Curnutte JT, Orkin SH. Human neutrophil cytochrome b light chain (p22-phox). Gene structure, chromosome location, and mutation in cytochrome-negative autosomal recessive chronic granulomatous disease. J Clin Invest 1990; 86:1729–1737.

47. Lomax KJ, Leto TL, Nunoi H, Gallin JI, Malech HL. Recombinant 47-kilodalton cytosol factor restores NADPH oxidase in chronic granulomatous disease. Science 1989; 245:409–412.

48. Volpp BD, Nauseef WM, Donelson JE, Moser DR, Clark RA. Cloning of the cDNA and functional expression of the 47 kilodalton cytosolic component of human neutrophil respiratory burst oxidase. Proc Natl Acad Sci USA 1989; 86:7195–7199.

49. Leto TL, Lomax KJ, Volpp BD, Nunoi H, Sechler JMG, Nauseef WM, Clark RA, Gallin JI, Malech JT. Cloning of a 67 kD neutrophil oxidase factor wtih similarity to a noncatalytic region of p60$^{c\text{-}src}$. Science 1990; 248:727–730.

50. Clark RA, Malech JL, Gallin JI, Nunoi H, Volpp BD, Pearson DW, Nauseef WM, Curnutte JT. Genetic variants of chronic granulomatous disease: Prevalence of deficiencies of two cytosolic components of the NADPH oxidase system. N Engl J Med 1989; 312:647–652.

51. Sechler JMG, Malech HL, White CJ, Gallin JI. Recombinant human interferon gamma reconstitutes defective phagocyte function in patients with

chronic granulomatous disease of childhood. Proc Natl Acad Sci USA 1988; 85:4874–4878.

52. Ezekowitz RA, Dinaur MC, Jaffe HS, Orkin SH, Newburger PE. Partial correction of the phagocytic defect in patients with X-linked chronic granulomatous disease by subcutaneous interferon gamma. N Engl J Med 1988; 319:146–151.

53. Buckley RH, Wray BB, Belmaker EZ. Extreme hyperimmunoglobulinemia E and undue susceptibility to infections. Pediatrics 1972; 49:59–70.

54. Del Prete G, Tiri A, Maggi E, De Carli M, Macchia D, Parronchi P, Rossi ME, Pietrogrande MC, Ricci M, Romagagni S. Defective in vitro production of gamma interferon and tumor necrosis factor by circulating T cells in the hyperimmunoglobulin E syndrome. J Clin Invest 1989; 84:1830–1835.

55. King CL, Gallin JI, Malech HL, Abramson SL, Nutman TB. Regulation of immunoglobulin production in hyperimmunoglobulin E recurrent-infection syndrome by interferon gamma. Proc Natl Acad Sci USA 1989; 86: 10085–10089.

56. Souillet G, Rousset F, de Vries JE. Alpha-interferon treatment of patient with hyper IgE syndrome. Lancet 1989; 2:1384.

57. Volberding PA, Mitsuyasu RT, Golando JP, Siegel RJ. Treatment of Kaposi's sarcoma with interferon alfa-2b (IntronA). Cancer 1987; 59(Suppl):620–625.

58. Abrams DI, Volberding PA. Alpha interferon therapy of AIDS-associated Kaposi's sarcoma. Semin Oncol 1986; 13(Suppl):437–447.

59. Kovacs JA, Deyton L, Davey R, Falloon J, Zunich K, Lee D, Metcalf JA, Bigley JW, Sawyer LA, Zoon KC. Combined zidovudine and interferon-a therapy in patients with Kaposi sarcoma and the acquired immunodeficiency syndrome (AIDS). Ann Intern Med 1989; 111:28–287.

60. Lane CH, Davey V, Kovacs JA, Feinberg J, Metcalf JA, Herpin B, Walker R, Deyton L, Davey RT, Falloon J, Polis MA, Salzman NP, Basler M, Masur H, Fauci AS. Interferon-alpha in patients with asymptomatic human immunodeficiency virus (HIV) infection. A randomized, placebo-controlled trial. Ann Intern Med 1990; 112:805–811.

61. Harshorn KL, Vogt MW, Chou TC, Blumberg RS, Byington R, Schooley RT, Hirsch MS. Synergistic inhibition of human immunodeficiency virus in vitro by azidothymidine and recombinant alpha A interferon. Antimicrob Agents Chemother 1987; 31:168–172.

62. Berglund O, Engman K, Ehrnst A, Anderson J, Lidman K, Akerlund B, Sonneborg A, Strannegard O. Combined treatment of symptomatic HIV-1 infection with native interferon-alpha and zidovudine. J Infect Dis 1991; 163:710–715.

63. Borack MJ, Pollard RB. An open label study of the safety and efficacy of co-administration of zidovudine and recombinant IFN-beta (abstract). (Fifth International Conference on AIDS) 405.

64. Smith KA. T-cell growth factor. Immunol Rev 1980; 51:337–357.

65. Gupta S. Interleukins: Molecular and biological characteristics. In: Gupta S, Talal N, eds. Immunology of Rheumatic Diseases. New York: Plenum Press; 1985:109–139.

66. Smith KA, Cantrell DA. Interleukin 2 regulates its own receptor. Proc Natl Acad Sci USA 1985; 82:864–868.

67. Green WC, Depper JM, Kronke M, Leonard WJ. The human interleukin-2 receptor: Analysis of structure and function. Immunol Rev 1986; 92:29–48.
68. Rijkers GT, Scharenberg GM, Van Dongess JM, Neijens HJ, Zegers BJM. Abnormal signal transduction in a patient with SCID. Pediatr Res 1991; 29:306–309.
69. Weinberg K, Parkman R. Severe combined immunodeficiency due to a specific defect in the production of interleukin-2. N Engl J Med 1990; 322:1718–1723.
70. Dopfer R, Niethammer D, Peter HH, Kniep E-M, Monner DA, Muhlradt PF. In vitro effect of IL-2 on lymphocyte subpopulation in a child with combined immunodeficiency. Immunobiology 1984; 167:452–461.
71. Pahwa R, Paradise C, Pahwa S, Chatila T, Day NK, Geha R, Schwartz SA, Slade H, Oyaizu N, Good RA. Recombinant IL-2 therapy in severe combined immunodeficiency disease. Proc Natl Acad Sci USA 1989; 86:5069–5073.
72. Buckley R, Schiff S, Markert L, Gerber P, Paradise C. Recombinant human interleukin-2 (rIL-2) therapy in primary immunodeficiency. J Allergy Immunol 1989; 83:296.
73. Doi S, Saiki O, Hara T, Sugita, Ha-Kawa K, Tanaker T, Hara H, Negoro S, Yabuuchi H, Kishimoto S. Administration of recombinant IL-2 augments the level of serum IgM in an IL-2 deficient patient. Eur J Pediatr 1989; 148:630–633.
74. Sneller MC, Strober W. Abnormal lymphokine gene expression in patients with common variable immunodeficiency. J Immunol 1990; 144:3762–3769.
75. Spickett GP, Farrant J. The role of lymphokines in common variable hypo-gammaglobulinemia. Immunol Today 1989; 10:192–194.
76. Cunningham-Rundles C. IL-2 deficiency in primary immunodeficiency: Exploration of recombinant IL-2 as a potential in vivo treatment. In: Gupta S, Griscelli C, eds. New Concepts in Immunodeficiency Diseases. London: John Wiley; 1993: 391–416.
77. Gupta S. Therapy of the acquired immunodeficiency syndrome and AIDS-related syndromes. TIPS 1986; 7:393–397.
78. Volberding P, Moody DJ, Beardslee D, Bradley EC, Wofsy CB. Therapy of acquired immunodeficiency syndrome with recombinant interleukin 2. AIDS Res Hum Retroviruses 1987; 3:115–124.
79. McMahon D, Armstrong J, Pazin G, Rinald C, Hung X, Tripoli C, Whiteside T, Herberman R, Ho M. Safety, tolerance, and immunological study of rIL-2 and zidovudine in patients with AIDS and ARC (abstract #1345). 31st ICAAC 323, 1991.
80. Schwartz DH, Skowron G, Merigan TC. Safety and effects of interleukin-2 plus zidovudine in asymptomatic individuals infected with human immunodeficiency virus. J AIDS 1991; 4:11–23.

Index